Lung Cancer Screening

Gregory C. Kane • Julie A. Barta
Ronald E. Myers • Nathaniel R. Evans III

Editors

Lung Cancer Screening

A Population Approach

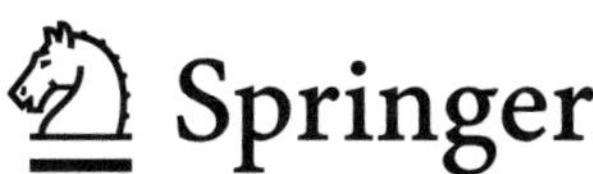 Springer

Editors
Gregory C. Kane
Department of Medicine
Thomas Jefferson University
Philadelphia, PA, USA

Ronald E. Myers
Medical Oncology
Thomas Jefferson University
Philadelphia, PA, USA

Julie A. Barta
Department of Medicine
Thomas Jefferson University
Philadelphia, PA, USA

Nathaniel R. Evans III
Department of Surgery
Thomas Jefferson University
Philadelphia, PA, USA

ISBN 978-3-031-33598-3   ISBN 978-3-031-33596-9   (eBook)
https://doi.org/10.1007/978-3-031-33596-9

This Springer imprint is published by the registered company Springer Nature Switzerland AG
The registered company address is: Gewerbestrasse 11, 6330 Cham, Switzerland

Foreword

Despite the recent remarkable progress in cancer research with improvements in prevention, diagnosis, therapeutic interventions, and survivorship, the United States (US) continues to struggle with inequities across the cancer care continuum. Disparities exist throughout all levels of the social-ecological model and persist across all cancer types. The causes of these inequities are vast and include structural racism, discrimination, stigma, poverty, distrust of the healthcare system, lack of access, and other social determinants of health. For lung cancer, which is the leading cause of cancer mortality in the United States, disease screening is a newer strategy for early detection and expands the armamentarium of well-established cancer screenings.

This book has a bold aim and focuses on a learning community model to address disparities and inequities in lung cancer, early identification and screening for individuals at risk through community intervention, outreach, and greater awareness and understanding of community needs and resources. This concept represents a phase shift in US lung cancer care. Heretofore, lung cancer preventive and treatment strategies failed to achieve equitable impact on mortality rates, especially with regard to issues of race, poverty, and stigma. As a result, lung cancer mortality rates, as reported by the American Cancer Society and described further in this treatise, are greater for Black men compared to White men and Black women compared to White women {Siegel, 2023 #740}.

As a national leader, Dr. Gregory Kane is a highly regarded pulmonary physician. As a frequent lecturer during American College of Physicians programs, Chairman of the Department of Medicine at the Sidney Kimmel Medical College, teacher and clinician, he demonstrates leadership in multiple aspects of Medicine. He has organized a superb group, including Nathaniel Evans, MD, Director of the Division of Thoracic Surgery and Co-Lead of the Lung Cancer, Screening and Nodules Program of the Korman Respiratory Institute; Ronald Myers, D.S.W., Ph.D., Division Director of Population Science in Medical Oncology; and Julie Barta, MD, Assistant Professor of Medicine and Lead of the Lung Cancer, Screening and Nodules Program of the Korman Respiratory Institute, each in their respective areas of expertise, to produce this superb premise. This book can serve as an information source for trainees, or a reference and update by primary care and other specialties and subspecialists to address the latest information in increasing screening and early diagnosis in lung cancer.

In this book, the group addresses inequities in lung cancer screening at the outset as an essential primary care metric by leading national healthcare quality organizations. As such, this represents the first time that the United States is working toward an equitable rollout of a new early detection and prevention strategy. The authors of this book, each heavily engaged in the work of a cancer screening for those from the academic and clinical care perspectives, are congratulated for integrating a robust public health perspective and for addressing underserved and often overlooked populations, and health inequities at the outset.

The reader will also notice important partnerships, which have the potential to form the cornerstone for new community-based interventions utilizing partnerships that have real-world impact and spur change at a community level. The authors also focus on the engagement of primary care and community health navigators working synchronously with lung cancer screening programs, essential relationships necessary to achieve the population impact.

The tools and approaches featured in this remarkable book can help transform the implementation of lung cancer screening to serve all populations using a community-based strategy. The challenge ahead is whether we as a nation can move swiftly and adroitly enough so that lung cancer is no longer the menace of the last century, and all underserved, and often overlooked, groups benefit equally.

Department of Medical Oncology   Edith Peterson Mitchell
Center to Eliminate Cancer Disparities
Sidney Kimmel Cancer Center at Jefferson
Philadelphia, PA, USA

Contents

Part IV Taking Care of the Patient

Part V Engaging the Community

Part VI Determining Impact at the Population Level

Part VII On the Horizon: What Lies Ahead in Lung Cancer Screening

Contributors

Neha Agarwal Pulmonary and Critical Care Sciences, University of Colorado, Aurora, CO, USA

Rita Axelrod Department of Medical Oncology, Sidney Kimmel Cancer Center, Thomas Jefferson University, Philadelphia, PA, USA

Bracken Babula Department of Medicine, Thomas Jefferson University, Philadelphia, PA, USA

Julie A. Barta Department of Medicine, Thomas Jefferson University, Philadelphia, PA, USA

Sydney C. Beache Department of Surgery, Washington University in St. Louis, St. Louis, MO, USA

Lisa A. Bevilacqua Division of Thoracic and Esophageal Surgery, Department of Surgery, Thomas Jefferson University Hospital, Philadelphia, PA, USA

Rickie Brawer Department of Medical Oncology, Thomas Jefferson University, Philadelphia, PA, USA

Sandra E. Brooks Independent Consultant and Faculty, Institute for Healthcare Improvement, Philadelphia, PA, USA

Beth Careyva Department of Family Medicine, Lehigh Valley Health Network, Allentown, PA, USA

Humberto Choi Cleveland Clinic, Respiratory Institute, Cleveland, OH, USA

William Curry Department of Family and Community Medicine and Department of Public Health Sciences, Penn State Health, Hershey, PA, USA

Melissa DiCarlo Department of Medical Oncology, Thomas Jefferson University, Philadelphia, PA, USA

Patricia M. Doykos The Bristol Myers Squibb Foundation, New York, NY, USA

Debra Dyer Department of Radiology, National Jewish Health, University of Colorado Denver, Denver, CO, USA

Nathaniel R. Evans III Department of Surgery, Thomas Jefferson University, Philadelphia, PA, USA

Heather Bittner Fagan Department of Family and Community Medicine, Christiana Care Health System, Wilmington, DE, USA

James H. Finigan Pulmonary and Critical Care Medicine, National Jewish Health, Denver, CO, USA

Jude Francis Information Services and Technology—Enterprise Analytics, Thomas Jefferson University Hospital, Philadelphia, PA, USA

Zachary French Department of Medical Oncology, Sidney Kimmel Cancer Center, Thomas Jefferson University, Philadelphia, PA, USA

Teresa Giamboy Jefferson Health Northeast, Sidney Kimmel Cancer Center at Torresdale, Thomas Jefferson University, Philadelphia, PA, USA

Tyler Grenda Division of Thoracic and Esophageal Surgery, Department of Surgery, Thomas Jefferson University, Philadelphia, PA, USA

Erin A. Hirsch Division of Medical Oncology, Department of Medicine, University of Colorado School of Medicine, Aurora, CO, USA

Amy G. Huebschmann Division of General Internal Medicine, Department of Medicine, University of Colorado School of Medicine, Aurora, CO, USA

Kathleen Jarrell Department of Surgery, Thomas Jefferson University Hospital, Philadelphia, PA, USA

Jennifer Johnson Department of Medical Oncology, Sidney Kimmel Cancer Center, Thomas Jefferson University, Philadelphia, PA, USA

Hee-Soon Juon Department of Medical Oncology, Thomas Jefferson University, Philadelphia, PA, USA

Gregory C. Kane Department of Medicine, Thomas Jefferson University, Philadelphia, PA, USA

Stephen K. Klasko Thomas Jefferson University and Jefferson Health, Philadelphia, PA, USA

Karen E. Knudsen Sidney Kimmel Cancer Center, Thomas Jefferson University, Philadelphia, PA, USA

American Cancer Society, Atlanta, GA, USA

Priscilla L. Ko The Bristol Myers Squibb Foundation, New York, NY, USA

Prarthna Chandar Kulandaisamy Division of Pulmonary, Critical Care, and Allergy, Department of Medicine, Jane and Leonard Korman Respiratory Institute, Thomas Jefferson University, Philadelphia, PA, USA

Jennifer Elston Lafata Division of Pharmaceutical Outcomes and Policy, Eshelman School of Pharmacy and UNC Lineberger Comprehensive Cancer Center, University of North Carolina at Chapel Hill, Chapel Hill, NC, USA

Ana Maria Lopez Department of Medical Oncology, Sidney Kimmel Cancer Center, Thomas Jefferson University, Philadelphia, PA, USA

Peter Mazzone Cleveland Clinic, Respiratory Institute, Cleveland, OH, USA

Russell K. Mcintire Department of Population Health, Thomas Jefferson University, Philadelphia, PA, USA

Cole Miller Sidney Kimmel Medical College, Thomas Jefferson University, Philadelphia, PA, USA

Ronald E. Myers Department of Medical Oncology, Thomas Jefferson University, Philadelphia, PA, USA

Division of Population Science, Department of Medical Oncology, Thomas Jefferson University, Philadelphia, PA, USA

Christine Neslund-Dudas Division of Thoracic and Esophageal Surgery, Department of Surgery, Thoms Jefferson University, Philadelphia, PA, USA

Olugbenga Okusanya Division of Thoracic and Esophageal Surgery, Department of Surgery, Thomas Jefferson University, Philadelphia, PA, USA

Kristine Pham Department of Medical Oncology, Thomas Jefferson University, Philadelphia, PA, USA

Sarah Reed Jefferson Health, Philadelphia, PA, USA

Brooke Ruane Department of Medicine, Jane and Leonard Korman Respiratory Institute, Thomas Jefferson University, Philadelphia, PA, USA

Ayako Shimada Department of Pharmacology and Experimental Therapeutics, Division of Biostatistics, Thomas Jefferson University, Philadelphia, PA, USA

Christine S. Shusted Division of Pulmonary and Critical Care Medicine, Department of Medicine, Sidney Kimmel Medical College at Thomas Jefferson University, Philadelphia, PA, USA

Randa Sifri Department of Family and Community Medicine, Thomas Jefferson University, Philadelphia, PA, USA

Brian Stello Department of Family Medicine, Lehigh Valley Health Network, Allentown, PA, USA

Jamie L. Studts Division of Medical Oncology, Department of Medicine, University of Colorado School of Medicine, Aurora, CO, USA

Baskaran Sundaram Department of Radiology, Thomas Jefferson University Hospital, Philadelphia, PA, USA

Channing E. Tate Division of General Internal Medicine, Department of Medicine, University of Colorado School of Medicine, Aurora, CO, USA

Nina A. Thomas Division of Pulmonary Sciences and Critical Care, Department of Medicine, University of Colorado School of Medicine, Aurora, CO, USA

Brian M. Till Department of Surgery, Thomas Jefferson University Hospital, Philadelphia, PA, USA

Maria Werner-Wasik Department of Radiation Oncology, Thomas Jefferson University, Philadelphia, PA, USA

Sung Whang Division of Thoracic and Esophageal Surgery, Department of Surgery, Philadelphia, PA, USA

Charnita Zeigler-Johnson Cancer Prevention and Control, Communicyt Outreach and Engagement, Fox Chase Cancer Center, Philadelphia, PA, USA

Part I
Introduction

Chapter 1
The Promise of Lung Cancer Screening

Gregory C. Kane

Background

Lung cancer is the single most common cause of cancer mortality in men and women, according to the American Cancer Society. It has been the most common cause of cancer death for men since the mid-1950s and, not to be out-done, lung cancer became the most common cause of cancer death in women in the 1980s, reflecting the uptick of smoking among women in the second half of the last century [1]. Startling to comprehend, there are more deaths from lung cancer each year in the United States than from colon, breast, and prostate cancers combined. The promise of lung cancer screening, then, is straightforward – *to reduce the impact of this deadly cancer in our community through prevention, screening, and more effective treatment.* While previous attempts to address cancer deaths, such as the "War on Cancer" launched by the Nixon administration in the 1970s, were ambitious; today, we have the actual tools to make an impact [2]. With the availability of effective tools, including new approaches to decreasing smoking rates, specialized imaging for early detection, and new treatment modalities for advanced tumors with high-impact molecular and immunologic therapeutics; we are truly poised for success, and already the mortality has been falling. In this third decade of the twenty-first century, we are achieving measurable progress against this devastating killer. The progress against lung cancer is measured in human lives – lives of mothers and fathers, brothers and sisters, sons and daughters, friends and neighbors, and colleagues and cousins [1]!

The advent of lung cancer screening (LCS) comes late to the pantheon of cancer screening presently employed in the United States. Currently, the four other solid

G. C. Kane (✉)
Department of Medicine, Thomas Jefferson University, Philadelphia, PA, USA
e-mail: Gregory.Kane@Jefferson.edu

© The Author(s), under exclusive license to Springer Nature Switzerland AG 2023
G. C. Kane et al. (eds.), *Lung Cancer Screening*,
https://doi.org/10.1007/978-3-031-33596-9_1

tumor cancers with effective screening programs include breast, prostate, cervix, and colon. The approaches for these four cancers utilize mammography and breast examination (both self-exam and those conducted by healthcare professionals), prostate-specific antigen determination and digital examination of the prostate, pelvic examination with Pap smear, and a myriad of techniques, but principally colonoscopy, for reducing the impact of colorectal cancer. Among these four, colorectal cancer reduction and cervical cancer reduction have been the most remarkable, as has the public information campaign to assure that eligible persons actually get screened [3, 4]. Only more recently has the United States Preventive Services Task Force (USPSTF) approved the modern approach to LCS. The reasons for this are complex, but lacking a high-resolution imaging technique prior to the deployment of modern multi-slice CT scanners has certainly been chief among these reasons. Historical efforts employing routine Chest X-ray as the imaging technique proved capable of detecting cancer – just not at an early stage. As a result, there was not a reliable or significant impact on the outcome. One unfortunate consequence of this result may have been a delay in embracing the possibility, and now reality, that LCS with CT scanning could prove so effective in finding cancers and saving lives.

One difference, between LCS and cancer screening for other tumors, is that LCS is a process rather than a single step or initiative [5]. This is due to the frequency of benign lung nodules detected in up to one-quarter of smokers undergoing CT scanning. In order to distinguish the presence or absence of suspicious CT scan findings, it is necessary to obtain a follow-up scan among those who undergo an initial screening. This distinguishing feature places a unique burden on screening programs. Not only is it essential to enroll patients, but patients must be followed over time at the proper intervals. And while colonoscopy must be performed at regular, but less frequent intervals; it is not necessary to repeat the procedure in a short interval to understand the significance of any of the findings, as is the cae with the initial low-dose CT (LDCT). A second difference is that only LDCT scanning can identify other findings that might prove helpful to the person undergoing screening. These include coronary calcifications, incidental tumors in the liver, adrenals or kidneys, and other lung diseases. A final difference is that LCS is being implemented in the era of striving for health equity. Never before, has a new cancer prevention strategy been implemented when the differential impact across all Americans was so critical and actually mattered! While some might choose to label these aspects of LCS as "challenges," many of the myriad of health professionals engaged in LCS prefer to view them as opportunities – opportunities to build programs within high-reliability healthcare entities, opportunities to infuse methods and reporting with quality and opportunities to succeed in reaching vulnerable populations to achieve health equity.

Today, the stage is set for achieving success in the battle against lung cancer. We have the public health and clinical tools to prevent smoking and help smokers quit. We have LDCT machinery, which can reliably detect cancers at an early stage, and we have effective treatment options based on the explosion of cancer research in the last two decades. The final measure of success will be the implementation by programs and providers serving patients in communities rural and urban, rich and poor, and high or low in healthcare literacy – all communities, but especially those communities where there is a disproportionate impact of smoking-related mortality.

Causes of Lung Cancer

While lung cancer can occur in nonsmokers and a number of nonsmoking-related causes are well-appreciated, including radon and asbestos; the chief cause of lung cancer is cigarette smoking [6]. Despite clear evidence of harm, approximately 14% of the adult population smoked cigarettes in 2019. There is reason for optimism, however, as this figure is down from 20.9% in 2005 [7]. Curiously, despite the high cost of tobacco products, smoking remains prevalent among the poor [8]. It is important to note that any progress in reducing smoking, not only impacts lung cancer incidence and mortality but affects numerous other causes of premature death. Since smoking is responsible for nearly one in five deaths in the United States from cancers at other sites and early cardiovascular disease, including stroke, the impact across a number of diseases could be substantial [7].

With high levels of income disparity in the United States, it is becoming clear for several reasons that smoking particularly affects the poorest communities. These reasons include the availability of tobacco products, levels of stress in these populations, and lack of health education [8]. Understanding the varying rates of smoking among communities and factors impacting smoking in the poorest communities will be essential for a national strategy to reduce the use of tobacco products and smoking, of which LCS is just one part.

One of the key elements of the current strategy to reduce lung cancer deaths is the mandatory inclusion of smoking cessation counseling in every LCS program. This distinguishes LCS efforts from mammography in that the current approach combines *prevention* through reducing the principal risk factor with imaging for *early detection*. Most programs must rely on certified tobacco-cessation counseling specialists or other health professionals for this component, and it is best when this service is delivered with shared-decision making. It is imperative that LCS programs incorporate high-quality smoking cessation counseling to achieve this aim. This approach was, indeed, part of the National Lung Screening Trial (NLST) and is required by Medicare for payment of LDCT scans [9, 10].

The Tools of Modern Medicine Are Coming Together

In the last decade, the first trial of its kind to use CT imaging – the NLST – demonstrated an impact on lung cancer mortality through annual LDCT screening for high-risk smokers and former smokers who quit less than 15 years previously [9]. In 2013, the USPSTF endorsed the use of LCS. Just 2 years later, in 2015, the Centers for Medicare and Medicaid Services added LCS as a preventive service benefit [10].

The success of this LDCT technique was born of the remarkable revolution we have seen in computerized cross-sectional imaging with greater and greater resolution, empowering radiologists and clinicians to detect nodules as small as 2–3 mm routinely as well as enabling routine follow up to detect growing lesions. Coupled with current tumor biology for lung cancers [11] where malignant epithelial carcinomas typically double in volume over 30–365 days; malignant lesions can be identified early with ease by observing growth over critically selected study intervals as short as 3 months for larger lesions and 6–12 months for smaller lesions. The NLST established a clear impact on enrollee survival, though programs must closely follow screening guidelines to match these outcomes.

Surprisingly, in the years since the publication of the NLST, efforts to expand LCS have been limited by low rates of screening uptake. In 2015, 4 years after the publication of the NLST, just 6% of eligible persons were being screened [12]. In recent years and despite the wide availability of CT scanning in our communities, rates have increased to just 16% in 2020 [13]. Moreover, the uptake of LCS has been sporadic across states and regions of the United States and has not been aligned with lung cancer mortality [13]. Indeed, LCS may have only approached the standard of care in all communities as of 2018, as the American Academy of Family Physicians (AAFP) concluded that the evidence (a single study, the National Lung Screening Trial) was not sufficient to advocate for screening given the narrow benefit window, costs and side effects of annual LDCT. This clearly has contributed to slowing the uptake. By comparison, breast and colon cancer which have lower overall mortality in the United States have screening rates of approximately 70% [14]. Thus, it is clear that much work lies ahead if we are to fully realize the promise of this new screening process.

Overcoming Barriers

The reasons for slow uptake are poorly understood. The stigma associated with smoking and lung cancer may be a contributor as some high-risk individuals might choose not to seek LCS due to fears or limited understanding of the benefit [15]. Myths concerning the effectiveness of modern treatments may also play a role. Some patients may have a high degree of fatalism with regard to surgery for lung cancer; believing that they will die of lung cancer regardless of early detection. These patients might avoid referral unless educational efforts address these myths. With a growing awareness of the social determinants of health [16], it is essential that health systems use outreach to educate, encourage, and enroll patients from communities with high smoking rates. Another reason for slow uptake may relate to the disproportionate enrollment of vulnerable patients in LCS programs, where health literacy and the comfort level with the screening process, and the healthcare system as a whole, may not be high. For example, in the NLST, less than 5% of enrolled patients were black. To achieve widespread screening, it is imperative to address all communities and build trust in our communities.

While CMS has added LCS as a preventive service benefit, there are few mandatory measures of implementation currently affecting healthcare systems or primary care physicians, which might stand to encourage the use of and referral for LCS. The inclusion of such measures in healthcare scorecards could have a further impact on progress toward higher rates of LCS uptake. It is essential that healthcare systems take the lead in measuring and reporting progress and milestones.

Given the low uptake despite the wide availability of CT scanning, it is essential to identify barriers and dismantle these barriers to expand LCS so that it can truly impact lung cancer mortality in our communities. We plan to address these issues in detail in the upcoming chapters of this book.

Realizing the Promise of Lung Cancer Screening

The potential for LCS is enormous if implemented consistently with CMS guidelines. These include the incorporation of smoking cessation counseling, shared decision making so that eligible persons understand the risks and benefits as well as the need for annual screening as part of a process, and finally, the use of LDCT to limit radiation exposure. The impact on our communities, if we can meet this challenge, will be substantial, allowing older Americans to enjoy retirement.

This book is intended to be a comprehensive guide to LCS for clinicians, healthcare systems, community leaders, and public health officials with the hope of creating a more equitable LCS landscape designed to favorably impact lung cancer-related outcomes in all communities. We will feature population approaches as relying on individual operators will simply not bring the necessary forces and organization to achieve high-quality results.

Simply stated, the promise of LCS is to impact the mortality from lung cancer in every community across the United States. Today, with tools to seriously address smoking cessation and dramatically improve early detection, we can make a huge difference. For our families and communities, it is time for this impact to be fully realized.

References

1. Siegel RL, Miller KD, Fuchs HE, Jemal A. Cancer statistics, 2022. CA Cancer J Clin. 2022;72(1):7–33.
2. Sporn MB. The war on cancer: a review. Ann N Y Acad Sci. 1997;833:137–46.
3. Benard VB, Thomas CC, King J, Massetti GM, Doria-Rose VP, Saraiya M. Vital signs: cervical cancer incidence, mortality, and screening - United States, 2007–2012. MMWR Morb Mortal Wkly Rep. 2014;63(44):1004–9.
4. QuickStats: death rates* from colorectal cancer,(†) by age group - United States, 1999–2019. MMWR Morb Mortal Wkly Rep. 2021;70(35):1233.
5. Shusted CS, Barta JA, Lake M, Brawer R, Ruane B, Giamboy TE, et al. The case for patient navigation in lung cancer screening in vulnerable populations: a systematic review. Popul Health Manag. 2019;22(4):347–61.
6. Smith RA, Glynn TJ. Epidemiology of lung cancer. Radiol Clin N Am. 2000;38(3):453–70.
7. The health consequences of smoking-50 years of progress: a report of the surgeon general. Reports of the Surgeon General. Atlanta GA; 2014.
8. Shusted CS, Kane GC. Linkage between poverty and smoking in Philadelphia and its impact on future directions for tobacco control in the city. Popul Health Manag. 2020;23(1):68–77.
9. The National Lung Cancer Screening Research Team. Reduced lung-cancer mortality with low-dose computed tomographic screening. N Engl J Med. 2011;365(5):395–409.

10. Moyer VA. Screening for lung cancer: U.S. Preventive Services Task Force recommendation statement. Ann Intern Med. 2014;160(5):330–8.
11. Wilson DO, Ryan A, Fuhrman C, Schuchert M, Shapiro S, Siegfried JM, et al. Doubling times and CT screen–detected lung cancers in the Pittsburgh Lung Screening Study. Am J Respir Crit Care Med. 2012;185(1):85–9.
12. Jemal A, Fedewa SA. Lung cancer screening with low-dose computed tomography in the United States—2010 to 2015. JAMA Oncol. 2017;3(9):1278–81.
13. Yong PC, Sigel K, Rehmani S, Wisnivesky J, Kale MS. Lung cancer screening uptake in the United States. Chest. 2020;157(1):236–8.
14. Fedewa SA, Kazerooni EA, Studts JL, Smith RA, Bandi P, Sauer AG, et al. State variation in low-dose computed tomography scanning for lung cancer screening in the United States. J Nat Cancer Inst. 2020;113(8):1044–52.
15. Chambers SK, Dunn J, Occhipinti S, Hughes S, Baade P, Sinclair S, et al. A systematic review of the impact of stigma and nihilism on lung cancer outcomes. BMC Cancer. 2012;12(1):184.
16. Daniel H, Bornstein SS, Kane GC, Carney JK, Gantzer HE, Henry TL, et al. Addressing social determinants to improve patient care and promote health equity: an American College of Physicians Position Paper. Ann Intern Med. 2018;168(8):577–8.

Chapter 2
A Brief History of Lung Cancer Screening

Julie A. Barta

Background

The current era of lung cancer screening builds upon several decades of work in the early detection of lung cancer, which is the most common cause of cancer death both in the United States and worldwide [1]. Several studies examining screening by chest X-ray and sputum cytology demonstrated no reduction in lung cancer mortality. A major turning point in the field occurred in 2006 with the publication of the International Early Lung Cancer Action Program (I-ELCAP) study, which demonstrated a stage shift in lung cancer diagnosis with low-dose CT screening of high-risk individuals [2]. Since this time, LCS research has rapidly moved forward with subsequent randomized controlled trials including the National Lung Screening Trial (NLST) and the Dutch Belgian Randomized Lung Cancer Screening Trial (NELSON) which demonstrated significant lung cancer mortality benefit, and ultimately garnering support from professional societies, preventive services experts, payers, and other organizations.

Lung Cancer Screening by Chest X-Ray and Sputum Cytology

Several early studies of chest X-ray screening with or without sputum cytology, carried out in the 1970s, failed to demonstrate a lung cancer mortality benefit with these methods. For instance in the Memorial Sloan-Kettering Study, Melamed and colleagues randomized 10,040 men over 45 years old with current smoking status

J. A. Barta (✉)
Department of Medicine, Thomas Jefferson University, Philadelphia, PA, USA
e-mail: Julie.barta@jefferson.edu

G. C. Kane et al. (eds.), *Lung Cancer Screening*,
https://doi.org/10.1007/978-3-031-33596-9_2

(>1 pack per day) to annual chest X-ray or dual screening (annual chest X-ray and sputum cytology every 4 months) [3]. Although individuals in the dual screening group were found to have lung cancer earlier than those in the X-ray only group, the total number of prevalence and incidence cancers was not significantly different between the two groups, and importantly there was no difference in overall survival or lung cancer mortality [3]. Similarly, Frost and colleagues in 1982 found no improvement in lung cancer mortality with the addition of sputum cytology to annual chest X-ray screening [4]. In contrast to these studies, the Mayo Lung Project was designed to evaluate dual screening vs. usual care, which entailed providing advice about annual X-rays and sputum cytology screening for lung cancer. This trial also found no significant difference in lung cancer mortality rates between the dual screening and usual care arms [5]. However, the Mayo Lung Project was noted to have several limitations including that the of prevalence cancers were not evaluated in the randomized comparison, nearly half of the usual care group obtained annual chest X-rays, and there was relatively low adherence with the screening protocol in the dual screening group [6].

The more recent Prostate, Lung, Colorectal, and Ovarian Cancer Screening Trial (PLCO) was the only randomized controlled trial to compare annual chest X-ray for 3 years with no screening for lung cancer [7]. The PLCO enrolled 154,901 average-risk participants (including current-, former-, and never-smokers). After 13 years of follow-up, there were no significant differences in lung cancer incidence, mortality, or stage at diagnosis between the two groups. Even among subgroup analyses of current and former smokers, who had higher lung cancer incidence than nonsmokers, there was no difference in lung cancer incidence or mortality among screening vs. control groups [7]. This large trial, with high adherence rates and low crossover in the control arm, provided definitive evidence that annual chest radiographic screening did not reduce lung cancer mortality relative to no screening. Notably, the PLCO trial's independent data and safety monitoring board recommended reporting the results early, providing additional context for the NLST, which had been published just a few months prior [8].

Lung Cancer Screening by CT Scan: Initial Studies

Initial studies of LDCT screening for lung cancer were led by the I-ELCAP investigators. Henschke and colleagues initially enrolled 1000 current and former smokers at least 60 years old to undergo annual LDCT using a single cohort, non-comparative design. On baseline screening, they found a lung cancer prevalence rate four times higher than that with chest X-ray, with 85% of screen-detected lung cancers diagnosed at stage I disease [9]. Subsequently, an expanded, international cohort of 31,567 individuals was studied [2]. This group included participants as young as 40 years old and utilized a broad definition of lung cancer risk for inclusion, such as smoking history, occupational factors, and secondhand smoke exposure. With up to 6 years of follow-up after screening, the investigators found again that 85% of individuals with screen-detected lung cancer had stage I disease, and the estimated 10-year survival rate in this subgroup was 88% [2]. The I-ELCAP investigators described that LDCT screening could detect curable, stage I lung cancer in a high proportion of individuals, leading to a high rate of survival. However, despite high rates of lung cancer-specific survival, I-ELCAP and other studies did not demonstrate a predicted reduction in lung cancer mortality [10].

The NLST, published in 2011, was the largest randomized, controlled trial comparing LDCT to chest X-ray, enrolling 53,454 individuals between ages 55 and 74 with at least 30 pack-years of smoking [8]. It included current smokers as well as those who had quit within 15 years. In the NLST, participants received 3 years of annual screening by either LDCT or by chest X-ray. At a median follow-up of 6.5 years, those in the LDCT arm experienced a 20% relative reduction in lung cancer mortality, as well as a 7% reduction in all-cause mortality. The adherence rate with three rounds of annual screening was over 90%. Twenty-four percent of LDCT scans were noted to be abnormal (defined as a lung nodule ≥ 4 mm), with lung cancer confirmed in just 3.6% of these abnormal scans [8]. Critiques of the NLST include its comparison of LDCT vs. chest X-ray (instead of no screening), and small differences in adherence and work-up of screen-detected nodules between the study arms. Despite this, the NLST set the stage for rapid advancement in the field of lung cancer screening.

Smaller prospective studies preceding the NLST also compared LDCT with chest X-ray among United States and international cohorts and similarly found that CT scans identified more early stage lung cancer, but none demonstrated a reduction in lung cancer mortality [11–13]. Following the NLST, several studies in Europe examined LDCT vs. no screening, with varying protocols for inclusion criteria and screening interval, but these trials were underpowered to detect a mortality difference with LDCT [14–18].

Nelson and Beyond

After the publication of the NLST, the United States Preventive Services Task Force (USPSTF) gave a "B" recommendation in support of LCS in 2013, and the Centers for Medicare and Medicaid Services (CMS) followed with a decision memo adding LCS as a preventive service benefit in 2015 [19, 20]. For patients, endorsement from these organizations was critical to expanding access to LCS, and for healthcare institutions, this marked a pivotal point in the development and growth of LCS programs across the country. Both the USPSTF and CMS have published revised statements in support of broadening eligibility criteria for the purpose of improving health equity among previously under-screened populations [21, 22].

The NELSON trial, published in 2020, demonstrated results remarkably similar to the NLST [23]. Over 15,000 individuals were randomized to LDCT screening with increasing intervals between scans vs. a control group, which received no screening. Notably, 84% of participants were men, and smoking intensity requirements were lower than that of the NLST, with a minimum history of 15–20 cigarettes a day for 25–30 years. At 10 years of follow-up, there was 24% decrease in lung cancer mortality among individuals undergoing LDCT screening. In a small subgroup of female participants from NELSON, there was an even greater reduction in lung cancer mortality with screening. Moreover, NELSON also demonstrated high discriminatory power for lung cancer diagnosis using volumetric measurements to characterize screen-detected lung nodules [24].

The most recent prospective clinical trial in the LCS field is the International Lung Screening Trial, which aimed to compare the effectiveness of USPSTF 2013 criteria with the $PLCO_{m2012}$ six-year lung cancer risk model in selecting individuals for annual lung cancer screening with LDCT scan [25]. Tammemagi and colleagues demonstrated that a $PLCO_{m2012}$ risk score of 1.7% had greater efficiency for enrolling high-risk patients into lung cancer screening. Specifically, the $PLCO_{m2012}$-eligible group had a statistically significantly higher cancer detection rate compared with USPSTF-eligible individuals. However, the patients selected for LCS based on individual risk were older in age, had more comorbidities, and a shorter life expectancy.

Conclusion

Lung cancer screening research and clinical trials over the past half-century have paved the way for significant advances in the field, and specifically the reduction of lung cancer mortality. While this progress has led to one of the most exciting periods in cancer screening, many questions remain. Areas of active investigation include testing methods for community outreach to improve LCS uptake, improving accuracy of lung cancer risk prediction among vulnerable populations, defining strategies for effective LCS implementation, and evaluating the role of molecular biomarkers in LCS. With the ultimate goal of improving the lives of all patients at risk for lung cancer, the future of screening remains as tantalizing as ever.

References

1. Sharma D, Newman TG, Aronow WS. Lung cancer screening: history, current perspectives, and future directions. Arch Med Sci. 2015;11(5):1033–43.
2. Henschke C, Yankelevitz DF, Libby DM, Pasmantier MW, Smith JP, Miettinen OS. Survival of patients with stage I lung cancer detected on CT screening. N Engl J Med. 2006;355(17):1763–71.
3. Melamed MR, Flehinger BJ, Zaman MB, Heelan RT, Perchick WA, Martini N. Screening for early lung cancer: results of the memorial Sloan-Kettering study in New York. Chest. 1984;86(1):44–53.
4. Frost JK, Ball WC, Levin ML, Tockman MS, Baker RR, Carter D, et al. Early lung cancer detection: results of the initial (prevalence) radiologic and cytologic screening in the Johns Hopkins study. Am Rev Respir Dis. 1984;130(4):549–54.

5. Fontana RS, Sanderson DR, Taylor WF, Woolner LB, Miller WE, Muhm JR, et al. Early lung cancer detection: results of the initial (prevalence) radiologic and cytologic screening in the Mayo Clinic study. Am Rev Respir Dis. 1984;130(4):561–5.
6. Humphrey LL, Teutsch S, Johnson M. Lung cancer screening with sputum cytologic examination, chest radiography, and computed tomography: an update for the U.S. Preventive Services Task Force. Ann Intern Med. 2004;140(9):740–53.
7. Oken MM, Hocking WG, Kvale PA, Andriole GL, Buys SS, Church TR, et al. Screening by chest radiograph and lung cancer mortality: the prostate, lung, colorectal, and ovarian (PLCO) randomized trial. JAMA. 2011;306(17):1865–73.
8. Aberle DR, Adams AM, Berg CD, Black WC, Clapp JD, Fagerstrom RM, et al. Reduced lung-cancer mortality with low-dose computed tomographic screening. N Engl J Med. 2011;365(5):395–409.
9. Henschke CI, McCauley DI, Yankelevitz DF, Naidich DP, McGuinness G, Miettinen OS, et al. Early Lung Cancer Action Project: overall design and findings from baseline screening. Lancet. 1999;354(9173):99–105.
10. Bach PB, Jett JR, Pastorino U, Tockman MS, Swensen SJ, Begg CB. Computed tomography screening and lung cancer outcomes. JAMA. 2007;297(9):953–61.
11. Swensen SJ, Jett JR, Hartman TE, Midthun DE, Mandrekar SJ, Hillman SL, et al. CT screening for lung cancer: five-year prospective experience. Radiology. 2005;235(1):259–65.
12. Diederich S, Wormanns D, Semik M, Thomas M, Lenzen H, Roos N, et al. Screening for early lung cancer with low-dose spiral CT: prevalence in 817 asymptomatic smokers. Radiology. 2002;222(3):773–81.
13. Pastorino U, Bellomi M, Landoni C, De Fiori E, Arnaldi P, Picchio M, et al. Early lung-cancer detection with spiral CT and positron emission tomography in heavy smokers: 2-year results. Lancet. 2003;362(9384):593–7.
14. Infante M, Cavuto S, Lutman FR, Passera E, Chiarenza M, Chiesa G, et al. Long-term follow-up results of the DANTE trial, a randomized study of lung cancer screening with spiral computed tomography. Am J Respir Crit Care Med. 2015;191(10):1166–75.
15. Wille MMW, Dirksen A, Ashraf H, Saghir Z, Bach KS, Brodersen J, et al. Results of the randomized Danish lung cancer screening trial with focus on high-risk profiling. Am J Respir Crit Care Med. 2015;193(5):542–51.
16. Pastorino U, Rossi M, Rosato V, Marchianò A, Sverzellati N, Morosi C, et al. Annual or biennial CT screening versus observation in heavy smokers: 5-year results of the MILD trial. Eur J Cancer Prev. 2012;21(3):308.
17. Becker N, Motsch E, Gross ML, Eigentopf A, Heussel CP, Dienemann H, et al. Randomized study on early detection of lung cancer with MSCT in Germany: results of the first 3 years of follow-up after randomization. J Thorac Oncol. 2015;10(6):890–6.
18. Field JK, Duffy SW, Baldwin DR, Whynes DK, Devaraj A, Brain KE, et al. UK lung cancer RCT pilot screening trial: baseline findings from the screening arm provide evidence for the potential implementation of lung cancer screening. Thorax. 2016;71(2):161.
19. Force USPST. USPSTF final recommendation statement: lung cancer screening. 2013. Available from: https://www.uspreventiveservicestaskforce.org/Page/Document/RecommendationStatementFinal/lung-cancer-screening.
20. Services CfMaM. Decision memo for screening for lung cancer with low-dose computed tomography (LDCT) (CAG-00439N). 2015. Available from: https://www.cms.gov/medicare-coverage-database/details/nca-decision-memo.aspx?NCAId=274.
21. Force USPST. Screening for lung cancer: US preventive Services task Force recommendation statement. JAMA. 2021;325(10):962–70.
22. Services CfMaM. Decision memo for screening for for lung cancer with low-dose computed tomography (LDCT) (CAG-00439R). 2022.
23. de Koning HJ, van der Aalst CM, de Jong PA, Scholten ET, Nackaerts K, Heuvelmans MA, et al. Reduced lung-cancer mortality with volume CT screening in a randomized trial. N Engl J Med. 2020;382:503–13.

24. Walter JE, Heuvelmans MA, de Jong PA, Vliegenthart R, van Ooijen PMA, Peters RB, et al. Occurrence and lung cancer probability of new solid nodules at incidence screening with low-dose CT: analysis of data from the randomised, controlled NELSON trial. Lancet Oncol. 2016;17(7):907–16.
25. Tammemägi MC, Ruparel M, Tremblay A, Myers R, Mayo J, Yee J, et al. USPSTF2013 versus PLCOm2012 lung cancer screening eligibility criteria (International Lung Screening Trial): interim analysis of a prospective cohort study. Lancet Oncol. 2022;23(1):138–48.

Chapter 3
Stigma and Fatalism in Lung Cancer

Lisa A. Bevilacqua, Nathaniel R. Evans III, and Olugbenga Okusanya

Stigma

Stigma Definition and Background

Health-related stigma is a common and well-described phenomenon, with a growing body of literature on the role of stigma in shaping how patients interact with the healthcare system. Stigma describes a negative and untrue set of beliefs or generalizations held by society toward an individual, group, or circumstance [1]. One component of health-related stigma that has been consistently identified is the role of blame toward individuals who have a preventable condition or engage in risky behaviors which may lead to a disease process [1]. Common and well-studied examples of such health-related stigma include the biases and assumptions associated with individuals with substance use disorders, mental illness, and HIV/AIDS. Individuals with these diseases have been shown to consistently receive poorer care, in part due to the stigma associated with their medical condition [2, 3].

L. A. Bevilacqua . O. Okusanya (✉)
Division of Thoracic and Esophageal Surgery, Department of Surgery,
Thomas Jefferson University Hospital, Philadelphia, PA, USA
e-mail: Lisa.Bevilacqua@Jefferson.edu; Olugbenga.Okusanya@Jefferson.edu

N. R. Evans III
Department of Surgery, Thomas Jefferson University, Philadelphia, PA, USA
e-mail: Nathaniel.Evans@Jefferson.edu

G. C. Kane et al. (eds.), *Lung Cancer Screening*,
https://doi.org/10.1007/978-3-031-33596-9_3

Stigma in Lung Cancer

Research into the stigma associated with a lung cancer diagnosis has grown significantly in the past decade [4, 5]. A lung cancer diagnosis is susceptible to stigmatization due to the perceived nature of this disease as being preventable by an individual's choices or behaviors. Cigarette smoking is a modifiable risk factor for the development of lung cancer, and this association is well-known both in medicine and among the general public. Smoking rapidly became a stigmatized behavior in the United States as part of an aggressive public health campaign [6]. As such, a diagnosis of lung cancer is linked in the public consciousness to smoking, and thus public perceptions of smoking as a "choice" or "behavior" contribute to stigma against patients with lung cancer [7]. Hamann et al. (2014) found that 95% of lung cancer patients they interviewed reported a perceived stigma associated with smoking, regardless of their actual smoking history [8]. Other studies have reported patient experiences in which an immediate assumption of a smoking history was made when revealing their diagnosis to family and friends [9]. These findings are especially notable when considering that 10–15% of newly diagnosed lung cancers occur in patients without a smoking history [10].

Compared to patients with other cancers, those with lung cancer report higher levels of stigma [11], psychological distress [6], and internalized shame [12]. In one study, a group of respondents demonstrated implicit bias against lung cancer as compared to breast cancer [13, 14]. In this study, participants responded to images representing lung cancer or breast cancer presented in random sequence and classified those images with words that represented positive or negative feelings. The authors found that participants were quicker to associate lung cancer images with negative concepts and breast cancer with positive concepts and slower in the opposite direction. These findings were held among all surveyed, including cancer patients, their caregivers, healthcare providers, and members of the public [14]. In one survey of patients with lung cancer, almost one-quarter of respondents felt that they were treated differently by healthcare providers because of the *type* of cancer they have [15]. Of those patients, smokers were more likely to report being treated differently than former and never smokers.

Furthermore, evidence supports that these experiences of stigma by patients with lung cancer are not simply perceptions [16]. One study found that among a random sample of healthy women, patients with lung cancer were considered "at least partly to blame" by 70% of respondents, approaching levels of blame for chlamydia (87%) and obesity (96%), but less than leukemia (9%), breast cancer (15%), bowel cancer (23%), or cervical cancer (37%) [17]. Even among physicians, there appears to be bias against lung cancer. One study found that primary care physicians were less likely to make specialist referrals for patients with advanced lung cancers versus advanced breast cancers [18]. When lung cancer patients were referred, it was more commonly for symptom control than cancer therapy.

A cross-sectional survey of the general public, oncologists, and people with lung cancer conducted in 2008 and 2018 found that over that decade, there had been no significant change in the percentage of the general public who believed that patients with lung cancer are "at least partially to blame" for their illness. However, there appeared to be improved awareness among oncologists in agreeing that stigma exists [9]. There also appears to be greater awareness of this stigma among patients with lung cancer. More patients believed there was a stigma associated with this disease over the timeframe studied. In this same group of patients, over half agreed that strangers and acquaintances had said or done things that blamed them for their illness and felt that friends/family would be more supportive if they had a different type of cancer [9].

Public perceptions of lung cancer as a disease that the patient is to blame can also be seen in the level of public engagement with efforts against lung cancer. In one sample of healthy adults without a cancer history, only 8% of those surveyed reported involvement with a lung cancer organization, compared to 18% for breast cancer organizations [19]. Among those surveyed, 59% also believed that patients with lung cancer "are at least partly to blame for their illness," with 31% also acknowledging that "lung cancer patients are treated differently than other cancer patients."

Additional evidence of the stigma associated with lung cancer can be seen in the relatively low funding rates that lung cancer receives compared to other cancers that are both less prevalent and less deadly. In 2020, lung cancer received approximately $447 million in NCI/NIH funding, compared to $788 million for breast cancer. Colorectal and prostate cancers received $319 and $264 million, respectively [20]. These findings have been replicated in the non-profit sector [21].

Structural factors also impact stigma against patients with lung cancer. It is well-established that tobacco companies have targeted people from low socioeconomic backgrounds and other marginalized groups. The tobacco industry also has a well-documented history of racism and has developed advertising tactics targeted at Black Americans to increase smoking rates [22]. Black and Hispanic neighborhoods are also more likely to have high distributions of tobacco retailers [23]. In addition, historically marginalized communities are less likely to be screened for tobacco use [24], receive physician advice to quit smoking [25], and receive tobacco cessation treatment [23]. Thus, when groups already marginalized and stigmatized within the healthcare system [23] are subject to more aggressive tobacco advertising and less counseling and screening, lung cancer stigma can be compounded. Unfortunately, few studies to date have investigated this complex relationship between lung cancer stigma and structural racism, poverty, and disparities in cancer outcomes.

Measuring Stigma

Two main instruments have been developed to assess stigma specifically in lung cancer. Cataldo et al. developed and validated the Cataldo Lung Cancer Stigma Scale (CLCSS) [26]. This 31-item Likert scale identifies four main domains: stigma and shame, social isolation, discrimination, and smoking. It has subsequently been shortened to a 21-item scale [27]. The Lung Cancer Stigma Inventory is another tool that has been developed and validated for use in measuring clinically significant levels of stigma in lung cancer [28]. In this model, Ostroff et al. develop a framework identifying three primary elements of lung cancer stigma from the patient's perspective: "(1) perceived stigma (how what others think and say is evaluated by the patient); (2) internalized stigma (how perceived stigma can affect patients through self-blame and guilt); and (3) constrained disclosure (how stigma limits discussions of lung cancer with others)." Several other instruments assessing stigma in multiple types of cancer have been used in the lung cancer literature [5].

Consequences of Stigma

The stigma against lung cancer has significant consequences for patients with this disease throughout the continuum of care, from diagnosis to treatment and through to survivorship [29, 30].

Delayed Presentation and Avoidance of Treatment

Despite lung cancer remaining the most common cause of cancer death in the United States [31], it continues to be routinely diagnosed at a late stage. This vicious cycle of late-stage diagnosis, in turn, contributes to the high mortality of this disease [32]. Several studies have found that lung cancer stigma is independently associated with delays in medical care-seeking behavior [33, 34]. In one study of patients at an academic thoracic practice in the United States, a positive correlation was noted between lung cancer stigma scores using the Cataldo scale and timing of medical help-seeking behavior, defined as days from symptom onset to when a patient called his or her primary care physician.

In other studies, a positive smoking status has been independently associated with delayed reporting of symptoms of lung cancer [35, 36], although many of these studies have been qualitative [37–39].

Quality of Life

Quality of life has been established as an independent predictor of survival for cancer patients [40]. Multiple studies have found that stigma is associated with poorer quality of life in lung cancer. One report found that even after controlling for sex, age, anxiety, and depression, lung cancer stigma still accounted for differences in quality of life [41]. Furthermore, stigma, depression, and quality of life did not differ by smoking status in this study. This association between stigma and quality of life has been replicated in diverse populations in the United States and abroad [42, 43].

Depression/Anxiety/Psychological Distress

Stigma has also been associated with adverse psychosocial outcomes, including depression, anxiety, and psychosocial distress among patients with lung cancer [28]. One study of 95 patients currently receiving chemotherapy showed a positive association between stigma and depressive symptoms, even after accounting for relevant demographic and clinical factors [27]. Depressive symptoms were also associated with social rejection, financial insecurity, internalized shame, and social isolation in this sample. Another study found a positive correlation between stigma and anxiety, depression, and lung cancer symptom severity. Furthermore, stigma explained a significant percentage of the variance in lung cancer symptom severity beyond that of anxiety, depression, and patient age.

In one longitudinal study of patients with lung cancer in Australia, there was a positive correlation between psychological distress and lung cancer stigma approximately 6 months after diagnosis, which did not exist at 3 months [44]. This contrasts with another longitudinal study of patients receiving active medical treatment of their lung cancer, which found that higher levels of stigma predicted significant declines in emotional well-being at 6 and 12 weeks, as well as declines in physical/functional well-being at the 6-week time point [45].

Interventions to Reduce Stigma

Despite the increasing awareness of the role of stigma in lung cancer diagnosis, psychosocial experiences, and outcomes over the past two decades, there has been limited research on interventions targeting this issue [46]. Hamann et al. advocated for a multilevel approach to addressing stigma and the barriers it creates at all phases of care, including prevention, screening, diagnosis, treatment, and survivorship [30].

One small pilot study of 14 patients assessed a Psychological Wellness Intervention based on Cognitive Behavioral Theory that included psychoeducation, skills in stress reduction, problem-solving, cognitive challenging, and enhancing relationship support [47]. This intervention was delivered by telephone delivered in six weekly 50–55-min sessions. The authors found that scores for psychological distress, cancer-related distress, depression, and stigma improved over time. These findings have not yet been replicated in larger samples or when compared to a control group not receiving an intervention.

Some interventions have also been aimed at the level of the healthcare provider. Banerjee et al. (2021) recently reported on using a communication skills module for 50 providers who treat patients with lung cancer [48]. The healthcare providers who participated in this intervention reported improvement in their self-efficacy in empathic communication. Further work is needed to determine if this intervention with providers translates into improved communication with and outcomes for patients.

Conclusions

Lung cancer stigma remains a persistent problem at the individual, healthcare provider, and societal level. Stigma creates barriers to care, including screening, open communication, and pursuit of treatment. Despite increasing recognition of these problems in the scientific literature, limited interventions have been developed to target stigma and its impact on lung cancer outcomes. Furthermore, although lung cancer remains the leading cause of cancer deaths in the United States, it remains underfunded in both the government and private sectors.

Fatalism

Fatalism is defined as the belief that events are predetermined and thus cannot be controlled [49]. Within the medical field, "cancer fatalism" has been described as "the belief that death is inevitable when cancer is present" and has been identified as a barrier to screening and treatment [50]. This phenomenon has also been linked to the concept of "therapeutic nihilism" and is closely related to experiences of healthcare stigma [29]. In one systematic review of the literature on stigma and nihilism in lung cancer, multiple qualitative studies reported a sense of fatalism (i.e., lung cancer is a fatal disease) among patients with a lung cancer diagnosis, although it was noted that there have been few studies that empirically quantify this association [29].

For example, one qualitative study investigating reasons for patient refusal of physicians' recommendations found that one of the reasons why patients with lung cancer refused was that they believed the treatment was futile [51]. Another interview-based study found that lung cancer was perceived as an uncontrollable disease among current, former, and never smokers from low socioeconomic backgrounds [39]. Within this sample, levels of fatalism were higher among smokers compared with nonsmokers, with almost half of current smokers agreeing that lung cancer is "a death sentence." In another UK survey, 20% of active smokers believed they had smoked too long to benefit from any lung cancer screening program, and 44% that they would invariably get lung cancer sometime during their life [39]. The finding of higher fatalism scores among current smokers compared to former and nonsmokers has been replicated in other studies [52].

Among providers treating patients with lung cancer, fatalism has been associated with variation in treatment options that healthcare professionals offer however these studies have also mainly been qualitative [29]. Other studies have attempted to quantify the impact of fatalistic beliefs on attitudes toward lung cancer among providers. One study of US-based pulmonologists and thoracic surgeons found that providers whose beliefs were categorized as "pessimistic" were significantly less likely to believe in a survival benefit for chemotherapy in addition to radiotherapy for unresectable locally advanced non-small cell lung cancer. In this study, pessimism was defined as underestimating 5-year survival for stage I disease. Interestingly, pulmonologists were more likely to underestimate the survival benefit when compared to surgeons, as were those who trained before 1980 compared to after [53]. Importantly, this study was done in 2000, and more contemporary beliefs on the futility of treatment for lung cancer as treatment paradigms have improved have not been investigated.

Social-demographic variables have been associated with differences in fatalism. Berghamo et al. (2013) surveyed 357 patients with lung cancer in New York City. Patients who identified as Black or Hispanic were significantly more likely to endorse fatalistic views and medical mistrust. These views were also more common among patients with late-stage lung cancer [54]. The authors hypothesized that this might partially explain the disparities in cancer stage at diagnosis.

In one study of colorectal and lung cancer patients, women, patients with lower educational attainment, and lower income all reported significantly more fatalistic beliefs [52]. Consistent with Berghamo et al., White patients reported the lowest levels of fatalism compared to Black, Hispanic, and Asian patients. Fatalistic views did not differ between cancer sites (lung versus colon); however, they differed by stage of cancer.

Cultural differences in beliefs and attitudes toward cancer may also contribute to fatalism regarding the role of surgery in the treatment of lung cancer. One well-described belief is the idea that operating on (cutting into) cancer can expose it to air, thus contributing to spread of the cancer. Patients who hold this belief have been shown to have less willingness to undergo surgery [55]. This belief is most commonly reported among women, rural patients, and Asian, African-American, and Latino/a patients and has been described in several cancer populations, including lung, bowel, and breast [55–57].

Thus, cancer fatalism, much like stigma, is multifactorial and contributes to disparities in cancer outcomes through reduced screening, delayed care, and pursuit of fewer/less aggressive treatment options.

References

1. Link BG, Phelan JC. Conceptualizing stigma. Annu Rev Sociol. 2001;27(1):363–85.
2. van Boekel LC, Brouwers EPM, van Weeghel J, Garretsen HFL. Stigma among health professionals towards patients with substance use disorders and its consequences for healthcare delivery: systematic review. Drug Alcohol Depend. 2013;131(1):23–35.
3. Berger BE, Ferrans CE, Lashley FR. Measuring stigma in people with HIV: psychometric assessment of the HIV stigma scale. Res Nurs Health. 2001;24(6):518–29.
4. Chapple A, Ziebland S, McPherson A. Stigma, shame, and blame experienced by patients with lung cancer: qualitative study. BMJ. 2004;328(7454):1470.
5. Webb LA, McDonnell KK, Adams SA, Davis RE, Felder TM. Exploring stigma among lung cancer survivors: a scoping literature review. Oncol Nurs Forum. 2019;46(4):402–18.
6. Evans-Polce RJ, Castaldelli-Maia JM, Schomerus G, Evans-Lacko SE. The downside of tobacco control? Smoking and self-stigma: a systematic review. Soc Sci Med. 2015;145:26–34.

7. Stuber J, Galea S, Link BG. Smoking and the emergence of a stigmatized social status. Soc Sci Med. 2008;67(3):420–30.

8. Hamann HA, Ostroff JS, Marks EG, Gerber DE, Schiller JH, Craddock Lee SJ. Stigma among patients with lung cancer: a patient-reported measurement model. Psychooncology. 2014;23(1):81–92.

9. Rigney M, Rapsomaniki E, Carter-Harris L, King JC. A 10-year cross-sectional analysis of public, oncologist, and patient attitudes about lung cancer and associated stigma. J Thorac Oncol. 2021;16(1):151–5.

10. Siegel DA, Fedewa SA, Henley SJ, Pollack LA, Jemal A. Proportion of never smokers among men and women with lung cancer in 7 US states. JAMA Oncol. 2021;7(2):302–4.

11. LoConte NK, Else-Quest NM, Eickhoff J, Hyde J, Schiller JH. Assessment of guilt and shame in patients with non-small-cell lung cancer compared with patients with breast and prostate cancer. Clin Lung Cancer. 2008;9(3):171–8.

12. Ernst J, Mehnert A, Dietz A, Hornemann B, Esser P. Perceived stigmatization and its impact on quality of life - results from a large register-based study including breast, colon, prostate and lung cancer patients. BMC Cancer. 2017;17:741.

13. Greenwald AG, Banaji MR. Implicit social cognition: attitudes, self-esteem, and stereotypes. Psychol Rev. 1995;102(1):4–27.

14. Sriram N, Mills J, Lang E, Dickson HK, Hamann HA, Nosek BA, et al. Attitudes and stereotypes in lung Cancer versus breast cancer. PLoS One. 2015;10(12):e0145715.

15. Weiss J, Yang H, Weiss S, Rigney M, Copeland A, King JC, et al. Stigma, self-blame, and satisfaction with care among patients with lung cancer. J Psychosoc Oncol. 2017;35(2):166–79.

16. Marlow LAV, Waller J, Wardle J. Does lung cancer attract greater stigma than other cancer types? Lung Cancer. 2015;88(1):104–7.

17. Marlow LAV, Waller J, Wardle J. Variation in blame attributions across different cancer types. Cancer Epidemiol Biomarkers Prev. 2010;19(7):1799–805.

18. Wassenaar TR, Eickhoff JC, Jarzemsky DR, Smith SS, Larson ML, Schiller JH. Differences in primary care clinicians' approach to non-small cell lung cancer patients compared with breast cancer. J Thorac Oncol. 2007;2(8):722–8.

19. Weiss J, Stephenson BJ, Edwards LJ, Rigney M, Copeland A. Public attitudes about lung cancer: stigma, support, and predictors of support. J Multidiscip Healthc. 2014;7:293–300.

20. National Institute of Health. Estimates of funding for various research, condition, and disease categories (RCDC) [Internet]. 2021 [cited 2022 Feb 6]. Available from: https://report.nih.gov/funding/categorical-spending#/

21. Kamath SD, Kircher SM, Benson AB. Comparison of cancer burden and nonprofit organization funding reveals disparities in funding across cancer types. J Natl Compr Cancer Netw. 2019;17(7):849–54.

22. Subbaraman N. How cigarettes became a civil-rights issue. Nature. 2021;598(7881):407–8.

23. American Heart Association. Structural racism & tobacco [Internet]. 2020 [cited 2022 Feb 22]. Available from: https://www.heart.org/-/media/Files/About-Us/Policy-Research/Fact-Sheets/Tobacco-and-Clean-Air/Structural-Racism-and-Tobacco-Fact-Sheet.pdf.

24. Tobacco use screening and counseling during physician office visits among adults—National Ambulatory Medical Care Survey and National Health Interview Survey, United States, 2005–2009 [Internet]. [cited 2022 Feb 22]. Available from: https://www.cdc.gov/mmwr/preview/mmwrhtml/su6102a7.htm.

25. Browning KK, Ferketich AK, Salsberry PJ, Wewers ME. Socioeconomic disparity in provider-delivered assistance to quit smoking. Nicotine Tob Res. 2008;10(1):55–61.

26. Cataldo JK, Slaughter R, Jahan TM, Pongquan VL, Hwang WJ. Measuring stigma in people with lung cancer: psychometric testing of the Cataldo lung cancer stigma scale. Oncol Nurs Forum. 2011;38(1):E46–54.

27. Carter-Harris L, Hall LA. Development of a short version of the Cataldo lung cancer stigma scale. J Psychosoc Oncol. 2014;32(6):665–77.

28. Ostroff JS, Riley KE, Shen MJ, Atkinson TM, Williamson TJ, Hamann HA. Lung cancer stigma and depression: validation of the lung cancer stigma inventory. Psychooncology. 2019;28(5):1011–7.
29. Chambers SK, Dunn J, Occhipinti S, Hughes S, Baade P, Sinclair S, et al. A systematic review of the impact of stigma and nihilism on lung cancer outcomes. BMC Cancer. 2012;12:184.
30. Hamann HA, Ver Hoeve ES, Carter-Harris L, Studts JL, Ostroff JS. Multilevel opportunities to address lung cancer stigma across the cancer control continuum. J Thorac Oncol. 2018;13(8):1062–75.
31. Cancer facts & figures 2021. 1930;72.
32. Ellis PM, Vandermeer R. Delays in the diagnosis of lung cancer. J Thorac Dis. 2011;3(3):183–8.
33. Carter-Harris L, Hermann CP, Schreiber J, Weaver MT, Rawl SM. Lung cancer stigma predicts timing of medical help–seeking behavior. Oncol Nurs Forum. 2014;41(3):E203–10.
34. Scott N, Crane M, Lafontaine M, Seale H, Currow D. Stigma as a barrier to diagnosis of lung cancer: patient and general practitioner perspectives. Prim Health Care Res Dev. 2015;16(6):618–22.
35. Smith SM, Campbell NC, MacLeod U, Lee AJ, Raja A, Wyke S, et al. Factors contributing to the time taken to consult with symptoms of lung cancer: a cross-sectional study. Thorax. 2009;64(6):523–31.
36. Kotecha J, Clark A, Burton M, Chan WY, Menzies D, Dernedde U, et al. Evaluating the delay prior to primary care presentation in patients with lung cancer: a cohort study. BJGP Open. 2021;5(2):BJGPO.2020.0130.
37. Tod AM, Craven J, Allmark P. Diagnostic delay in lung cancer: a qualitative study. J Adv Nurs. 2008;61(3):336–43.
38. Cassim S, Chepulis L, Keenan R, Kidd J, Firth M, Lawrenson R. Patient and carer perceived barriers to early presentation and diagnosis of lung cancer: a systematic review. BMC Cancer. 2019;19(1):25.
39. Quaife SL, Marlow LAV, McEwen A, Janes SM, Wardle J. Attitudes towards lung cancer screening in socioeconomically deprived and heavy smoking communities: informing screening communication. Health Expect. 2017;20(4):563–73.
40. Ganz PA, Lee JJ, Siau J. Quality of life assessment. An independent prognostic variable for survival in lung cancer. Cancer. 1991;67(12):3131–5.
41. Brown Johnson CG, Brodsky JL, Cataldo JK. Lung cancer stigma, anxiety, depression, and quality of life. J Psychosoc Oncol. 2014;32(1):59–73.
42. Maguire R, Lewis L, Kotronoulas G, McPhelim J, Milroy R, Cataldo J. Lung cancer stigma: a concept with consequences for patients. Cancer Rep. 2019;2(5):e1201.
43. Chambers SK, Baade P, Youl P, Aitken J, Occhipinti S, Vinod S, et al. Psychological distress and quality of life in lung cancer: the role of health-related stigma, illness appraisals and social constraints. Psychooncology. 2015;24(11):1569–77.
44. Rose S, Boyes A, Kelly B, Cox M, Palazzi K, Paul C. Lung cancer stigma is a predictor for psychological distress: a longitudinal study. Lung cancer stigma is a predictor for psychological distress. Psychooncology. 2021;30(7):1137–44.
45. Williamson TJ, Choi AK, Kim JC, Garon EB, Shapiro JR, Irwin MR, et al. A longitudinal investigation of internalized stigma, constrained disclosure, and quality of life across 12 weeks in lung cancer patients on active oncologic treatment. J Thorac Oncol. 2018;13(9):1284–93.
46. Hamann HA, Williamson TJ, Studts JL, Ostroff JS. Lung cancer stigma then and now: continued challenges amid a landscape of Progress. J Thorac Oncol. 2021;16(1):17–20.
47. Chambers SK, Morris BA, Clutton S, Foley E, Giles L, Schofield P, et al. Psychological wellness and health-related stigma: a pilot study of an acceptance-focused cognitive behavioural intervention for people with lung cancer. Eur J Cancer Care (Engl). 2015;24(1):60–70.
48. Banerjee SC, Haque N, Bylund CL, Shen MJ, Rigney M, Hamann HA, et al. Responding empathically to patients: a communication skills training module to reduce lung cancer stigma. Transl Behav Med. 2021;11(2):613–8.

49. Shen L, Condit CM, Wright L. The psychometric property and validation of a fatalism scale. Psychol Health. 2009;24(5):597–613.
50. Powe BD, Finnie R. Cancer fatalism: the state of the science. Cancer Nurs. 2003;26(6):454–67.
51. Sharf BF, Stelljes LA, Gordon HS. 'A little bitty spot and I'm a big man': patients' perspectives on refusing diagnosis or treatment for lung cancer. Psychooncology. 2005;14(8):636–46.
52. Lyratzopoulos G, Liu MP-H, Abel GA, Wardle J, Keating NL. The association between fatalistic beliefs and late stage at diagnosis of lung and colorectal cancer. Cancer Epidemiol Biomark Prev. 2015;24(4):720–6.
53. Schroen AT, Detterbeck FC, Crawford R, Rivera MP, Socinski MA. Beliefs among pulmonologists and thoracic surgeons in the therapeutic approach to non-small cell lung cancer. Chest. 2000;118(1):129–37.
54. Bergamo C, Lin JJ, Smith C, Lurslurchachai L, Halm EA, Powell CA, et al. Evaluating beliefs associated with late-stage lung cancer presentation in minorities. J Thorac Oncol. 2013;8(1):12–8.
55. James A, Daley CM, Greiner KA. "Cutting" on cancer: attitudes about cancer spread and surgery among primary care patients in the USA. Soc Sci Med. 2011;73(11):1669–73.
56. Lannin DR, Mathews HF, Mitchell J, Swanson MS, Swanson FH, Edwards MS. Influence of socioeconomic and cultural factors on racial differences in late-stage presentation of breast cancer. JAMA. 1998;279(22):1801–7.
57. Ramírez AS, Rutten LJF, Oh A, Vengoechea BL, Moser RP, Vanderpool RC, et al. Perceptions of cancer controllability and cancer risk knowledge: the moderating role of race, ethnicity, and acculturation. J Cancer Educ. 2013;28(2):254–61.

Chapter 4
Training in Shared Decision Making About Lung Cancer Screening: Patient Eligibility Assessment, Education, and Decision Counseling

Melissa DiCarlo, Kristine Pham, and Ronald E. Myers

Background

Persons eligible for lung cancer screening (LCS) under current United States Preventive Services Task Force (USPSTF) guidelines include adults who are 50 to 80 years of age, have at least a 20-pack-year smoking history, and either currently smoke or have formerly smoked but quit within the past 15 years [1]. Recently revised Centers for Medicare and Medicare Services (CMS) guidelines provide coverage to individuals who satisfy criteria that align with USPSTF guidelines, except for limiting age eligibility to those between 50 and 77 years of age [2]. Inclusion of a shared decision-making (SDM) requirement makes LCS unique in Centers for Medicare and Medicaid (CMS) coverage for cancer screening. CMS specifies that SDM should involve the identification of patients who are eligible for LCS, the use of a decision aid to educate patients about screening risks and benefits, informing patients about initial and repeat LCS, along with diagnostic follow-up, and helping patients clarify their personal preference related to screening. It is important that practice providers, patient navigators, care coordinators, and others learn how to assess patient eligibility for screening, educate patients about screening, and engage patients in SDM about LCS [3].

M. DiCarlo (✉) · K. Pham
Department of Medical Oncology, Thomas Jefferson University, Philadelphia, PA, USA
e-mail: Melissa.DiCarlo@Jefferson.edu; Kristine.Pham@Jefferson.edu

R. E. Myers
Medical Oncology, Thomas Jefferson University, Philadelphia, PA, USA
e-mail: Ronald.Myers@Jefferson.edu

The Need for Training in Shared Decision Making About Lung Cancer Screening

Brenner et al. [4] recorded 14 physician–patient conversations about initiating LCS. Half of the encounters involved primary care providers. Qualitative analyses of conversation transcripts focused on patient involvement in decision making, time spent discussing SDM, evidence of decision-aid use, and SDM quality. Findings indicated that patient involvement in decision making was very low (6 on a scale of 0 to 100), less than 1 min was devoted to discussing LCS screening, there was no evidence of decision-aid use, and none of the conversations met the lowest threshold of skill criteria used to assess decision quality (8 out of 12 SDM behaviors). More recently, Nishi et al. [5] recently reported on a study that involved 266 consenting patients who were determined to be eligible for LCS and were recruited from two academic tertiary care centers in the south-central United States. All study participants underwent LCS and completed a survey questionnaire that included items to assess their involvement in the SDM process, knowledge of LCS, receipt of LCS educational materials, knowledge about LCS, and decisional conflict related to screening. Survey data analysis showed that 87% of participants reported that they were involved in the screening decision process. However, only 41% provided correct responses to survey knowledge questions and 34% reported decisional conflict about screening.

In a recent review, Müller et al. [6] found that a number of training programs have been developed to educate healthcare providers about the need for SDM related to many important health care decisions, but few have focused on imparting knowledge and skills actually needed to engage patients in SDM. Légaré et al. [7] observed that this limitation helps to explain why providers often do not engage their patients in SDM about their care, and that training strategies should not only increase provider knowledge, but also must enhance provider skills and confidence in SDM performance [8, 9]. There is little information in the literature on the impact of training providers to engage patients in SDM about LCS and on the effect of training on LCS rates in clinical practice.

In a study that involved physician training in SDM for prostate cancer screening, Volk et al. [10] enrolled 49 primary care physicians to complete an online training course that used case-based learning. The course prepared participants to encourage patients to ask questions about screening, provide guidance to patients about decision making, tailor information about screening to patient needs, and establish a decision-making partnership. Using post-training data, the authors found that over 90% of providers correctly identified the steps in the SDM process, 65% said they felt very confident in their capacity to explore a patient's values related to screening, and more than 70% reported that they intended to engage their eligible patients in SDM about screening in the future.

Lowenstein et al. [11] recently reported on a study conducted in three radiology clinics in a large academic medical center, where nursing and advanced practice providers were trained to use an interactive tablet to conduct an in-office SDM session with patients who presented at the clinic for LCS. Through the analysis of 26 audio-recorded sessions, the authors determined that most elements of SDM required by CMS were reviewed by the nonphysician providers. Furthermore, they found that among 30 patients who completed an SDM session with a trained provider, patient knowledge about LCS increased significantly.

Hoffman et al. [12] have highlighted the importance of training primary care physicians and non-physicians who "can help to ensure patient engagement, deliver consistent and comprehensive information, and support tobacco cessation … (and) increase value-concordant decisions and satisfaction with the decision process." To address this need, the National Lung Cancer Roundtable, Thomas Jefferson University, the College of Chest Physicians, and the GO2 Foundation have developed a comprehensive lung cancer screening SDM training program.

Developing a Lung Cancer Screening Shared Decision-Making Training Program

Beginning in 2018, the National Lung Cancer Roundtable, Thomas Jefferson University, and the American College of Chest Physicians initiated the process of bringing together physicians, researchers, instructional designers, and public health professionals from around the nation to begin developing a training short course for providers on SDM about LCS. Initial discussions led to the development of a unique online training program designed to prepare primary care providers, nurses, and others to engage patients in all aspects of SDM about LCS as defined by CMS coverage guidelines. This collaboration, which also involved the GO2 Foundation for Lung Cancer, was designed to a self-directed, accredited, online training program that includes three modules, which prepare to learner (1) assess patient eligibility for lung cancer screening, (2) educate patients about lung cancer and lung cancer screening, and (3) help patients make a well-informed decision about screening. This unique program, *Shared Decision Making in Lung Cancer Screening*, can be accessed online at the following site:

https://www.chestnet.org/Store/Products/Standard-Products/eLearning/Shared-Decision-Making-in-Lung-Cancer-Screening.

Module 1 is titled, *Assessment of Eligibility for Lung Cancer Screening*. The objective of this module is to help learners to identify eligible patients based on CMS and USPSTF guidelines, calculate pack-years of cigarette smoking history, and complete necessary documentation in the electronic medical record (EMR). The module meets the objectives by guiding learners through CMS and USPSTF eligibility criteria, suggesting prompts for initiating a discussion with patients about smoking history. In addition, the module provides a simple formula for the learner to use in calculating pack-years of smoking exposure. In addition, the module guides the learner through four case-based scenarios to enhance pack-year calculation skills. In each of these scenarios, a patient story is presented and prompts are given to facilitate the discussion of smoking history. After each instance, the learner is asked to determine the patient screening eligibility status. Feedback is provided to the learner in order to reinforce the correct determination. Furthermore, this module guides the learner to enter patient smoking history data and screening eligibility status in the patient's EMR. Module 1 includes a pretest and a posttest that ask questions to assess learner knowledge before and after completing this part of the training program.

Module 2 is titled, *Education about Lung Cancer Screening*. This module presents the learner with information on lung cancer risk, initial and repeat screening, and the potential benefits and harms of screening. Information on the importance of tobacco treatment is also provided. The objective of this module is to educate providers on LCS, so that they can educate their patients about this important preventive health behavior. The module first reviews the relative risk of smoking and cancers, providing learners with baseline understanding of smoking exposure and cancer risk. The presentation of this information is followed by an overview of the importance of annual low-dose computed tomography (LDCT) screening for lung cancer. In addition, the module provides guidance on how LDCT screening can be described to patients. Moreover, the module identifies potential risks of screening and highlights the importance of tobacco treatment and available tobacco treatment resources for persons who currently smoke and those who have quit smoking.

The module also gives the provider access to LCS infographisc that can be shared with patients and can be used as an educational tool. One of the LCS infographics provides basic information about the LCS process. The other infographic, which is shown in the figure below, presents more detailed information about the likelihood of being diagnosed with early stage lung cancer in the absence of screening in the presence of LCS. In addition, this tool includes information about the likelihood of being recommended for annual screening (given a normal screening result) and of being referred for diagnostic follow-up after screening (given an abnormal screening result). The information also presents important information about the potential for over-diagnosis, the safety of LDCT screening, screening-related costs, and the importance of tobacco treatment. Finally, the infographic encourages patients to indicate their level of interest in LCS and let their healthcare provider know how they feel about screening. Module 2 includes pretest and posttest questions intended to assess knowledge before and after completing this section of the training program.

Module 3 of the training program, *Support for Making a Decision about Lung Cancer Screening*, serves as an introduction to SDM about LCS. Objectives of this module are to enable learners to understand what constitutes shared decision making, elicit patient values related to LCS, determine patient screening preference, develop a patient-specific screening action plan, and document the patient's screening preference and action plan in the EMR. Importantly, the module provides guidance on how to conduct a screening decision counseling session [13] that involves not only providing information about LCS but also completing an exercise that involves eliciting reasons that patients may have to be screened or not to be screened. This exercise involves eliciting personal reasons/goals that motivate the patient to and not to screen. The learner finds out how to elicit and clarify reasons/ goals that are important to the patient. Past research has shown that there are a variety of cognitive, affective, and social factors that affect personal preference for choosing one option over another [14, 15]. These factors may be described as fears, worries and concerns, importance or convenience, susceptibility or risk, efficacy or accuracy, and social support and influence.

In accordance with the categories listed here, examples of reasons/goals a patient may have to screen include the following: (1) "I'm worried about having cancer and I want to know," (2) "Screening won't take much time," (3) "My smoking history puts me at risk," (4) "I believe screening can help find out if I have a problem," and (5) "My daughter wants me to screen." Similarly, patients may express reasons/ goals that influence why they don't want to have LDCT screening, such as the following: (1) "I'm afraid of finding out that I have lung cancer," (2) "I'm too busy to go in for screening," (3) "I stopped smoking, so I'm not at risk," (4) "I've heard that screening generates a lot of false positives," and (5) "My friends think screening is a bad idea." Specific patient scenarios included in the module show the learner how to help patients identify their top reasons, elicit the level of influence each reason has on their decision, weigh the relative importance of the reason, clarify the patient's screening preference, and develop a screening plan that is concordant with that preference. The program provides learners allows the learner to download a "fillable" PDF document displayed below that they can use to facilitate structured SDM conversations with patients about LCS.

Going forward, we plan to include access in the training program to an online interactive decision counseling tool (the Jefferson Decision Counseling Guide) that can be used to guide the SDM conversation and assess SDM quality. This tool uses patient responses to compute a patient's LCS preference score and screening decision and can serve to document the encounter and the screening decision.

Updated 3/20/2023

Decision Counseling Guide for Lung Cancer Screening

People have reasons/goals that favor **being screened (Option A)** and **NOT being screened (Option B)** for lung cancer. Encourage the patient to talk about their reasons/goals related to the options and clarify their preference.

STEP ONE: Help the patient identify their reasons/goals related to each option, select the most important reasons/goals (up to a total of 3) and rank those in order of importance (1= most important, 2 = 2nd most important, 3 = 3rd most important). Then, enter the top 3 reasons/goals in **STEP TWO**.

Reasons/Goals related to **being screened**   Reasons/Goals related to **NOT being screened**

_______________________________   _______________________________

_______________________________   _______________________________

_______________________________   _______________________________

STEP TWO: Ask the patient how much more they think <u>one option</u> can help to address their top reason(s)/goal(s) <u>than the other option</u>. Example: *"I understand you want [to find out if you have lung cancer]. How much more do you think being screened can help [to find out if you have lung cancer] than not being screened?"* If there is only one reason/goal, complete this step and go to **STEP FOUR**. If there are two or three reasons/goals, complete this step and proceed to **STEP THREE** and then **STEP FOUR**.

Compare and Score the Options

Top 3 Reasons/Goals	About the Same	A Little More	Some- what More	Much More	Very Much More	Overwhelmingly More
1. _____________________	☐	☐	☐	☐	☐	☐
2. _____________________	☐	☐	☐	☐	☐	☐
3. _____________________	☐	☐	☐	☐	☐	☐

STEP THREE: Ask the patient how much more important <u>one reason/goal</u> is <u>than another</u>. Example: *"How much more important is it to find out if you have lung cancer than to avoid radiation exposure?"* If there are 2 reasons/goals, enter how much more important 1 is compared to 2. If there are 3 reasons/goals, enter the importance of 1 compared to 2, 2 compared to 3, and 1 compared to 3.

Compare and Score the Reasons/Goals

Top 3 Reasons/Goals Compared	About the Same	A Little More	Some- what More	Much More	Very Much More	Overwhelmingly More
1. compared to 2.	☐	☐	☐	☐	☐	☐
2. compared to 3.	☐	☐	☐	☐	☐	☐
1. compared to 3.	☐	☐	☐	☐	☐	☐

STEP FOUR: Ask the patient to indicate what they want to do about screening on a scale of 0 to 10 (0 = I really don't want to be screened, 5 = I'm unsure about being screened, 10 = I really want to be screened). Enter the result and develop an action plan based on this result.

I don't want to be screened					I'm unsure				I want to be screened	
0	1	2	3	4	5	6	7	8	9	10
☐	☐	☐	☐	☐	☐	☐	☐	☐	☐	☐

As in other modules of the training program, Module 3 includes a pretest and a posttest questions designed to assess learner knowledge before and after completing this section of the training program. Finally, the training program includes an evaluation that learners are asked to complete. The evaluation captures information on learner perspectives related to each module. More specifically, items are included to determine overall effectiveness and the extent to which objectives were achieved. Items were also included to assess whether the learner's practice is likely to change based on the content and materials that are part of the training program and whether the individual's SDM skills and performance are likely to change. Furthermore, the evaluation instrument asked the learner to identify impediments to implementation of SDM in practice and to provide feedback on the training experience.

Evaluating SDM Quality

It has been recognized that there is a need for high-quality SDM performance in healthcare [16, 17]. As described by Brenner et al. [4] and others, this need is apparent in relation to conversations about LCS that take place between providers and patients. In the Lung Cancer Screening Shared Decision Making Training Program, we address this problem by using data from the online Jefferson Decision Counseling Guide to evaluate five aspects of the physician–patient encounter. Specifically, the online tool allows the provider to document the following: (1) patient education about LCS, (2) the clarify of patient reasons to and not to have screening, (3) the uniqueness of patient reasons to and not to have screening, (4) the concordance of patient preference and choice to or not to screen, and (5) development of an action plan.

The Jefferson Decision Counseling Guide allows for access to any educational resource or materials during the conversation. As previously discussed, it is important to ensure that the patient is educated about the risks and benefits of lung cancer screening, and for the provider to address any concerns that may arise. Before proceeding to the next step, the provider is required to indicate "yes" or "no" when prompted if educational materials were reviewed with the patient. Once the patient reviews information about screening, the provider elicits the patient's reasons for and against screening. Then, the provider guides the patient through the process of identifying their top three reasons, elicits the effect of each reason on the decision to or not to screen, asks the patient to rank the reasons in terms of importance, and determines the relative importance of the reasons. The provider uses the Jefferson Decision Counseling Guide to execute an algorithm that computes the patient's preference score, a continuous measure ranging from 0 to 100, with a higher score indicating a preference for screening.

Finally, the Jefferson Decision Counseling Guide is designed to generate a SDM quality score that ranges from 0 to 5, with 0 (zero) being a low-quality decision counseling session and 5 being a high-quality decision counseling session. The score is based on whether the following components of SDM were completed: patient education, elicitation of clear patient reasons influencing preference, identification of unique patient reasons influencing preference, determination of a patient preference that is concordant with the patient choice, and development of a preference-related action plan. Each of these components is scored 1 = Completed or 0 = Not Completed.

Disseminating the Lung Cancer Screening SDM Training Program

The Lung Cancer Screening SDM Training Program development team has embarked on the process of disseminating the program. This process involved the initial release online program and planning for dissemination in Jefferson Health and other health systems.

Initial Release of the SDM Training Program. The current Lung Cancer Screening Shared Decision Making Training Program was launched in June 2021 by the American College of Chest Physicians (CHEST), in conjunction with Thomas Jefferson University. This event was announced by a press release, and information about how to access was disseminated to CHEST organization membership. After the program release, Thomas Jefferson University and the Center for Health, Law, and Policy Innovation (CHLPI) at Harvard University organized an online webinar titled, *Engaging a Learning Community to Achieve the Promise of Lung Cancer Screening.* This webinar, which was sponsored by Dialogue4Health, included a presentation and panel discussion on the role health systems can play in promoting quality SDM and increasing LCS. Participants were also informed about the online Lung Cancer Screening Shared Decision-Making Training program.

SDM Training Program Dissemination in Health Systems. Primary care practices in Jefferson Health, a large health system that serves diverse patient populations in southeastern Pennsylvania, New Jersey, and Delaware. Beginning in 2022, we initiated work with health system leadership to identify points of contact with primary care practices. We are working with these key players to develop effective modes of communication that can be used to engage each of the organizations five campuses and practices/providers (e.g., email blast, live information session, grand rounds presentations, etc.). As part of this process, we are exploring challenges and opportunities related to disseminating information about the training program, designing strategies that can maximize provider awareness and uptake of the training program, and collecting data on training program completion (including program pretest, posttest, and evaluation data), SDM performance, and LCS rates before and after program dissemination.

We have also engaged leadership from other health systems to identify opportunities for disseminating the Lung Cancer Screening Shared Decision-Making Program. In this regard, we plan to contact organizational leaders of Federally Qualified Health Centers (FQHCs) in the area. FQHC providers play a key role in delivering preventive health care to vulnerable patient populations, including many individuals who are at risk for being diagnosed with lung cancer and are eligible for LCS. Following the model outlined above, we will work with FQHC leadership to identify and engage the points of contact who can help develop a plan to disseminate the SDM program to providers in FQHC practices. Again, this plan will involve tracking the dissemination process, provider uptake of training, SDM performance, and LCS rates before and after dissemination occurs.

Conclusion

Currently, few health systems support programs designed to train healthcare providers in SDM about LCS. This situation contributes to poor-quality SDM performance and disappointingly low LCS rates. In our view, both SDM and LCS rates can be improved substantially through SDM training.

The potential impact that investing in such training is substantial, as indicated by Shih et al. [18]. In this study, the authors identified two cohorts of persons who were 55 to 64 years of age and were privately insured and underwent LDCT screening between 2016 and 2017 to determine the extent to which SDM about LCS was implemented and the effect of SDM on screening. In the first cohort, SDM documentation reached 8%, and LDCT screening rates were also 8%. The second cohort included persons who had SDM documented at the time of an office visit. In this cohort, the LDCT screening reached 62%. Given that LCS rates across the United States are lower than 20% [19], the potential impact health system support for SMD training on LCS rates in diverse patient populations in substantial.

We are in the early stages of disseminating the SDM training program described above. Plans for dissemination include advertising the program to primary care providers across Jefferson and other health systems in Philadelphia. We also aim to offer training to providers in Federally Qualified Health Centers (FQHC) in the area. In addition, we are taking steps to identify geographic areas in which lung cancer mortality rates and cigarette smoking rates are high. In these areas, we intend to implement intensive efforts to promote SDM training for providers in practice. Moreover, we intend to assess SDM training program participation, SDM performance, and LCS rates before and after training. If embraced by health systems across the country, this approach offers a unique opportunity to increase high-quality SDM, raise LCS rates, reduce the burdens of lung cancer morbidity and mortality, and increase equity in lung cancer care.

Finally, it is important to note that in addition to developing the Lung Cancer Screening Shared Decision-Making Training program, we have developed an approach to measuring the quality of SDM of SDM performance. Following recommendations made by Alston et al. [20], this approach involves assessing whether patients have been exposed to information about the screening decision to be made, documenting if patients have been given the opportunity to express their reasons for and against having an LDCT screening test; clarifying the patient's preference related to screening; and engaging patients in the process of developing a preference-concordant action plan related to screening.

Implementing an SDM training process and applying a rigorous process of evaluating the quality of SDM about LCS are important elements of an overall program of increasing SDM quality and health equity in lung cancer screening [21]. It is important to note that while current LCS guidelines are clear about recommending, and even requiring SDM (CMS guidelines) prior to initial screening, they are vague about the nature and content of SDM performance. That is, the guidelines recommend the presentation of information about the benefits and harms of LCS, the frequency of screening, and the follow-up of positive test results. However, they do not explain that SDM involves more than simply providing information. It also involves a discussion of patient values, clarification of patient preference, and the development of a plan to operationalize that preference. It is hoped that these elements of the SDM process and some standards for SDM quality assessment will be included in future iterations of USPSTF and CMS guidelines for LCS.

References

1. US Preventive Services Task Force, Krist AH, Davidson KW, Mangione CM, Barry MJ, Cabana M, et al. Screening for lung cancer: US preventive services task force recommendation statement. JAMA. 2021;325(10):962–70.
2. Syrek Jenson T, Chin J, Baldwin J, Evans M, Long K, Li C, et al. Screening for lung cancer with low dose computed tomography (LDCT) [Internet]. cms.gov. 2022 [cited 2022 Mar 10]. Available from: https://www.cms.gov/medicare-coverage-database/view/ncacal-decision-memo.aspx?proposed=N&ncaid=304.
3. Tanner NT, Silvestri GA. Shared decision-making and lung cancer screening: let's get the conversation started. Chest. 2019;155(1):21–4.
4. Brenner AT, Malo TL, Margolis M, Elston Lafata J, James S, Vu MB, et al. Evaluating shared decision making for lung cancer screening. JAMA Intern Med. 2018;178(10):1311–6.
5. Nishi SPE, Lowenstein LM, Mendoza TR, Lopez Olivo MA, Crocker LC, Sepucha K, et al. Shared decision-making for lung cancer screening: how well are we "sharing"? Chest. 2021;160(1):330–40.
6. Müller E, Strukava A, Scholl I, Härter M, Diouf NT, Légaré F, et al. Strategies to evaluate healthcare provider trainings in shared decision-making (SDM): a systematic review of evaluation studies. BMJ Open. 2019;9(6):e026488.
7. Légaré F, Adekpedjou R, Stacey D, Turcotte S, Kryworuchko J, Graham ID, et al. Interventions for increasing the use of shared decision making by healthcare professionals. Cochrane Database Syst Rev. 2018;7:CD006732.
8. Légaré F, Brouillette M-H. Shared decision-making in the context of menopausal health: where do we stand? Maturitas. 2009;63(3):169–75.
9. Carter-Harris L, Slaven JE, Monahan PO, Shedd-Steele R, Hanna N, Rawl SM. Understanding lung cancer screening behavior: racial, gender, and geographic differences among Indiana long-term smokers. Prev Med Rep. 2018;10:49–54.

10. Volk RJ, Shokar NK, Leal VB, Bulik RJ, Linder SK, Mullen PD, et al. Development and pilot testing of an online case-based approach to shared decision making skills training for clinicians. BMC Med Inform Decis Mak. 2014;14:95.

11. Lowenstein LM, Godoy MCB, Erasmus JJ, Zirari Z, Bennett A, Leal VB, et al. Implementing decision coaching for lung cancer screening in the low-dose computed tomography setting. JCO Oncol Pract. 2020;16(8):e703–25.

12. Hoffman RM, Reuland DS, Volk RJ. The Centers for Medicare & Medicaid services requirement for shared decision-making for lung cancer screening. JAMA. 2021;325(10):933–4.

13. Myers RE. Decision counseling in cancer prevention and control. Health Psychol. 2005;24(4S):S71–7.

14. Tiro JA, Vernon SW, Hyslop T, Myers RE. Factorial validity and invariance of a survey measuring psychosocial correlates of colorectal cancer screening among African Americans and Caucasians. Cancer Epidemiol Biomark Prev. 2005;14(12):2855–61.

15. Flight IH, Wilson CJ, McGillivray J, Myers RE. Cross-cultural validation of the preventive health model for colorectal cancer screening: an Australian study. Health Educ Behav. 2010;37(5):724–36.

16. Sepucha K, Ozanne EM. How to define and measure concordance between patients' preferences and medical treatments: a systematic review of approaches and recommendations for standardization. Patient Educ Couns. 2010;78(1):12–23.

17. Langford AT, Kang SK, Braithwaite RS. When does nonadherence indicate a deviation from patient-centered care? Am J Manag Care. 2021;27(5):e141–4.

18. Shih TC-T, Xu Y, Lowenstein LM, Volk RJ. Implementation of shared decision making for lung cancer screening among the privately insured nonelderly. Medical Decison Making Policy & Practice, 2021;6(1):2381468320984773. https://doi.org/10.1177/2381468320984773.

19. Zahnd WE, Eberth JM. Lung cancer screening utilization: a behavioral risk factor surveillance system analysis. Am J Prev Med. 2019;57(2):250–5.

20. Alston C, Berger Z, Brownlee S, Elwyn G, Fowler Jr. FJ, Hall LK, Montori VM, Moulton B, Paget L, Haviland-Shebel B, Singerman R, Walker J, Wynia MK, Henderson D. Shared decision-making strategies for best care: patient decision aids. NAM Perspectives. Discussion Paper, National Academy of Medicine, Washington, DC; 2014. https://doi.org/10.31478/201409f.

21. Newsome M. We must improve equity in cancer screening. Scientific American; 2021.

Chapter 5
Smoking Cessation in a Lung Cancer Screening Program

Brooke Ruane

Background

Tobacco use is the leading preventable cause of disease and all-cause mortality in the United States [1, 2]. Cigarettes are responsible for over seven million deaths worldwide and 480,000 deaths in the United States yearly [3, 4]. In 1964, the United States Surgeon General released a landmark report on the harmful effects of smoking. Since then, there have been worldwide initiatives to end tobacco use [1]. Research dedicated to better understanding tobacco use has significantly contributed to the improvement of smoking cessation initiatives and treatment options. Nicotine addiction and dependence is the main reason smokers continue to smoke. Smoking cessation must be approached as an addiction, with comprehensive interventions addressing the psychological and physiological aspects of addiction. Smoking cessation within a LCS program could broaden the impact of LCS, further reducing mortality and risk of smoking-related diseases. This chapter will examine nicotine addiction and dependence, review pharmacologic and behavioral strategies to address nicotine addiction, and the importance of smoking cessation within a LCS program.

Nicotine and Tobacco

Nicotine is a highly addictive chemical substance, naturally found in the tobacco plant. It has been shown to be more addictive than heroin, cocaine, marijuana, and other illicit drugs [5].

B. Ruane (✉)
Department of Medicine, Jane and Leonard Korman Respiratory Institute, Thomas Jefferson University, Philadelphia, PA, USA
e-mail: Brooke.Ruane@Jefferson.edu

Nicotine is present in all forms of tobacco products, along with thousands of other chemicals and toxins that are created and released by the combustion of tobacco. These toxins are inhaled when tobacco is burned and used in the form of a cigarette. Surprisingly, nicotine itself does not have the same risks as other chemicals in tobacco and tobacco smoke. Despite what many think, many diseases and deaths in smokers are related to the mix of these chemicals, not the nicotine itself [6]. However, nicotine is the primary inducer of tobacco dependence and may result in compulsive behavior or an addiction. The paramount driver of continued tobacco use is nicotine addiction [6]. Not all smokers are diagnosed as nicotine dependent; however, the incidence of diagnosis is higher than any other substance use disorder [7].

The tobacco industry has been working for decades to continually improve and intensify the rapid delivery of nicotine without regard for the downstream health impact. Tobacco companies discovered that adding the corrosive substance ammonia increased nicotine absorption, making cigarettes even more addictive than prior iterations of cigarettes [1, 2, 8].

Chemicals in Cigarettes

One cigarette, when lit and activated, contains a mix of over 7000 chemicals, including toxic metals, poisonous gases, and carcinogens. There are at least 70 known carcinogens in cigarettes, such as formaldehyde, which is used to embalm bodies, and vinyl chloride, which is used to make pipes [2].

Not all chemicals found in a cigarette are added in the manufacturing process. Some substances, like nicotine, are naturally occurring in the plant itself. Other potentially harmful chemicals, such as cadmium, lead, and nitrates, are absorbed from the soil and fertilizer as the tobacco plant grows and remains in the tobacco leaves when they are processed and turned into cigarettes [5]. Additional chemical compounds form due to combustion during the burning of a cigarette. As a result, harmful chemicals may develop throughout the lifecycle of a cigarette; growing, manufacturing, or burning [5].

Over the years, the tobacco industry has redesigned the cigarette to help increase sales and improve profit margins. The "light" or "ultralight" cigarettes were designed after the link between tar and cancer risk was identified [5, 8, 9]. Features of these light cigarettes include cellulose acetate filters to trap tar and reduce intake, highly porous cigarette paper to allow toxic chemicals to escape, ventilation holes in the filter tip to dilute smoke with air, and different tobacco blends thought to decrease smoke yield of polynuclear aromatic hydrocarbons (PAHs) [9]. When all these features were combined and machine measured, they produced a lower yield of tar than the smoke from a regular cigarette [9].

Light cigarettes were marketed as containing fewer chemicals and less tar, as well as carrying a reduced risk of disease. However, individuals smoking light cigarettes are at the same risk of developing smoking-related cancers and diseases as their regular cigarette-smoking counterparts [9]. Studies indicate that the same features that reduce tar yield also lessen nicotine yield. To compensate for the lower nicotine yield, smokers must take deeper, larger, and more frequent puffs or increase their cigarette intake to achieve a comparable nicotine level [9]. Despite features of light cigarettes appearing less harmful due to decreased tar levels, machine-measuring does not take overcompensation due to lesser nicotine levels into consideration; therefore, smokers of light cigarettes inhale more tar, nicotine, and chemicals than machine-based numbers indicate [9].

Chemicals in Other Tobacco Products

The cigarette is not the only tobacco product with potentially harmful chemicals, other products include hookah, smokeless tobacco, and e-cigarettes. Hookah smoke has been found to contain carbon monoxide, metals, and carcinogens [10]. Additionally, hookah smokers may be at a higher risk of absorption of these toxic chemicals than cigarette smokers. This risk is associated with the length of time for a "hookah session" [10, 11]. A 1-h hookah session produces as much smoke as several packs of cigarettes, inhaling 100–200 times the amount of smoke in a single cigarette [5, 10, 11].

Smokeless tobacco has been found to contain at least 4000 chemicals, with as many as 30 linked to cancer [5, 12]. Heavy metals including cadmium, lead, and nickel, in addition to other harmful substances such as formaldehyde, and N-Nitrosonornicotine (NNN) have all been found in smokeless tobacco [5, 10]. NNN is a known carcinogen in animals and may be linked to increased cancer risk in humans [5, 13, 14]. Furthermore, smokeless tobacco is proven to cause esophageal, pancreatic, and oral cancer [5, 15].

E-cigarettes are the most recent "tobacco product" with a variety of models released in the last decade. Marketed as a "safer" alternative to smoking, yet containing many of the same chemicals and toxins as cigarettes. While not all, most contain nicotine and have also been found to contain formaldehyde, acrolein, and acetaldehyde [1, 5]. The combination of these chemicals is linked to irreversible lung damage [5]. Additionally, e-cigarettes are often flavored with chemical compounds such as diacetyl and acetoin. While these chemicals are safe to ingest, inhaling these compounds is associated with interstitial lung disease [5, 16].

Biological Basis of Nicotine Dependence

Nicotine acts on the brain and nervous system, easily crossing the blood-brain barrier and then diffusing into brain tissue. Nicotine is a selective binder to nicotinic cholinergic receptors (nAChRs) in the brain and other tissues [17]. It imitates the action of the natural neurotransmitter acetylcholine by binding to those "nicotine receptors." This results in a release of neurotransmitters, predominately dopamine, norepinephrine, acetylcholine, serotonin (5-HT), GABA, glutamate, and endorphins [17], stimulating various responses and behaviors after intake.

The most crucial reward pathway in the brain is the mesolimbic dopamine system, composed of the ventral tegmental area (VTA) and nucleus accumbens (NAc) [18]. The VTA-NAc pathway involves reward and mediating the reinforcing actions of drug abuse. Dopamine is the neurotransmitter responsible for emotion, motivation, feelings of pleasure, and VTA-NAc pathway activation [17, 18].

When nicotine receptors located in the VTA and NAc are stimulated, they release large quantities of dopamine, activating the mesolimbic dopamine system [18]. Addictive substances and behaviors provide shortcuts to the brain's reward system by flooding it with dopamine. This process is critical for drug-induced rewards and is responsible for reinforcing behaviors similar to other dependence-producing drugs [18]. Nicotine use alters the brain structure and function of neurotransmitters, including dopamine, norepinephrine, serotonin (5-HT), glutamate, gamma-aminobutyric acid (GABA), and endogenous opioid peptides, which are associated with the development of psychiatric disorders [18]. Habitual nicotine use results in an increase in active nicotine receptor sites, resulting in nicotine tolerance and dependence [18].

Cognitive Management of Dependence

The majority of cigarette smokers (68%) want to quit smoking entirely [1]. However, quitting smoking successfully is exceedingly difficult. Nicotine addiction is a mental and physical disease with compulsive behaviors. Prior to the twentieth century, smoking cessation was approached as a habit, not an addiction [2, 18]. The pharmacologic and behavioral process changes that determine nicotine addiction are like those seen with heroin and cocaine addiction. Cigarettes are designed for addiction, delivering more nicotine faster than seen in previous eras [2]. The simple design of the cigarette allows nicotine in toxic substances inhaled into the pulmonary alveolar sacs to rapidly enter blood capillaries via simple diffusion, travel via the pulmonary veins to the left atrium, enter the left ventricle and be pumped immediately through the aortic arch to the central nervous system. Nicotine alters brain structure and function, resulting in cravings that intensify with prolonged use [2, 7]. Smokers become dependent on the physical action of smoking, in addition to the physiological dependence, and continue to smoke despite knowing the negative health effects and wanting to quit. Smokers feel intense compulsions to continue to smoke, in addition to feeling trapped in a pattern of repetitive and senseless thinking.

When initiating smoking cessation treatment, it is important to evaluate what level of nicotine dependence may be present in the smoker. High levels of nicotine dependence are associated with an increased risk of difficulty quitting, distress, and relapse [1, 19]. Additionally, smokers with high nicotine dependence have a greater success rate with nicotine replacement therapy (NRT) [1, 20]. Therefore, nicotine dependence levels should be evaluated, allowing for treatment options and tailoring of recommendations based on the level of dependence. Several questionnaires can be utilized to measure nicotine dependence, including the Fagerstrom Test for Nicotine Dependence, Wisconsin Inventory of Smoking Dependence and Motives, and Smokeless Tobacco Dependence Scale [17].

Nicotine dependence must be treated as an addiction, with counseling and behavioral approaches, as well as medications for withdrawal symptoms. A comprehensive approach to tobacco-cessation must address pharmacology, conditioned factors, personality, and social settings [18]. A publication by Jiloha et al. states that pharmacological treatment for smoking cessation should both block the positive reinforcing effects of nicotine as well as prevent or reduce the development of withdrawal symptoms. Pharmacotherapy should also target the receptor subtypes involved in nicotine addiction without affecting the receptors that, if activated, would produce unwanted adverse effects.

In the United States, it is common to browse for smoking cessation treatments and receive infinite results. However, the Food and Drug Administration (FDA) currently has only approved a handful of treatment modalities for smoking cessation; including nicotine replacement therapy (NRT) (transdermal patch, gum, nasal spray, inhaler, and lozenges); bupropion (Zyban, Wellbutrin), varenicline (Chantix) [20].

Nicotine Replacement Therapies

At least half of adult smokers (55.1%) attempt to quit smoking each year, with thousands struggling with quitting daily [7]. Evidence-based cessation counseling, in conjunction with medications, is the most efficacious intervention and is proven to increase rates of long-term cessation. Although both cessation counseling and medication can be effective, the dual modality methodology is superior [1, 7]. Despite this evidence, less than one-third of smokers of those attempting to quit report using medications or counseling when quitting smoking [1, 7].

Nicotine dependence is what makes quitting so tricky and leads to most smokers having multiple quit attempts [21]. Many smokers may have at least 30 or more quit attempts before successfully quitting [22]. Because all smoking cessation treatment strategies should approach nicotine as an addiction, a dual-tack approach is best, which addresses both the physical (urges, withdrawal) and psychological (mental, emotional) aspects of dependence. NRTs work to address physical aspects of addiction [15], while behavioral programs, such as 1–800-QUIT-NOW or smoking cessation counseling programs, aim to address the psychological aspects of addiction [23].

NRTs work directly and indirectly by enhancing natural gratification signals, thereby helping to manage chronic withdrawal and sudden compulsions. The main mechanism of action of an NRT is the stimulation of nicotinic receptors in the ventral tegmental area of the brain and the consequent release of dopamine in the nucleus accumben [24]. NRTs deliver lower plasma concentrations that rise more slowly than conventional cigarettes, decreasing the behaviorally reinforcing effects of smoking [1]. Additionally, NRTs work to satisfy the physiological need for a reward [1, 18].

NRTs have shown to be effective and may double one's chances at smoking cessation [15]. There are six different forms of NRT products: transdermal patches, lozenges, gums, nasal sprays, inhalers, and sublingual tablets [1, 25]. The nicotine patch, also known as "the controller medication," delivers a steady dose of nicotine over 16–24 h to maintain a continuous nicotine level in the blood and prevent cravings from peaking [1, 26]. All other NRT products are "short-acting" and achieve lower levels of nicotine in the blood than nicotine patches. Therefore, they are mainly prescribed for "breakthrough cravings" and are used every 1–2 h as needed for withdrawal symptoms [1, 26]. When used in combination with patches, short-acting NRTs act to provide an additional spike in nicotine levels in the blood, like that of a cigarette.

There are only two prescription medications approved by the FDA to treat nicotine addiction, varenicline and bupropion. Varenicline is a selective $alpha_4$-$beta_2$ neuronal nicotinic acetylcholine receptor partial agonist and antagonist, which works to block the effects of nicotine on the brain while also providing some receptor stimulation [27]. Its mechanism of action inhibits dopaminergic activation produced through smoking, decreases cravings, reduces withdrawal symptoms, and prevents nicotine stimulation of the mesolimbic dopamine system which is associated with nicotine addiction [27]. The American Thoracic Society (ATS) clinical practice guidelines strongly recommend varenicline for smoking cessation over the nicotine patch and bupropion [28]. Additionally, there are recommendations to initiate varenicline even in adults not ready to quit [28].

Bupropion is an atypical antidepressant that was initially developed to treat depression and later found to be effective in smoking cessation [25]. Bupropion is a norepinephrine/dopamine reuptake inhibitor and can decrease the function of nAChRs by acting as an antagonist of the receptors [1]. As an nAChR antagonist, it alters nicotine-mediated dopamine responses, which likely causes antismoking activity [18].

Lung Cancer and Smoking

The risks of disease and death related to tobacco use have been well documented for more than a century. Smoking is the number one cause of lung cancer. However, despite this knowledge, lung cancer is still the most common tobacco-related cause of cancer mortality in the United States [2]. Cigarettes contain notorious carcinogens, toxins, and chemicals. Repeated exposure to these chemicals through tobacco smoke stresses healthy cells, causing damage and altering their normal growth and function, thus starting a path toward cancer formation [2]. Typically, the immune system protects individuals from cancer by sending out tumor fighters to attack cancer cells. However, the same toxins within the cigarette that stress healthy cells weaken tumor-fighting cells. Without tumor fighters, these abnormal cancer cells continue to grow and spread. Therefore, not only does tobacco smoke causes cancer, but then it inhibits the body from fighting the cancer with its own immune system [2].

Even after a cancer diagnosis, 64% of patients continue to smoke [29]. Smoking cessation is critical amongst this population as poorer outcomes in cancer patients have been linked to tobacco use. It directly impacts the overall effectiveness of treatment, quality of life, and long-term survival [29]. In addition to promoting tumor growth, tobacco smoke may decrease chemotherapy benefits [2]. Therefore, smoking after cancer diagnosis increases the failure of treatment across all types of cancer [30]. Smokers with cancer have a lower quality of life, as well as an increase in symptoms during and following chemotherapy infusions compared to nonsmokers with cancer [31]. There is also an increased chance of second primary cancer with continued tobacco use.

Smoking Cessation Within a Lung Cancer Screening Program

Lung cancer screening with low-dose computed tomography (LDCT) has been demonstrated to decrease lung cancer mortality and overall mortality in high-risk individuals [32]. Individuals who qualify for screening are not only at an increased risk for lung cancer, but also at risk for other cancers and diseases. Furthermore, those undergoing screening and continuing to smoke are at even higher risk.

Smoking cessation counseling along with SDM, are CMS requirements for all current smokers in order to receive reimbursement for screening. LCS programs have an opportunity to further improve the impact of LCS by integrating smoking cessation within their programs as many individuals who undergo screening are current smokers. Studies indicate an increase in smoking cessation following a screen-detected abnormality on LDCT [33]. The SDM process and screening results review process are opportunities to encourage smoking cessation [33]. Integrating smoking cessation within LCS further improves smoking-related morbidity and mortality [33].

Thomas Jefferson University Hospital, a major urban, academic medical center, has a nursing-driven centralized lung cancer screening program. The program relies heavily on a multidisciplinary model to provide the best possible patient care; however, our core team is comprised of an advanced practice provider, two master tobacco treatment specialist-certified nurse navigators, and a dedicated coordinator. After referral to the program, an eligibility assessment including an extensive smoking history is conducted by the program coordinator. After patients sit down with our highly trained specialized nurse navigators for a shared decision-making session with smoking cessation counseling when applicable. If a patient agrees to undergo screening with a LDCT, the program offers an extensive result review, as well as concierge scheduling of follow-up tests, procedures, and appointments, if applicable. In addition to our high-quality, evidence-based workflow, our LCS program has worked diligently to develop a more comprehensive and standardized approach to smoking cessation. Along with tobacco cessation counseling during SDM, our tobacco treatment protocol includes follow-up counseling at the time of LCS results review, additional support at an optional 2-week appointment, and/or ongoing telephone counseling as requested by patients. Furthermore, we provide all patients who are interested in a prescription for tobacco cessation medication and other treatment options.

An effective smoking cessation program must have a comprehensive approach to treating nicotine addiction at both the psychological and physiological root of the dependence. Often, healthcare professionals feel they do not have time to address all aspects of patient care in addition to tobacco cessation with their patients. LCS programs have a unique opportunity to provide one-to-one tobacco counseling with patients who are at increased risk for negative health outcomes associated with tobacco use.

Conclusion

Smoking cessation is known to decrease the risk of lung cancer mortality, all-cause mortality, as well as reduce the incidence of diseases including chronic obstructive pulmonary disease (COPD), heart disease, and cerebrovascular disease. Smoking cessation at any age has short-term and long-term benefits including increasing life expectancy. Even among individuals considered senior citizens ($\geq$65 years), cessation can increase the life expectancy by years [2]. Additionally, even just decreasing one's daily cigarette consumption is linked to increased health benefits, such as decreases in COPD and asthma symptoms, and reduced progression of peripheral vascular disease [34]. All healthcare providers should initiate smoking cessation discussions with smokers at each point of contact, regardless of specialty. Unfortunately, the increasing complexity of patient care and time constraints for office appointments provide barriers for the proper initiation of smoking cessation. LCS programs are not only dedicated to early detection but also prevention of lung cancer. Therefore, programs have been well-positioned to be the champions of smoking cessation. Furthermore, CMS requires smoking cessation counseling of all current smokers undergoing SDM for LCS. Smoking cessation is multifaceted process and requires a comprehensive approach that addresses the physiological and psychological aspects of addiction, while providing support and nonjudgmental space to discuss the challenges of quitting smoking. The integration of evidence-based smoking cessation counseling and treatment in LCS programs would amplify the benefits of LCS, further improving long-term patient outcomes.

References

1. U.S. Department of Health and Human Services. Smoking cessation. A report of the surgeon general. Atlanta, GA: U.S. Department of Health and Human Services, Centers for Disease Control and Prevention, National Center for Chronic Disease Prevention and Health Promotion, Office on Smoking and Health; 2020.

2. U.S. Department of Health and Human Services (USDHHS). A report of the surgeon general: how tobacco smoke causes disease: what it means to you (Consumer Booklet). Atlanta, GA: U.S. Department of Health and Human Services, Centers for Disease Control and Prevention, National Center for Chronic Disease Prevention and Health Promotion, Office on Smoking and Health; 2010.
3. WHO report on the global tobacco epidemic, 2017—executive summary: monitoring tobacco use and prevention policies. Available at: https://www.who.int/tobacco/global_report/2017/executive-summary/en/.
4. World Health Organization Report on the Global Tobacco Epidemic. Warning about the dangers of tobacco. Geneva: World Health Organization; 2021.
5. U.S. Food & Drug Administration. Chemicals in tobacco products and your health (internet). Chemicals in tobacco products and your HEALTH. 2021. Available from: https://www.fda.gov/tobacco-products/health-effects-tobacco-use/chemicals-tobacco-products-and-your-health.
6. The health consequences of smoking—50 years of progress: a report of the surgeon general. Rockville, MD: US Public Health Service; US Department of Health and Human Services; 2014.
7. Centers for Disease Control and Prevention (US), National Center for Chronic Disease Prevention and Health Promotion (US), Office on Smoking and Health (US). Atlanta, GA: Centers for Disease Control and Prevention (US); 2010.
8. Rabinoff M, Caskey N, Rissling A, Park C. Pharmacological and chemical effects of cigarette additives. Am J Public Health. 2007;97(11):1981–91.
9. National Cancer Institute. Risks associated with smoking cigarettes with low machine-measured yields of tar and nicotine. Bethesda, MD: National Cancer Institute; 2001. Smoking and Tobacco Control Monograph 13.
10. Food and Drug Administration (FDA). Harmful and potentially harmful constituents in tobacco products and tobacco smoke: established list. Fed Regist. 2012;77(64):20034–7.
11. Centers for Disease Control and Prevention. Hookahs (Internet). Centers for Disease Control and Prevention. 2016. Available from: https://www.cdc.gov/tobacco/data_statistics/fact_sheets/tobacco_industry/hookahs/index.htm
12. National Cancer Institute (NCI), Centers for Disease Control and Prevention (CDC). Smokeless tobacco and public health: a global perspective. Bethesda, MD: U.S. Department of Health and Human Services, Centers for Disease Control and Prevention and National Institutes of Health, National Cancer Institute. NIH Publication No. 14-7983; 2014.
13. Stephens WE, Calder A, Newton J. Source and health implications of high toxic metal concentrations in illicit tobacco products. Environ Sci Technol. 2005;39(2):479–88.
14. U.S. Department of Health and Human Services (USDHHS). How tobacco smoke causes disease: the biology and behavioral basis for smoking-attributable disease: a report of the surgeon general. Atlanta, GA: U.S. Department of Health and Human Services, Centers for Disease Control and Prevention, National Center for Chronic Disease Prevention and Health Promotion, Office on Smoking and Health; 2010.
15. American Cancer Society. Cancer prevention & early detection facts & figures 2017–2018. Atlanta: American Cancer Society; 2017.
16. Allen J, Flanigan SS, LeBlanc M, et al. Flavoring chemicals in e-cigarettes: diacetyl, 2,3-pentanedione, and acetoin in a sample of 51 products, including fruit-, candy-, cocktail-flavored e-cigarettes. Environ Health Perspect. 2016;124:733–9. https://ehp.niehs.nih.gov/15-10185/. Accessed March 27, 2018.
17. Widysanto A, Combest FE, Dhakal A, et al. Nicotine addiction. (Updated 2021 Nov 23). In: StatPearls (Internet). Treasure Island, FL: StatPearls Publishing; 2022. Available from: https://www.ncbi.nlm.nih.gov/books/NBK499915/.
18. Jiloha RC. Biological basis of tobacco addiction: implications for smoking-cessation treatment. Indian J Psychiatry. 2010;52(4):301–7. Available from: https://www.ncbi.nlm.nih.gov/pmc/articles/PMC3025154/.
19. Piper M, McCarthy D, Bolt D, Smith S, Lerman C, Benowitz N, et al. Assessing dimensions of nicotine dependence: an evaluation of the Nicotine Dependence Syndrome Scale (NDSS)

and the Wisconsin Inventory of Smoking Dependence Motives (WISDM). Nicotine Tob Res. 2008;10(6):1009–20.

20. Stead LF, Perera R, Bullen C, Mant D, Hartmann-Boyce J, Cahill K, et al. Nicotine replacement therapy for smoking cessation. Cochrane Database Syst Rev. 2012;11:CD000146.

21. Bhatt G, Goel S, Soundappan K, Kaur R. Theoretical constructs of smoking cessation among current tobacco smokers in India: a secondary analysis of Global Adult Tobacco Survey-2 (2016-2017). BMJ Open. 2022;12(1):e050916. https://doi.org/10.1136/bmjopen-2021-050916.

22. Chaiton M, Diemert L, Cohen JE, Bondy SJ, Selby P, Philipneri A, Schwartz R. Estimating the number of quit attempts it takes to quit smoking successfully in a longitudinal cohort of smokers. BMJ Open. 2016;6(6):e011045. https://doi.org/10.1136/bmjopen-2016-011045. PMID: 27288378; PMCID: PMC4908897.

23. CDC Tobacco Free. 1-800-QUIT-NOW: 15 years of helping people quit (internet). Ctr Dis Control Prev 2021. Available from: https://www.cdc.gov/tobacco/features/quitlines/index.html.

24. Molyneux A. Nicotine replacement therapy (published correction appears in BMJ. 2004 Mar 20;328(7441):686). BMJ. 2004;328(7437):454–6. https://doi.org/10.1136/bmj.328.7437.454.

25. Roddy E. Bupropion and other non-nicotine pharmacotherapies. BMJ. 2004;328(7438):509–11. https://doi.org/10.1136/bmj.328.7438.509.

26. Wadgave U, Nagesh L. Nicotine replacement therapy: an overview. Int J Health Sci. 2016;10(3):425–35.

27. Singh D, Saadabadi A. Varenicline. (Updated 2021 Aug 6). In: StatPearls (Internet). Treasure Island, FL: StatPearls Publishing; 2022. Available from: https://www.ncbi.nlm.nih.gov/books/NBK534846/.

28. Leone FT, Zhang Y, Evers-Casey S, Evins AE, Eakin MN, Fathi J, et al. Initiating pharmacologic treatment in tobacco-dependent adults. An official American Thoracic Society clinical practice guideline. Am J Respir Crit Care Med. 2020;202(2):e5–31.

29. Tseng TS, Lin HY, Moody-Thomas S, et al. Who tended to continue smoking after cancer diagnosis: the national health and nutrition examination survey 1999–2008. BMC Public Health. 2012;12:784. https://doi.org/10.1186/1471-2458-12-784.

30. Office of the Surgeon General, Assistant Secretary for Health (ASH). Health consequences of smoking, surgeon general fact sheet (Internet). HHS.gov. 2014. Available from: https://www.hhs.gov/surgeongeneral/reports-and-publications/tobacco/consequences-smoking-factsheet/index.html.

31. Peppone LJ, Mustian KM, Morrow GR, et al. The effect of cigarette smoking on cancer treatment-related side effects. Oncologist. 2011;16(12):1784–92. https://doi.org/10.1634/theoncologist.2011-0169.

32. The National Lung Screening Trial Research Team. Reduced lung-cancer mortality with low-dose computed tomographic screening. N Engl J Med. 2011;365(5):395–409.

33. Tammemägi MC, Berg CD, Riley TL, Cunningham CR, Taylor KL. Impact of lung cancer screening results on smoking cessation. J Natl Cancer Inst. 2014;106(6):dju084. https://doi.org/10.1093/jnci/dju084.

34. Begh R, Lindson-Hawley N, Aveyard P. Does reduced smoking if you can't stop make any difference? BMC Med. 2015;13(1):257.

Chapter 6
Why Health Equity Is So Important in Lung Cancer Screening?

Gregory C. Kane and Stephen K. Klasko

In her landmark book, Medical Apartheid, Harriet Washington catalogs a history of disparate medical care in the United States dating to the very founding of our nation [1]. The documented transgressions are an abomination and are only matched in modern history by the medical experimentation of physicians associated with the Third Reich in Nazi Germany during World War II. Of course, the distinguishing feature of the history that Washington so clearly brings to the light of day is that the abuses against both slaves and free Blacks went on for more than 200 years, whereas the perpetrators of Nazi atrocities occurring between 1933 and 1945 were brought to justice through the Nuremberg trials soon after the conclusion of World War II with the Doctor's Trials ending in August 1947 [2].

One of us (GCK) considered this history when looking a former Tuskegee Airman in the eye for an initial pulmonary evaluation at the Jefferson-National Jewish Health Korman Respiratory Institute in Philadelphia (part of Jefferson Health). Well aware of the Tuskegee experiment, this physician was humbled by Mr. Ramsey King's (not his real name) ability to forgive the past and find gratitude in his heart and his life. It is hard for us to imagine today that we live in a country that would deny local residents (the black community of Tuskegee Alabama) who were serving to protect the country, essential and available treatment for an infection in the name of "research." The standard and simple therapy for syphilis, penicillin, was withheld in a misguided effort to contribute additional and unnecessary information to our understanding of the natural history of syphilis. Fast forward to the present, even today, as I examined Mr. King, I was mindful of the medical

G. C. Kane (✉)
Department of Medicine, Thomas Jefferson University, Philadelphia, PA, USA
e-mail: Gregory.Kane@Jefferson.edu

S. K. Klasko
Thomas Jefferson University and Jefferson Health, Philadelphia, PA, USA

G. C. Kane et al. (eds.), *Lung Cancer Screening*,
https://doi.org/10.1007/978-3-031-33596-9_6

47

establishment's role in providing not only disparate care, but unethical and criminal withholding of treatment. It was a sobering experience, indeed, to acknowledge the sins of organized medicine while at the same time, trying to earn the trust of a military service hero as well as a father, soldier, and airman. If Harriet Washington's collection of past wrongs is not enough, recent events in the United States since the COVID-19 pandemic have further highlighted the need for health equity all across this nation. One of us (SKK) was responsible during the pandemic for the largest health system in a major urban community, Philadelphia, with among the greatest poverty in the African-American community. Asking the descendants of these "experiments" to "trust the science" added a whole new challenge in the fight against COVID-19.

In this chapter, we will use the convention outlined by Richard Rothstein in his landmark book entitled The Color of Law [3]. Thus, the term "we" will refer to the collective of the members of the healthcare system workforce, including administrative and clinical leaders, physicians, nurses, respiratory therapists, medical assistants, navigators, and public health professionals. As Rothstein declared in the preface: "As the citizens of this democracy, we, all of us, white, black, Hispanic, Asian, Native American and others, bear a collective responsibility to enforce our Constitution and to rectify past violations whose effects endure." When using the word, we, our meaning is that this is what we, collectively must and should be doing in order to achieve health equity in lung cancer screening (LCS) and so many other health care services in the United States. In order to ensure an equitable future, it is our collective responsibility as physicians, healthcare professionals of all types, and healthcare leaders to practice and teach a brand of medicine that provides health assurance for all in an equitable manner.

As the ravages of COVID-19 exposed raw emotions all across the globe, racial and ethnic disparities were examined in the United States with greater focus than in any time since the late 1960s. While the events around the murder of George Floyd in Minneapolis, Minnesota catalyzed a national reckoning with white privilege and racial injustice, healthcare organizations also joined the dialogue and recommitted to addressing disparities in health and healthcare delivery. Data from the Robert Wood Johnson Foundation and Virginia Commonwealth University have highlighted stark differences in health outcomes between US neighborhoods, in some cases separated by as few as five miles, but with life expectancy discrepancies that would reach 20 years. This is true in Philadelphia and nearly as disparate in other major cities in the United States [4]. For example, in Philadelphia, the average survival in Society Hill (Zip code 19107) is 88 years, while just five miles away in the Strawberry Mansion section of the city (Zip code 19121) the average life expectancy is just 68 years. Imagine looking at two newborns in the Jefferson University Hospital nursery and recognizing that one will live until 3010 while the other will die well before the end of the century… totally based on the zip code to which they are going home. It turns out that one of the most direct causes of life expectancy in the United States is the neighborhood where you were born [4]! When considered afresh, these disparities have galvanized what we must do to provide more equitable healthcare and address the social determinants of health as well if we are to give all

Americans, no matter the color of their skin or socioeconomic status, an equal opportunity for life, liberty and the pursuit of happiness in this country [5, 6].

Lung cancer screening (LCS), as a newly prescribed screening service, recently endorsed by the United States Preventive Services Task Force (USPSTF) provides a new and important opportunity for organized American medicine to address health equity for all and demonstrate that we have learned from the past and re-committed ourselves to a more equitable future. Specifically, LCS is an opportunity to impact all communities equitably [7]. As the most recent cancer among the top causes of cancer death to be added to the USPSTF list of recommended screenings (cervical, breast, prostate, and colon); there is an exciting opportunity to measure and report our progress and take an accounting of the impact of LCS on overall lung cancer mortality. The exciting aspect of this transcends the numbers, namely, to start understanding lung cancer mortality in specific populations nationally and within individual cities and even within specific zip codes. This will require new approaches and new partnerships as well as a new spirit in American healthcare. It will also be a "wake up call" around an aspect of health care that we have known academically but rarely acted on, namely, that most of a patient's health is determined by what happens in the home, not what happens in the doctor's office.

So then, what is health equity? The definition is more challenging than it may seem and requires multiple vantage points. The United States Department of Health and Human Services as well as the CDC have defined health equity as "the attainment of the highest level of health for all people" [8]. The Robert Wood Johnson Foundation has described health equity as meaning "that everyone has a fair and just opportunity to be as healthy as possible." This requires removing obstacles to health such as poverty, discrimination, and their consequences, including powerlessness and lack of access to good jobs with fair pay, quality education and housing, safe environments, and health care" [9]. On balance, Dr. Camara Jones of the Morehouse School of Medicine has referred to health equity as "the assurance of the conditions of optimal health for all people" [9]. Regardless of which definition we choose to feature, the bottom line is that now is the time to help all people in all communities to achieve their best health, by understanding and addressing the root causes of disease and dysfunction.

Unfortunately, from the outset of LCS, we have been plagued by the mistakes of the past and find ourselves playing "catch up". The pivotal study which highlighted the success of lung cancer screening and reducing mortality [10] only included approximately 4 1/2% African-Americans in its enrollment. Thus, this pivotal study limited the true insights we could draw upon from the African-American population. Since that time, it has been necessary for subsequent investigators to explore the nuances and lessons to overcome that underrepresentation. Recently published studies have provided evidence of progress, but further work is required [11].

Fortunately, many modern healthcare leaders have taken on the mantle of addressing health equity in their communities. One of the authors of this chapter (SKK) developed a number of healthcare initiatives impacting Philadelphia while leading Jefferson Health as President and CEO from 2013 through 2021. Jefferson developed the Philadelphia Collaborative for Health Equity and committed the majority of its philanthropic efforts to reducing disparities. At the same time, the CEO committed 25% of his personal incentive to targeted health equity initiatives. Jefferson's efforts led to investments from individuals and corporations with the aim of reducing disparities in heart disease and stroke among immigrant and under-served populations, as well as similar initiatives in cancer therapeutics and lung cancer screening among others.

This approach is not unique. Cincinnati Children's Hospital, for example, is a referral pediatric academic Medical Center that has addressed community issues such as reading proficiency. This certainly is not a traditional metric directly related to the financial bottom line of the organization, to address specific social determinants of health, namely, education and health literacy [12]. At Jefferson Health's academic center, the Thomas Jefferson University Hospital, early efforts at lung cancer screening achieved a substantial impact among the African-American community with more than 40% of LCS scans performed among this self-identified demographic [11]. If this can be accomplished in the poorest city in the United States with one of the highest smoking rates, [13] it would be expected that we could see this type of success in other communities.

The senior administrations of Jefferson and Cincinnati Children's approached health equity as an important aspect of their success and set the tone for other health systems striving to address health equity in their own communities. In essence, they and others started a movement that made clear that the institution's success was partly dependent on its outreach to all segments of its community and the health of the most underserved members of that community.

Central to an equitable approach are several factors: equitable outreach (actively reaching and serving sub-populations within a particular region), motivation and commitment to not repeating the mistakes of the past, and conscious efforts to overcome bias and adjust methodology to meet a particular patient population's expectations. Historically, academic centers, often located in the heart of our poorest cities, have been content to allow those who choose to present for screening or other services to undergo such procedures, rather than making inroads into the most vulnerable communities. As Arnold Relman, former editor of the New England Journal of Medicine has described, the healthcare system in the United States has gone through three tectonic shifts. These have included "the Era of Expansion," "the Era of Cost Containment," and most recently "the Era of Assessment and Accountability" [14]. Now, we must seek new approaches with the goal of reaching vulnerable patients who may be most at risk for mortality related to some common diseases. Noting that Relman often railed against the "medical-industrial complex," it would be remarkably fitting for us to refer to this new re-examination and new dialogue among Academic Medical Center's as the dawn of "the Era of Health Equity" [15].

To be sure, reaching such communities takes unique efforts to create trust and acceptance. We cannot achieve health equity without building trust in our communities. While the meaning of trust is readily understood and felt by members of each community, these authors have chosen to define trust by a mathematical formula. Trust is equal to the sum of credibility, reliability, and intimacy while inversely related to self-interest [16]. Surprisingly, to those of us in healthcare, this methodology was derived from professionals in the financial industry and was first displayed as a formula:

$$\text{Trust} = \frac{\text{Credibility} + \text{Reliability} + \text{Intimacy}}{\text{Self} - \text{Interest}}$$

Lung cancer screening is an opportunity to alter our path in healthcare and define this generation's era of health equity. This opportunity could not have come at a more opportune time. Mortality disproportionately affects black men more than white men, and black women more than white women [17]. We will be judged by the next generation's assessment of how we respond to this challenge.

It is exciting that several organizations including the Bristol Myers Squibb Foundation have made a point to support a more equitable approach to Lung Cancer Screening and outreach to vulnerable populations. In Anne Arundel County, Maryland, healthcare teams are addressing disparities as core to their strategic mission. In rural North Carolina, leaders are literally bringing health equity to the poor through mobile screening units utilizing CT scanners in traveling buses. In Kentucky, leaders are addressing one the nation's highest statewide lung cancer mortality rates with an impressive and nationally leading approach to impact all persons, regardless of their community or skin color through "Kentucky LEADS." And in Maine, where there is a fatal combination of one of the highest lung cancer incidence rates and the reality that many residents face social determinants which challenge access, the Maine Lung Cancer Prevention and Screening initiative (Lung CAPS) has helped facilitate the growth of more equitable lung cancer screening [18].

Jefferson Health's partnership with the Bristol Myers Squibb Foundation has set an example for addressing vulnerable populations upfront and doing so with an awareness of bias, culture, the importance of building trust, and managing fear. As such, a program that looks to overcome inequity must work to overcome barriers, reflect, and engage the community.

Only in fully engaging the community can an academic health center deliver on the promise of lung cancer screening for all! It is a direct by-product of this relationship and the challenge that it engendered through a charitable grant, that Jefferson Health's academic center, the Thomas Jefferson University Hospital, excelled in early efforts of lung cancer screening to achieve a substantial impact among the African-American community with more than 40% of LCS scans performed among this key demographic with a higher-than-expected lung cancer mortality [11, 17].

In conclusion, health equity entails giving every person the opportunity to enjoy their maximum health status. To achieve that goal with respect to lung cancer and lung cancer mortality, a population approach to successful screening is essential. Such an approach would have its foundation in the epidemiology of lung cancer and utilize methods of community engagement and outreach to assure that no patient is left behind in the goal to prevent lung cancer and further reduce mortality through early detection. In this new Era of "Addressing Health Equity," health systems can lead the way. At Jefferson, the only way we can achieve our mission of "we improve lives" is if health equity and trust are at the center of all of our health assurance activities. Only in this way can we erase the stain of the Tuskegee era and slavery on this country's medical history.

References

1. Washington H. Medical apartheid: the dark history of medical experimentation on black Americans from colonial times to the present. Harlem Moon, Broadway Books; 2006.
2. Klee E. Auschwitz, die NS-Medizin und ihre Opfer. Frankfurt am Main: Fisher; 1997. D 805.5.A96 K54 1997.
3. Rothstein, Richard. The color of law. A forgotten history of how our government segregated America. WW Norton & Co. Ltd London.
4. Arias E, Escobedo LA, Kennedy J, Fu C, Cisewski J. U.S. Small-area life expectancy estimates project: methodology and results summary. National Center for Health Statistics. Vital Health Statistics. 2018;2(181):1–40.
5. Daniel H, Bornstein S, Kane GC, for the ACP Health and Public Policy Committee [others]. Addressing social determinants to improve patient care and promote health equity: an American College of Physicians Position Paper. Ann Intern Med. 2018;168(8):577–8. https://doi.org/10.7326/M17-2441.
6. Butkus R, Rapp K, Cooney TG, Engel LS, for the Health and Public Policy Committee American College of Physicians. Envisioning a better U.S. health care system for all: reducing barriers to care and addressing social determinants of health. Ann Intern Med. 2020;172:S50–9.
7. Moyer VA. Screening for lung cancer: U.S. Preventive Services Task Force recommendation statement. Ann Intern Med. 2014;160:330–8.
8. National Center for Health Statistics. Healthy people 2000 final review. Hyattsville, MD: Public Health Service; 2001.
9. https://www.rwjf.org/en/library/research/2017/05/what-is-health-equity-.html.
10. The national lung cancer screening research team. N Engl J Med. 2011;365:395–409. https://doi.org/10.1056/NEJMoa1102873.
11. Lake M, Shusted C, Juon H-S, Mcintyre RK, Zeigler-Johnson C, Evans NR, Kane GC, Barta J. Black patients referred to a lung cancer screening program experience lower rates of screening and longer time to follow-up. BMC Cancer. 2020;20:561. https://doi.org/10.1186/s12885-020-06923-0.
12. Karpf M. The role of academic health centers in addressing health equity and social determinants of health. Acad Med. 2019;94(9):1273–5. https://doi.org/10.1097/ACM.0000000000002834.
13. Shusted C, Kane GC. The linkage between poverty and smoking in Philadelphia and its impact on future directions for tobacco control in the city. Popul Health Manag. 2020;23(1):68–77. https://doi.org/10.1089/pop.2019.0006.
14. Relman AS. Assessment and accountability: the third revolution in medical care. N Engl J Med. 1991;319:1220–2.
15. Langer E. Arnold S. Relman, New England Journal of Medicine editor, dies at 91. Washington Post. 2014. ISSN 0190-8286. Retrieved 2020-02-25.
16. Maister DH, Green CH, Galford RM. The trusted advisor. New York, NY: Free Press; 2000.
17. Siegel RL, Miller KD, Fuchs HE, Jemal A. Cancer statistics, 2022. CA Cancer J Clin. 2022;72(1):7–33. https://doi.org/10.3322/caac.21708.
18. https://lungdiseasenews.com/2018/01/02/bristol-myers-squibb-foundation-funds-cancer-screening-philadelphia/. Accessed 12 Jan 2022.

Part II

Applying a Learning Community Model

Chapter 7
Engaging a Health System Learning Community to Increase Lung Cancer Screening

Ronald E. Myers, Melissa DiCarlo, Rickie Brawer, Hee-Soon Juon, Kristine Pham, Christine S. Shusted, Charnita Zeigler-Johnson, and Julie A. Barta

Background

As shown in randomized controlled trials, screening with low-dose computed tomography (LDCT) is an effective way to diagnose early lung cancer. In 2011, the National Lung Screening Trial (NLST) found a 20% relative reduction in lung

R. E. Myers (✉)
Medical Oncology, Thomas Jefferson University, Philadelphia, PA, USA
e-mail: Ronald.Myers@Jefferson.edu

M. DiCarlo · H.-S. Juon · K. Pham
Department of Medical Oncology, Thomas Jefferson University, Philadelphia, PA, USA
e-mail: Melissa.DiCarlo@Jefferson.edu; Hee-Soon.Juon@Jefferson.edu; Kristine.Pham@Jefferson.edu

R. Brawer
Department of Medical Oncology, Thomas Jefferson University, Philadelphia, PA, USA
e-mail: Rickie.Brawer@Jefferson.edu

C. S. Shusted
Division of Pulmonary and Critical Care Medicine, Department of Medicine, Sidney Kimmel Medical College at Thomas Jefferson University, Philadelphia, PA, USA
e-mail: Christine.Shusted@Jefferson.edu

C. Zeigler-Johnson
Cancer Prevention and Control, Communicyt Outreach and Engagement, Fox Chase Cancer Center, Philadelphia, PA, USA
e-mail: Charnita.Zeigler-Johnson@fccc.edu

J. A. Barta
Department of Medicine, Thomas Jefferson University, Philadelphia, PA, USA
e-mail: Julie.Barta@jefferson.edu

cancer mortality when screening with annual LDCT screening compared to single-view chest radiography [1]. A recent meta-analysis of lung cancer screening research studies has reinforced the finding that periodic LDCT screening can significantly reduce the cumulative 10-year lung cancer mortality rate [2].

The United States Preventive Services Task Force (USPSTF) initially issued guidelines supporting lung cancer screening with annual LDCT in 2013 [3], which have recently been revised and updated. Currently, the USPSTF recommends that asymptomatic adults who are between the ages of 50 and80 years have at least a 20 pack-year history of cigarette smoking, and currently smoke or have smoked and who quit within the past 15 years should make a shared decision with a healthcare provider about having annual LCS [4].

The Centers for Medicare and Medicaid Services (CMS) announced in 2015 that annual LCS would be covered as a preventive health care benefit for persons who are 55 to 77 years of age, have 30 pack-years of exposure to smoking, have not quit smoking with 15 years, and undergo shared decision making (SDM) about LCS [5]. Importantly, shared decision making (SDM) is required for coverage of LCS. These guidelines have recently been updated, expanding the age eligibility to 50 to 77 years, and reducing the period of cigarette smoking exposure to 20 pack-years [6].

Unfortunately, SDM and LCS occur infrequently in clinical practice [7–9] and statewide LCS rates are very low [7, 10–12]. Health systems in the United States are in a unique position to support the implementation of effective methods to increase SDM and LCS rates, and thereby reducing lung cancer mortality and related disparities.

A Model to Guide Formation of a Health System Learning Community

With support from a 5-year Bristol Myers Squibb Foundation grant, Jefferson Health (Jefferson), a large academic health system in Philadelphia, PA, developed the Lung Cancer Learning Community (LC2) Initiative. This project focused on increasing SDM and LCS in vulnerable populations by applying the Health System Learning Community (HSLC) Model, a framework developed with support from the Patient-Centered Outcomes Research Institute guide health system efforts to increase cancer screening [13].

The HSLC Model is a theory-based framework that integrates concepts from the Collective Impact Model (CIM) and the Interactive Systems Framework for Dissemination and Implementation (ISF) [14, 15]. The model extends the Exploration, Preparation, Implementation, and Sustainment (EPIS) framework described by Moullin et al. [16] by focusing on how to operationalize health system-based learning communities to effect change in routine care.

The HSLC posits that a learning community comprised of health organization leaders and important stakeholders can work together to identify major population health problems. This model calls for collaborative action to identify effective evidence-based intervention strategies that can address population health needs and determine how such strategies can be implemented. The model also offers steps that can be taken to engage collaborators in developing health intervention strategies, adapting those strategies to fit health system and population needs, implementing effective interventions in practice settings, and sustaining implementation in routine care.

At Jefferson, the LC2 Initiative seeks to achieve the following aims: **Aim 1**. Engage health system patients and providers, health plans, community organizations, and other stakeholders in an effort to increase SDM and LCS in vulnerable populations; **Aim 2**: Identify effective intervention strategies that can increase SDM and LCS in primary care practices that serve vulnerable patients; **Aim 3**: Catalyze health system, health plan, and community support for intervention implementation; and **Aim 4**. Evaluate learning community member engagement.

Aim 1: Engaging Patients, Providers, and Stakeholders.

As shown in Fig. 7.1, Jefferson initially formed a Strategic Management Team (SMT). The SMT includes individuals representing Jefferson's Department of Medicine, Department of Medical Oncology, Department of Radiology, and the Department Family and Community Medicine. This group, which is responsible for providing oversight of the learning community, meets every 2 weeks.

The SMT organized a Coordinating Team (CT) to lead the day-to-day activities of the learning community. The CT, which meets on a weekly basis, includes researchers, public health professionals, social workers, administrators, and staff from the health system's centralized LCS program. The SMT also formed a Steering Committee (SC), Patient and Stakeholder Advisory Committee (PASAC), Research and Evaluation Committee (REC), System Leadership Group (SLG), and a Policy Group.

Members of the SC include senior clinical leaders and representatives from major health plans in the area, state and local health departments, and community organizations. This group, which meets four times a year, is responsible for identifying intervention strategies that can reach vulnerable populations and for determining how to sustain the implementation of effective intervention in the health system.

The PASAC includes patients from vulnerable populations (African American and Asian primary care patients), primary care physicians, clinical care coordinators, oncology social workers, and representatives of community organizations. PASAC members meet four times a year in order to examine intervention materials and methods and recommend how intervention delivery can be adapted to fit the health system and address patient population needs. In effect, the PASAC represents the "voice" of those who will be directly affected by and involved in the implementation of recommended intervention strategies.

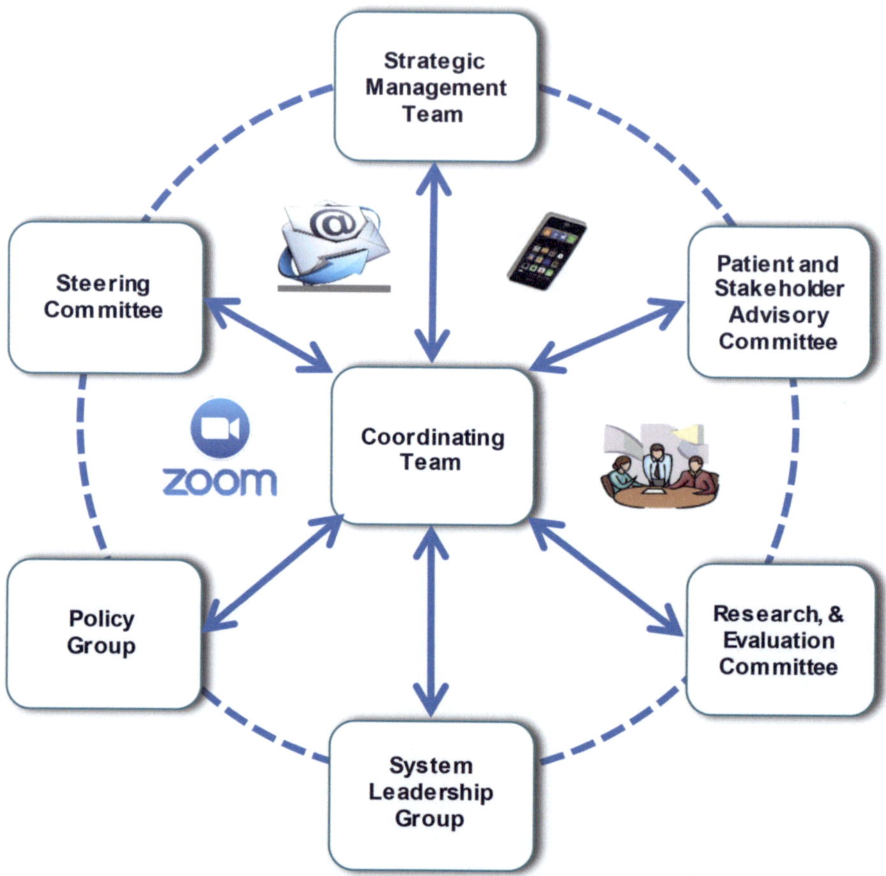

Fig. 7.1 Lung cancer learning community model

The REC is comprised of health system population science researchers, clinicians involved in LCS, and biostatistics support personnel. REC members meet once a month in meetings that focus on the implemention of research studies, collection of relevant data on intervention processes and outcomes, and analysis of collected data to determine the impact of interventions on SDM and LCS rates. This group also is charged with the responsibility of evaluating learning community member participation and engagement.

The System Leadership Group (SLG) includes health system leaders who are responsible for setting health system priorities and allocating resources for operationalizing those priorities. The SLG meets on an annual basis to review study progress and make decisions related to screening intervention implementation and maintenance.

Finally, the Policy Group brings together members of the SC, REC, and SLG who are experienced in carrying out cost analyses, developing value-based care arrangements, and advocacy. This group meets on an ad hoc basis to explore issues related to implementing SDM and LCS and develop proposals that can be operationalized at the health system level.

Aim 2. Identifying Effective Interventions.

Patient Outreach. Regarding **Aim 2**, the SC identified primary care patient outreach as a potentially effective strategy to increase SDM and LCS. The specific nature of patient outreach in LCS was informed by prior research on patient decision support and navigation methods [17–19] that have been effective in raising cancer screening rates among diverse patient populations [18, 19]. Specifically, the intervention strategy involved using health system electronic medical record (EMR) data to identify primary care patients who were potentially eligible for LCS who had a scheduled appointment to see their primary care provider, and engaging research coordinators in the delivery of an LCS telephone outreach contact (OC). Thus, OC involved delivery of mailed LCS education materials and a telephone outreach call to patients identified through EMR review.

SC members proposed delivery of OC to patients in primary care practices that served African American, Chinese, and Korean patients. The SC also recommended that selected patients should be mailed a copy of the patient educational booklet used by Jefferson's centralized screening center and a print decision aid that answered patient questions about LCS, screening efficacy, and the risks and benefits of LDCT. Furthermore, the SC suggested that this mailing should be followed by a care coordinator telephone contact to verify LCS eligibility, review mailed materials, and offer to schedule an LCS visit.

The SC also proposed that selected primary care patients should not only receive the mailed OC materials and outreach call, but should also be guided through SDM by the research coordinator during the telephone contact. It was decided that research coordinators would use the Decision Counseling Program©, an interactive online decision aid, to guide patients through LCS education and decision counseling (DC) sessions to verify screening eligibility, review educational materials, elicit personal values related to screening, and clarify screening preference. This combined intervention is referred to as OC-DC. Importantly, the SC recommended that in OC and OC-DC contacts, research coordinators should be authorized to help patients schedule a visit to the health system's centralized LCS center or encourage the patient to discuss screening with their primary care provider. The SC conveyed its recommendations and intervention materials to the PASAC and REC.

The PASAC reviewed OC and OC-DC print materials and decision counseling methods in order to determine how the interventions should be adapted to meet the needs of patients from vulnerable populations. In this regard, PASAC members recommended that the patient education materials be modified to ensure they were written at a sixth-grade reading level and were translated from English into Chinese and Korean languages. PASAC members also recommended that health system care

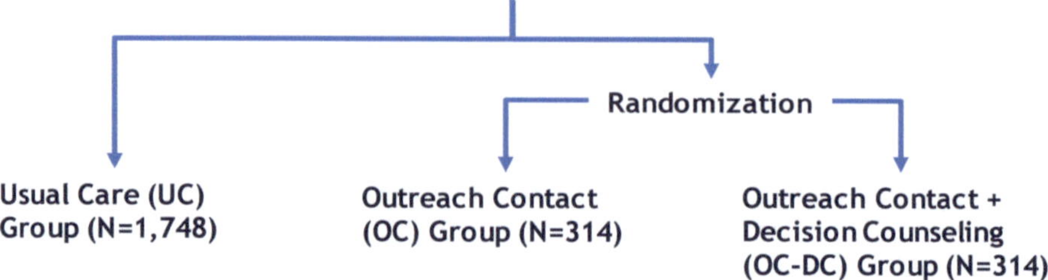

Fig. 7.2 Lung cancer screening outreach pilot study design

coordinators should be trained in DC and should have the capacity to conduct telephone DC sessions in the preferred language of each patient. The CT conveyed recommendations made by the SC and PASAC to the REC.

In accordance with this guidance, members of the REC developed a randomized trial (Fig. 7.2) that was approved by the Thomas Jefferson University Institutional Review Board. As described in a recent publication, [20] the pilot study was designed to determine LCS rates in the context of usual care and assess the impact of OC and OC-DC intervention strategies on LCS in four primary care practices that serve African American, Chinese, and Korean patients. In terms of intervention contacts, health system care coordinators sought to engage patients in the language preferred by patients in each practice. The pilot study, which was initiated in 2019, included 2376 patients through EMR inspection who were 50 to 80 years of age, were current or former smokers, and had not undergone LCS recently. As smoking pack-year data were lacking in the EMR for most patients, the patient sample included individuals who were deemed "potentially-eligible" for LCS. The CT worked with Jefferson IS&T personnel to identify patients for the pilot study and oversaw patient recruitment, randomization, and delivery of OC and OC-DC patient contacts.

A total of 1748 patients were assigned to a usual care Control Group, and 628 patients will be randomized either to an OC Group ($N = 314$) or an OC-DC Group ($N = 314$). At 90 days after enrollment, CT members reviewed EMR data to assess patient LCS. Data analyses showed that at baseline, patients in the Control Group, OC Group, and OC-DC Group has screening rates of 2%, 4%, and 7%, respectively. Together, the screening rate among patients in the combined OC and OC-DC Group was significantly higher than that of patients in the Control Group ($p = 0.001$). Among patients in the OC Group ($n = 31$) and the OC-DC Group ($n = 39$) who were determined to be eligible for screening, LCS rates were 29% and 39%, respectively.

Provider Support. The CT has worked with the National Lung Cancer Round Table and the American College of Chest Physicians® to advance provider education about SDM in LCS. This effort has resulted in the development of a free, accredited online training program, which is titled, "Shared Decision Making in Lung Cancer Screening." The program, which has been updated to reflect recent changes the United States Preventive Services Task Force and Centers for Medicaid and Medicare Services in LCS guidelines, will be launched in 2022. Importantly, health systems will be able to offer this program to all providers who are in a position to assess patient eligibility for LCS and engage eligible patients in SDM.

The new program includes three modules that offer training in (1) Assessment of patient eligibility for lung cancer screening and tobacco treatment, (2) Education of patients about lung cancer screening, and tobacco treatment, and (3) Support for SDM about lung cancer screening. Learners who complete all three modules will be able to identify individuals who are eligible for annual lung cancer screening, educate those who are eligible about the potential benefits and harms of screening, help them make a shared decision about screening, and inform those who smoke or who have stopped smoking about available tobacco treatment services.

Aim 3. Catalyzing Support for Collaborative Action

Jefferson engaged a representative of the Harvard University Center for Health, Law and Policy Innovation (CHLPI) in the Policy Group to help assess health system, health plan, and community views on how to increase SDM and LCS. To this end, the Policy Group developed a key-informant interview guide that could elicit interviewee views on fostering collaborative efforts to identify screening-eligible patients, facilitate educate providers and patients about LCS, implement effective intervention strategies, develop value-based arrangements that support SDM and LCS, and advocate for increased resources needed to sustain intervention implementation.

The Policy Group identified and targeted eight health system leaders and five health plan leaders for interviews. CT members conducted either an in-person or telephone-based interview with each designated participant. All interviews were audio recorded and were transcribed. Two CT research coordinators reviewed and coded the transcripts using NVivo software (QSR International, Burlington, MA, USA) to identify salient themes. A third CT member acted as a tiebreaker in instances where there was a difference of assigned code.

These qualitative analyses identified the following major themes: (1) Supporting a learning community infrastructure, (2) Sharing physician, patient, and community educational resources and effective intervention strategies, (3) Advocating for public/private investment in lung cancer screening, (4) Conducting cost analyses related to screening, (5) Using value-based contracting to support screening, and (6) Incentivizing provider assessment of screening eligibility. Each of these themes was defined as a proposal for collaborative action. Based on these findings, the Policy Group developed an online survey questionnaire designed to assess support for operationalizing the proposals.

Working with the Policy Group, the CT proceeded to identify leaders of the health system, leaders of area health plans, and representatives of area public and private health organizations and community organizations. An invitation to complete the survey was distributed to 12 health system leaders, six health plan leaders, representatives of three health organizations, and four community representatives

Table 7.1 Survey on support for call to action proposals ($N = 25$)

Collaborative action proposals	Support					
	Yes		No		Total	
Health plans and health systems should…	N	$\%$	N	$\%$	N	$\%$
Support a learning community infrastructure.	25	100.0	0	0.0	25	100.0
Share educational resources for physicians, patients, and the community.	25	100.0	0	0.0	25	100.0
Advocate for investment in lung cancer screening.	25	100.0	0	0.0	25	100.0
Conduct cost analyses related to screening.	23	92.0	2	8.0	25	100.0
Use value-based contracting to support screening.	21	84.0	4	16.0	25	100.0
Incentivize the assessment of screening eligibility.	20	80.0	5	20.0	25	100.0

via email. Follow-up emails and telephone reminders. We received a completed survey questionnaire for all 25 (100%) individuals who were invited to participate. Data analyses involved determining frequencies of response for each survey item.

Table 7.1 shows that there was unanimous support for the development of lung cancer learning communities in health systems, collaboration on patient screening education and intervention delivery, and advocacy to increase public and private investment in LCS. Twenty-three (92%) respondents supported collaboration on the conduct of cost analyses related to LCS; 21 (84%) expressed support for incorporating LCS in value-based contracting between the health system and payers; and, 20 (80%) felt it was important to incentivize the process of determining patient eligibility for LCS.

We have included these findings in the form of proposals presented in a white paper titled, "Engaging a Learning Community to Achieve the Promise of Lung Cancer Screening" [21]. The proposals, which are outlined below, serve as a "call to action" for health systems and lung cancer learning communities:

Proposal 1 Health systems should organize a lung cancer learning community that can guide collaborative efforts of the health system, health plans, and other stakeholders to increase shared decision making and screening, promote smoking cessation, and reduce disparities.

Proposal 2 Health system lung cancer learning communities should encourage health systems and health plans to identify individuals eligible for lung cancer screening and ensure that shared decision making, lung cancer screening, and smoking cessation services are offered at multiple "touchpoints" in care.

Proposal 3 Health system lung cancer learning communities should encourage health systems and health plans to conduct cost analyses to guide collaborative efforts to support shared decision making, screening, diagnostic follow-up, treatment, and smoking cessation.

Proposal 4 Health system lung cancer learning communities should advocate for increased public and private investment to identify and implement effective strategies that can increase shared decision making, lung cancer screening, and smoking cessation.

Aim 4. Evaluating Engagement Among Members of the Learning Community

As part of the LC2 initiative, Jefferson evaluated the engagement of learning community members in the activities described above. As shown in Table 7.2, we initially invited 102 members to participate in a total of 168 in-person or virtual meetings of the CT, SMT, SLG, SC, PASAC, REC, and PT. Participation was at least 70% for these groups, with the exception of the SC, which was 60%.

We also asked individuals who attended meetings to complete a survey questionnaire that included items from Wilder Collaboration Factors Inventory (CFI) [22, 23]. Learning community members completed the survey at three points in time (2018, 2019, and 2020). Specifically, the participant survey assessed perceptions related to the strength of engagement in the LC2 Initiative, using a Likert scale response set (Strongly Disagree = 1 to Strongly Agree = 5). The survey solicited responses in five domains: purpose of the learning community (two factors), member characteristics (four factors), process and structure (four factors), communication (two items), and resources (one factor). Mean scores were computed for each domain and constituent factors.

Table 7.3 shows that the LC2 Initiative provided strong support for participant understanding of learning community purpose, collaborative interactions with other members, and access to resources. In addition, participants felt that the learning community provided moderate to high levels of support for their engagement in guiding LC2 Initiative processes, outcomes assessment, and overall communication. A review of individual factors suggests that the learning community could be strengthened by devoting increased attention to increasing the representativeness of membership, facilitating greater discussion, clarifying member roles and responsibilities, and providing guidance related to the priorities and pacing of learning community activities.

Table 7.2 LC2 Initiative member participation by learning community component

Learning community component	Members N	Meetings N	Participation[a] (%)
Coordinating team	8	70	(77.5)
Strategic management team	5	36	(86.1)
System leadership group	13	3	(76.9)
Steering committee	23	6	(60.1)
Patient and stakeholder advisory committee	29	3	(70.3)
Research and evaluation committee	13	40	(70.0)
Policy team	11	8	(84.5)
Total	102	168	

[a]Average participation in each meeting/the total number of meetings

Table 7.3 Wilder CFI survey results among LC2 Members, 2018–2020

| | 2018 | | 2019 | | 2020 | |
| | $N = 41$ | | $N = 27$ | | $N = 35$ | |
Domains and factors	Mean	SD	Mean	SD	Mean	SD
Purpose	4.0	0.6	4.0	0.7	4.2	0.7
Concrete, attainable goals and objectives	4.0	0.8	4.0	0.7	4.1	0.8
Shared vision	4.0	0.6	4.1	0.7	4.2	0.7
Member characteristics	4.0	0.5	4.2	0.5	4.1	0.5
Mutual respect, understanding, and trust	4.1	0.6	4.5	0.5	4.4	0.5
Appropriate cross-section of members	3.9	0.6	4.1	0.7	3.8	0.6
Members see collaboration as in their self-interest	4.2	0.8	4.2	0.7	4.3	0.6
Ability to compromise	3.7	0.7	3.8	0.9	3.8	1.0
Process and structure	3.9	0.6	3.9	0.6	3.9	0.6
Members share a stake in both process and outcome	4.0	0.6	3.9	0.6	4.1	0.6
Flexibility	4.0	0.8	4.2	0.7	3.9	0.9
Development of clear roles and policy guidelines	3.6	0.8	3.6	0.8	3.5	0.9
Appropriate pace of development	3.8	0.7	3.8	0.7	3.9	0.7
Communication	3.9	0.7	4.0	0.7	3.9	0.8
Open and frequent communication	4.0	0.7	4.0	0.9	4.0	0.9
Established informal relationships and communication links	3.7	1.0	4.0	0.9	3.7	1.0
Resources	4.2	0.7	4.1	0.8	4.1	0.9
Skilled leadership	4.2	0.7	4.1	0.8	4.1	0.9

Scores ≥4.0 indicate areas of strength related to engagement; scores 3.0–3.9 indicate areas of moderate strength; and, scores <3.0 indicate areas of weakness

Conclusion

In accordance with the HSLC Model, Jefferson developed a health system-based learning community that is dedicated to increasing SDM and LCS in diverse patient populations, identifying an effective intervention that can increase SDM and LCS rates, and, developing strategies for advancing SDM and LCS in health systems. The LC2 Initiative described here represents the effort of one health system to embrace the challenge of catalyzing collaboration among multiple stakeholders to implement innovations that can change healthcare practice.

The multicomponent organizational structure of the LC2 Initiative addresses aspects of health system change described by Psek et al. [24] that include data analytics, people and partnerships, patient and family engagement, ethics and oversight, evaluation and methodology, funding, organization, prioritization, and deliverables. As described by Lessard et al. [25], this type of learning community can facilitate activities at multiple levels of a health system and involve individuals who represented health system, payer, and community perspectives.

Health systems have the opportunity to embrace the challenge of adopting and adapting a learning community strategy in order to advance SDM and LCS in diverse patient populations. If health systems accept this "call to action," we can we increase SDM and LCS substantially and achieve higher levels of equity in LCS.

References

1. National Lung Screening Trial Research Team, Aberle DR, Adams AM, Berg CD, Black WC, Clapp JD, et al. Reduced lung-cancer mortality with low-dose computed tomographic screening. N Engl J Med. 2011;365(5):395–409.
2. Hoffman RM, Atallah RP, Struble RD, Badgett RG. Lung cancer screening with low-dose CT: a meta-analysis. J Gen Intern Med. 2020;35(10):3015–25.
3. Moyer VA, U.S. Preventive Services Task Force. Screening for lung cancer: U.S. Preventive Services Task Force recommendation statement. Ann Intern Med. 2014;160(5):330–8.
4. US Preventive Services Task Force, Krist AH, Davidson KW, Mangione CM, Barry MJ, Cabana M, et al. Screening for lung cancer: US preventive services task force recommendation statement. JAMA. 2021;325(10):962–70.
5. CMS. Medicare coverage of screening for lung cancer with low dose computed tomography (LDCT). 2015 [cited 2018 May 10]. Available from: https://www.cms.gov/Outreach-and-Education/Medicare-Learning-Network-MLN/MLNMattersArticles/Downloads/mm9246.pdf.
6. Syrek Jenson T, Chin J, Baldwin J, Evans M, Long K, Li C, et al. Screening for lung cancer with low dose computed tomography (LDCT) [Internet]. cms.gov. 2022 [cited 2022 Mar 10]. Available from: https://www.cms.gov/medicare-coverage-database/view/ncacal-decision-memo.aspx?proposed=N&ncaid=304.
7. Huo J, Hong Y-R, Bian J, Guo Y, Wilkie DJ, Mainous AG. Low rates of patient-reported physician-patient discussion about lung cancer screening among current smokers: data from health information national trends survey. Cancer Epidemiol Biomark Prev. 2019;28(5):963–73.
8. Brenner AT, Malo TL, Margolis M, Elston Lafata J, James S, Vu MB, et al. Evaluating shared decision making for lung cancer screening. JAMA Intern Med. 2018;178(10):1311–6.
9. Byrne MM, Lillie SE, Studts JL. Lung cancer screening in a community setting: Characteristics, motivations, and attitudes of individuals being screened. Health Psychol Open. 2019;6(1):2055102918819163.
10. Rai A, Doria-Rose VP, Silvestri GA, Yabroff KR. Evaluating lung cancer screening uptake, outcomes, and costs in the united states: challenges with existing data and recommendations for improvement. J Natl Cancer Inst. 2019;111(4):342–9.
11. Richards TB, Soman A, Thomas CC, VanFrank B, Henley SJ, Gallaway MS, et al. Screening for lung cancer - 10 states, 2017. MMWR Morb Mortal Wkly Rep. 2020;69(8):201–6.
12. Fedewa SA, Bandi P, Smith RA, Silvestri GA, Jemal A. Lung cancer screening rates during the COVID-19 pandemic. Chest. 2022;161(2):586–9.
13. Myers RE, DiCarlo M, Romney M, Fleisher L, Sifri R, Soleiman J, et al. Using a health system learning community strategy to address cancer disparities. Learn Health Syst. 2018;2(4):e10067.
14. Chambers DA. The interactive systems framework for dissemination and implementation: enhancing the opportunity for implementation science. Am J Community Psychol. 2012;50(3–4):282–4.
15. Flood J, Minkler M, Hennessey Lavery S, Estrada J, Falbe J. The collective impact model and its potential for health promotion: overview and case study of a healthy retail initiative in San Francisco. Health Educ Behav. 2015;42(5):654–68.
16. Moullin JC, Dickson KS, Stadnick NA, Rabin B, Aarons GA. Systematic review of the exploration, preparation, implementation, sustainment (EPIS) framework. Implement Sci. 2019;14(1):1.

17. Myers RE, Bittner-Fagan H, Daskalakis C, Sifri R, Vernon SW, Cocroft J, et al. A randomized controlled trial of a tailored navigation and a standard intervention in colorectal cancer screening. Cancer Epidemiol Biomark Prev. 2013;22(1):109–17.
18. Myers RE, Sifri R, Daskalakis C, DiCarlo M, Geethakumari PR, Cocroft J, et al. Increasing colon cancer screening in primary care among African Americans. J Natl Cancer Inst. 2014;106(12).
19. Myers RE, Stello B, Daskalakis C, Sifri R, DiCarlo M, Johnson M, et al. Decision support and navigation to increase colorectal cancer screening among hispanic primary care patients. Cancer Epidemiol Biomark Prev. 2019;26(3):433.
20. DiCarlo M, Myers P, Daskalakis C, Shimada A, Hegarty S, Zeigler-Johnson C, Juon HS, Barta J, Myers RE. Outreach to primary care patients to increase lung cancer screening: a randomized trial. Prev Med Prev Med. 2022;159:107069.
21. Myers RE, Brawer R, DiCarlo M, Garber G, Giamboy T, Juon H-S, et al. Engaging a learning community to achieve the promise of lung cancer screening. 2021.
22. Ziff MA, Willard N, Harper GW, Bangi AK, Johnson J, Ellen JM. Connect to protect researcher-community partnerships: assessing change in successful collaboration factors over time. Glob J Community Psychol Pract. 2010;1(1):32–9.
23. Mattessich PW, Murray-Close M, Monsey BR. The Wilder Collaboration Factors Inventory: assessing your collaboration's strengths and weaknesses. 2001.
24. Psek W, Davis FD, Gerrity G, Stametz R, Bailey-Davis L, Henninger D, et al. Leadership perspectives on operationalizing the learning health care system in an integrated delivery system. EGEMS (Wash DC). 2016;4(3):1233.
25. Lessard L, Michalowski W, Fung-Kee-Fung M, Jones L, Grudniewicz A. Architectural frameworks: defining the structures for implementing learning health systems. Implement Sci. 2017;12(1):78.

Chapter 8
Different Approaches for Offering Lung Cancer Screening

Humberto Choi and **Peter Mazzone**

Background

The goal of lung cancer screening (LCS) is to reduce lung cancer deaths by early detection. Population LCS is not just the performance of a low-dose computed tomography (LDCT) scan. It is a complex program that aims to find a balance of maximizing mortality reduction, while avoiding potential harms from screening. A team effort involving multiple disciplines is necessary to offer high-quality LCS. There are different models of how a program can be organized to offer screening.

The processes involved in screening include identifying and scheduling appropriate individuals, conducting a shared decision making (SDM) visit, performing a LDCT scan, interpreting the scan and communicating the results, managing abnormal findings, and assuring adherence with diagnostic follow-up and the annual repeat screening exam. The role and extent of participation of the stakeholders differ depending on how the program is structured.

In this chapter, we will review the components of high-quality LCS, define LCS program models, discuss how program components could be addressed in each LCS program model, and review the role of a program coordinator or navigator.

H. Choi (✉) · P. Mazzone
Cleveland Clinic, Respiratory Institute, Cleveland, OH, USA
e-mail: choih@ccf.org; mazzonp@ccf.org

G. C. Kane et al. (eds.), *Lung Cancer Screening*,
https://doi.org/10.1007/978-3-031-33596-9_8

Components of a High-Quality Lung Cancer Screening Program

High-quality LCS maximizes the benefits of screening while reducing potential harms. Key components that should be present in every LCS program have been identified [1]. In any approach, the program should include the following components:

- Criteria for who is eligible for LCS: In accordance with the best evidence and current policy.
- Criteria for the frequency and duration of screening: In accordance with the best evidence and current policy.
- Plans for the performance of initial and repeat LDCT: Based on ACR-STR technical specifications [2].
- Structured reporting of LDCT results, including reporting of lung nodule findings: Based on current guidance (e.g., LungRADS), recommendations for follow-up, and reporting of significant non-nodule findings.
- Criteria for lung nodule size that is labeled as a test positive: In accordance with the best evidence and current recommendations (e.g., LungRADS).
- Lung nodule management algorithms and team: Following algorithms for small solid, large solid, and sub-solid lung nodules based on best evidence and current guidelines, and engagement of a multi-disciplinary team with lung nodule management expertise.
- Smoking cessation expertise: Either as part of the screening program or in concert with an established smoking cessation program.
- A means to promote patient and provider education: Focused on LCS, diagnostic follow-up, and tobacco treatment.
- A patient navigation and scheduling system: To promote outreach to eligible patients and ensure compliance with initial screening, diagnostic follow-up, and annual repeat screening recommendations.
- Data collection: To assist with patient tracking and management as well as to drive quality improvement initiatives.

In Table 8.1 we summarize the key components of an LCS program and how respective screening processes may be managed differently by centralized, decentralized, and hybrid approaches. We will define each of these approaches below.

Table 8.1 Lung cancer screening program components and processes in centralized, decentralized, and hybrid approaches

Components of a high-quality LCS program [1]	Program element	Centralized	Decentralized	Hybrid
Eligibility criteria in keeping with current recommendations and policy [3] Frequency and duration of screening in keeping with current recommendations and policy	*Clinical leadership*	PCP, pulmonologist, radiologist	–	PCP, pulmonologist, radiologist
	Identifying and enrolling individuals	PCP, specialists, EHR tools, population management system	PCP	PCP, population management system
	Scheduling	Structured scheduling system	Primary care office or radiology scheduler	Variable
	SDM	Dedicated program provider	PCP	PCP
LDCT performed based on ACR-STR technical specifications Structured reporting of LDCT results	*Imaging protocol*	Radiologist	Radiologist	Radiologist
	Structured report	Radiologist	Radiologist	Radiologist
	Communication of results	Dedicated program provider	PCP	PCP
	Non-nodule incidental findings	Non-cancer specialists	PCP with support of local specialists	PCP
Develop policy for lung nodule size that is labeled as a positive test Lung nodule management algorithms and multidisciplinary team	*Nodule evaluation algorithm*	Pulmonologist, interventional pulmonologist, radiologist, thoracic surgeon	PCP with the support of local thoracic specialists	Variable
	Tracking and ensuring follow-up	Dedicated coordinator/ navigator	PCP	PCP or dedicated coordinator/ navigator
Smoking cessation	*Offer tobacco treatment*	Trained program providers, dedicated smoking cessation program or referral to other programs	PCP or referral to smoking cessation programs	PCP, dedicated smoking cessation program or referral to other programs
Patient and provider education	*Program awareness*	Marketing team	–	Marketing team
Data collection, reporting and quality improvement	*Patient management system, regular data review*	IT specialist, program leadership team	–	IT specialist, program leadership
Other	*Administration*	Administrator	–	Variable

Centralized Model

Centralized programs generally have a dedicated team that is responsible for most or all processes related to LCS (Fig. 8.1). Centralized screening requires core clinical leadership, dedicated resources, and personnel to maintain the infrastructure and manage or support each step of the screening process.

A centralized program receives referrals from providers outside of the program or actively identifies screening-eligible individuals served by the health system. Program members perform SDM visits, orders, and schedules LDCT scans. The program is responsible for interpreting the LDCT scans, communicating results to patients and ordering providers, managing screen-detected findings, and tracking patients to ensure adherence with follow-up recommendations and annual repeat screening. A dedicated LCS coordinator or navigator, clinical leadership, multidisciplinary collaboration, clinical providers, schedulers, IT and administrative support, patient management and data collection systems, and marketing expertise are all components of a centralized screening program.

The Lung Cancer Screening Program at Cleveland Clinic is an example of a centralized model [4]. Our program was initially decentralized, but challenges involving the selection of screen-ineligible individuals, difficulties with timely communication and management of screening-detected findings and mandates to perform meaningful SDM visits and report data to a central registry, all supported a shift to a centralized model. The program became fully centralized in 2015. Clinical leadership of the program includes a pulmonologist and thoracic radiologist who

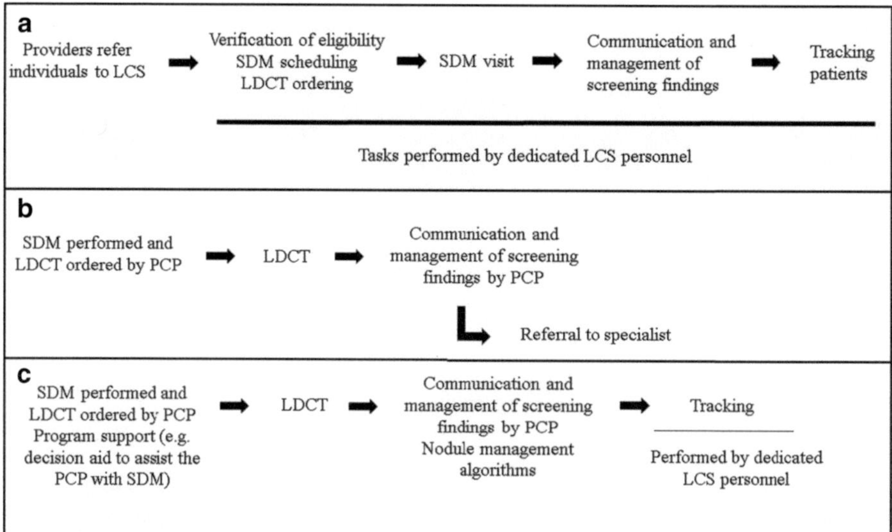

Fig. 8.1 Different approaches to offering lung cancer screening: (**a**) centralized model; (**b**) decentralized program; (**c**) hybrid program. *LCS* lung cancer screening, *LDCT* low dose computed tomography, *PCP* primary care provider, *SDM* shared decision making

provide oversight of the program. Infrastructure support includes program coordinators and schedulers.

Primary care providers within our health system have partnered with and referred individuals to the program. Scheduling systems have been developed so that the patient can be scheduled for their SDM visit as they leave their provider visit, can self-schedule their visit, or have the screening scheduling team assist with scheduling. The program coordinator assists in tracking scheduling progress and following individuals who completed an LDCT scan to ensure adherence with follow-up or annual repeat screening. Advanced practice providers (APPs) review eligibility criteria at the time of the SDM visit, where they also educate, support values-driven decisions, and offer tobacco cessation treatment. The relationship they develop with providers helps when they communicate LDCT results, and advise about the management of screen-detected findings. Regional physician champions assist the APP team with clinical management and outreach efforts at screening sites across our health system.

High-risk cases (e.g., Lung-RADS 4 cases) are reviewed at a weekly lung nodule management multidisciplinary meeting with a thoracic radiologist and pulmonologists specialized in lung nodule and lung cancer management. Lung cancer care is offered together with multidisciplinary collaboration that involves thoracic surgery, medical, and radiation oncology. Non-nodule-related findings on LDCT are also managed by our LCS team. Collaboration with non-cancer specialists is guided by care pathways developed to manage non-nodule incidental findings (e.g., thyroid nodules, adrenal nodules, coronary calcification, aortic aneurysms, and interstitial lung disease).

Information technology (IT) experts have assisted with building order sets, reports, and notes with extractable data elements. We use a commercially available software application to collect data from these reports and notes, report data to the ACR registry, and track individuals to maximize compliance with follow-up recommendations. A separate coordinator from the radiology department is responsible for the oversight of the registry and reporting to the American College of Radiology database. This coordinator also troubleshoots issues with CT scanners and facilitates communication between the clinical team and radiologists.

Decentralized and Hybrid Models

A decentralized LCS program performs and interprets LDCT scans, while identification of screen-eligible individuals, ordering LDCT scans, performing SDM, communication of scan results, management of nodule and non-nodule findings, and smoking cessation guidance are owned by the ordering provider (Fig. 8.1). Therefore, decentralized programs rely mostly on primary care providers (PCPs) (Table 8.1).

Hybrid LCS programs include some of the elements of both centralized and a decentralized approaches. Definitions of hybrid programs have varied, as there are different ways that a hybrid program incorporates centralized and decentralized processes (Table 8.1). A program in a large health system may have one central site performing screening with a centralized approach whereas peripheral sites screen with a decentralized approach. Other hybrid programs may have centralized resource support for some of the screening components related to the ordering providers who otherwise own the patients care (e.g., a population management system or program navigator, connection with a nodule, or smoking cessation program). The centralized team may also develop and share tools with the PCPs (e.g., decision aids to assist with SDM, nodule management algorithms, algorithms for the management of non-nodule findings, and connections to nodule management and smoking cessation programs).

Though high-quality care is possible in any of these approaches, a hybrid model is preferred to a fully decentralized program, whereas a centralized approach is not possible given the multiple demands put on primary care providers. It is important to highlight that centralized oversight and support within a hybrid program can be critical to ensuring that all of the components of high-quality screening program are in place. A centralized team can assist in scheduling individuals, make sure that they are eligible for screening, standardize smoking cessation practices, standardize screen-detected management, track and ensure adherence, maintain a registry, and population management. Other functions such as administration support, marketing, and IT support are also more easily performed by a centralized team.

Successful decentralized and hybrid models rely on PCPs who have the time and interest to take ownership of preventive cancer care. In these screening models, PCPs are responsible for SDM and the management of screen-detected findings, processes that could benefit from an established patient–provider relationship and the trust developed over time. The adoption of the Lung CT Screening Reporting and Data System (Lung-RADS) that provides standardized screening LDCT reporting and management recommendations assists in the interpretation of LDCT scans. However, the integration of a reliable network of engaged specialists with expertise in lung nodule and lung cancer care is essential considering the high rate of false-positive findings and non-nodule-related incidental findings [5].

A qualitative study that evaluated clinician perspectives noted that providers at less centralized programs felt that time to complete the many steps of LCS was the greatest barrier to screening their patients [6]. They identified that they needed assistance with verifying eligibility, ensuring insurance coverage, and tracking patients. These are the functions where central support such as that provided by a program coordinator can be impactful. Clinicians in LCS programs without a dedicated coordinator have to rely on calendar alerts, problem lists, and other methods to track patients [6].

Role of Patient Care Coordinators or Patient Navigators

The patient care coordinator or patient navigator is an important team member in all models of LCS. This is a role that impacts outcomes and promotes the retention of individuals in the program. The terms coordinator and navigator are used interchangeably in the literature to describe similar responsibilities given to the person in this role. Although the job title and specific tasks may differ among programs, the role typically involves ensuring that appropriate and eligible individuals are enrolled in screening, verifying insurance coverage, and tracking individuals to ensure adherence. Coordinators may also be responsible for conducting SDM, nodule management, diagnostic evaluation for potential cancer, and management of incidental findings [7]. The complexity of certain tasks makes this role well-suited for healthcare professionals who have a clinical background, such as nurses, nurse practitioners, or physician assistants. However, many tasks can be performed by non-clinical providers.

Large programs may have more than one coordinator, a mix of both clinical and non-clinical coordinators. In our program at Cleveland Clinic, the coordinators are not clinical providers. They assess eligibility criteria, make sure that individuals are scheduled and have follow-up, participate in outreach, patient retention, data collection, and scheduling coordination aspects of the program. In the Lung Cancer Screening Program at Cleveland Clinic, the APP team's responsibilities include: (1) performing SDM (i.e., verifying patient eligibility, educating patients about the benefits and harms of screening, ensuring that the screening decision reflects patient values and preference, and providing smoking cessation guidance), (2) tracking and managing the screening-detected findings, and arranging repeat screening. Some of these responsibilities may be performed in relation to LCS by individuals identified as patient care coordinators or patient navigators in other health systems.

A large, academic center evaluated the impact of the hiring of a full-time coordinator to a centralized screening program [8]. The coordinator (nurse practitioner) conducted SDM, tobacco treatment counseling, and tracked participants. In that program, adherence to screening increased from 22% to 66% after hiring the program coordinator.

Integration of Smoking Cessation Interventions

LCS is a "teachable moment" for smoking cessation interventions. CMS and the USPSTF recommend that smoking cessation counseling and interventions are integrated into LCS programs [9]. Smoking cessation maximizes the clinical benefit of LCS and its' cost-effectiveness [10].

The approach to smoking cessation is not different in the LCS setting than it is in any office setting. There are several smoking cessation resources that can assist in building a standardized approach [11–14]. The standardization of care is likely more consistent in centralized compared with decentralized programs. A study conducted at a decentralized LCS program in Seattle, Washington, demonstrated a low provision of smoking cessation resources to individuals who smoke [15]. In that study, only 20% of participants were referred to tobacco services, 29% were recommended nicotine replacement therapy and 17% received a prescription for smoking cessation aids. In addition, only 5% received both counseling services and cessation medication [15]. Interestingly, smoking cessation resources were more likely to be offered when LDCT was ordered by a PCP or a specialist compared to another generalist provider.

Undergoing screening alone is not enough to modify smoking behavior [16, 17]. Therefore a proactive and systematic strategy to offer smoking cessation is necessary. It is important for screening programs to develop their own smoking cessation resources or make referrals to established programs.

Determining the Best Approach to Offer Lung Cancer Screening

A high-quality LCS program can be successful in any setting with the appropriate support to provide all of the components of high-quality screening. The model adopted by a program depends on the clinical setting and available resources. In addition to clinical expertise, the level of interest and engagement of PCPs and specialists are factors that can determine a program success.

A policy statement from the American College of Chest Physicians and American Thoracic Society provides guidance on the components necessary to develop a high-quality program. [1] The principles are to carefully select individuals using accepted criteria, perform LDCT imaging, offer tobacco treatment, provide structured interpretation and reporting, and multidisciplinary management of pulmonary nodules and suspected cancers. Quality indicators related to the processes and outcomes of LCS have been proposed (Table 8.2) [18]. Regardless of the program model, these indicators can be used to measure the performance of an LCS program's delivery of high-quality care.

There are many benefits of a centralized approach. It has been demonstrated that a centralized model is more likely to include individuals who meet eligibility criteria and more likely to have screening participants adhere to annual repeat screening compared to a decentralized program [19]. A single-center study from a hybrid program that included centralized and decentralized approaches at different sites compared the outcomes between the two approaches [19]. Among the patients who were ineligible for screening, 90% were screened in the decentralized program. Adherence to annual repeat screening was 70% in the centralized program compared with 41% in the decentralized approach. Similar results were reported by Yim et al. [20] in a study that included five health systems. Adherence to annual repeat screening was lower in decentralized programs compared to centralized programs (34.8% vs 76.1%, respectively) in this study. Interestingly, black race was associated with 27% reduced adherence to annual repeat screening in decentralized programs, while no such effect was observed in centralized programs [19].

The PCP's perspectives are important when developing a program. PCPs routinely screen individuals for other types of cancers, such as breast, cervical, and colorectal cancers. In general, PCPs are supportive of LCS but there is variability on their role preferences [21]. There is also concern about the limited time and ability to counsel patients about LDCT screening, and about the high false-positive rates

Table 8.2 Proposed quality indicators related to processes and outcomes of lung cancer screening programs [18]

	Process and outcome metrics
Screening appropriateness	The percentage of individuals who complete LDCT screening for lung cancer who are screening eligible based on USPSTF criteria
Smoking cessation	The percentage of people who currently smoke who participate in LDCT scan screening who have documentation of a smoking cessation intervention
Compliance	The percentage of lung cancer LDCT scan screening eligible individuals who completed an LDCT scan examination and are identified as having lung-RADS category 1 or 2 findings who completed the next annual LDCT screening examination The percentage of individuals who completed an LDCT scan lung cancer screening examination and were identified as having a lung-RADS category 3 nodule in which a surveillance LDCT scan is performed at 6 months (±2 months) The percentage of individuals who completed an LDCT scan lung cancer screening examination and were identified as having a lung-RADS category 4 nodule in which a surveillance LDCT scan is performed at 3 months (±6 weeks) or additional diagnostic evaluation is performed within 3 months
Evaluation of concerning findings	The time in days from identification of a lung-RADS category 4B or X lung nodule or mass on an LDCT scan screening examination, in someone with lung cancer, to the diagnosis of lung cancer

LDCT low dose computed tomography, *Lung-RADS* lung CT Screening Reporting and Data System, *USPSTF* United States Preventive Services Taskforce

that may require specialist consultation [21]. A centralized model generally assumes the responsibility of most of the LCS process, ideally while maintaining good communication with PCPs to keep them engaged. In the decentralized approach, the presence of a coordinator can offset some of the responsibilities of PCPs such as assuring eligibility and follow-up.

Very few LCS programs have included rural areas. Often the areas where smoking rates and lung cancer burden are high may lack screening programs and some key specialists such as pulmonary, thoracic surgery, and radiologists with experience in screening, who are essential for a program to be successful [22]. It is important for programs in locations where some resources or personnel are not available to develop relationships with programs where their patients can receive these services. Mobile screening programs are alternatives for remote areas [23].

Conclusion

There are different LCS program models – centralized, decentralized, and hybrid. Each model can be successful when organized and supported to provide all of the components of high-quality screening. The structure of each LCS program will depend on available resources, the type of institution, and the skills of local providers. Although the approaches may differ, the principles of a high-quality LCS program are the same: careful patient selection, shared decision making, LDCT imaging with structured reporting, provide tobacco treatment, and multidisciplinary management of screen-detected findings.

References

1. Mazzone P, Powell CA, Arenberg D, Bach P, Detterbeck F, Gould MK, et al. Components necessary for high-quality lung cancer screening: American College of Chest Physicians and American Thoracic Society Policy Statement. Chest. 2015;147(2):295–303.
2. Available from: https://www.acr.org/-/media/ACR/Files/Practice-Parameters/CT-Thoracic.pdf.
3. Krist AH, Davidson KW, Mangione CM, Barry MJ, Cabana M, Caughey AB, et al. Screening for lung cancer: US Preventive Services Task Force recommendation statement. JAMA. 2021;325(10):962–70.
4. Mazzone P, Choi H, Azok J. Creating and scaling a high-quality lung cancer screening program. NEJM Catalyst Innovat Care Deliv 2020;1(5).
5. Janssen K, Schertz K, Rubin N, Begnaud A. Incidental findings in a decentralized lung cancer screening program. Ann Am Thorac Soc. 2019;16(9):1198–201.
6. Melzer AC, Golden SE, Ono SS, Datta S, Triplette M, Slatore CG. "We just never have enough time": clinician views of lung cancer screening processes and implementation. Ann Am Thorac Soc. 2020;17:1264.
7. Tanner NT, Brasher PB, Wojciechowski B, Ward R, Slatore C, Gebregziabher M, et al. Screening adherence in the veterans administration lung cancer screening demonstration project. Chest. 2020;158(4):1742–52.
8. Spalluto LB, Lewis JA, LaBaze S, Sandler KL, Paulson AB, Callaway-Lane C, et al. Association of a lung screening program coordinator with adherence to annual CT lung screening at a large academic institution. J Am Coll Radiol. 2020;17(2):208–15.
9. US Preventive Services Task Force Final Recommendation Statement. Lung cancer: screening. Available from: https://www.uspreventiveservicestaskforce.org/uspstf/recommendation/lung-cancer-screening.
10. Tanner NT, Kanodra NM, Gebregziabher M, Payne E, Halbert CH, Warren GW, et al. The association between smoking abstinence and mortality in the National Lung Screening Trial. Am J Respir Crit Care Med. 2016;193(5):534–41.
11. A clinical practice guideline for treating tobacco use and dependence: 2008 update. A U.S. Public Health Service report. Am J Prev Med. 2008;35(2):158–76.
12. Barua RS, Rigotti NA, Benowitz NL, Cummings KM, Jazayeri MA, Morris PB, et al. 2018 ACC expert consensus decision pathway on tobacco cessation treatment: a report of the American College of Cardiology Task Force on clinical expert consensus documents. J Am Coll Cardiol. 2018;72(25):3332–65.
13. Centers for Disease Control and Prevention. Smoking and tobacco use. Available from: https://www.cdc.gov/tobacco/
14. American Lung Association. Quit smoking. Available from: https://www.lung.org/quit-smoking.
15. Shen J, Crothers K, Kross EK, Petersen K, Melzer AC, Triplette M. Provision of smoking cessation resources in the context of in-person shared decision-making for lung cancer screening. Chest. 2021;160(2):765–75.
16. Slatore CG, Baumann C, Pappas M, Humphrey LL. Smoking behaviors among patients receiving computed tomography for lung cancer screening. Systematic review in support of the U.S. preventive services task force. Ann Am Thorac Soc. 2014;11(4):619–27.
17. Tammemagi MC, Berg CD, Riley TL, Cunningham CR, Taylor KL. Impact of lung cancer screening results on smoking cessation. J Natl Cancer Inst. 2014;106(6):dju084.

18. Mazzone PJ, White CS, Kazerooni EA, Smith RA, Thomson CC. Proposed quality metrics for lung cancer screening programs: a National Lung Cancer Roundtable Project. Chest. 2021;160(1):368–78.
19. Smith HB, Ward R, Frazier C, Angotti J, Tanner NT. Guideline-recommended lung cancer screening adherence is superior with a centralized approach. Chest. 2021;161:818.
20. Yim RR, Mitra N, Saia C, Neslund-Dudas C, Greenlee R, Burnett-Hartman A, Honda S, Simoff M, Schapira M, Croswell J, Meza R, Rizwoller D, Vachani A. Racial disparities in adherence to annual lung cancer screening and recommended follow-up care: a multicenter cohort study. Ann Am Thorac Soc. 2022;19(9):1561–9.
21. O'Brien MA, Llovet D, Sullivan F, Paszat L. Primary care providers' views on a future lung cancer screening program. Fam Pract. 2019;36(4):501–5.
22. Kale MS, Wisnivesky J, Taioli E, Liu B. The landscape of US lung cancer screening Services. Chest. 2019;155(5):900–7.
23. Headrick JR Jr, Morin O, Miller AD, Hill L, Smith J. Mobile lung screening: should we all get on the bus? Ann Thorac Surg. 2020;110(4):1147–52.

Chapter 9
Enhancing EMR Methods to Identify Patients Eligible for Lung Cancer Screening

Hee-Soon Juon, Sarah Reed, Ayako Shimada, Jude Francis, and Ronald E. Myers

Background

Lung cancer is by far the leading cause of cancer death among both men and women, making up almost 25% of all cancer deaths in the United States [1]. In 2022, there will be an estimated 236,740 cases of lung cancer and 130,180 deaths from the disease in the United States [1]. The number of new lung cancer cases continues to decrease, partly because people are quitting smoking. Also, the number of deaths from lung cancer continues to drop due to people stopping smoking and advances in early detection and treatment [1].

H.-S. Juon
Department of Medical Oncology, Thomas Jefferson University, Philadelphia, PA, USA
e-mail: Hee-Soon.Juon@Jefferson.edu

S. Reed
Jefferson Health, Philadelphia, PA, USA

Janus Health Technologies, Chicago, IL, USA
e-mail: sarah.reed@janus-ai.com

A. Shimada
Department of Pharmacology and Experimental Therapeutics, Division of Biostatistics, Thomas Jefferson University, Philadelphia, PA, USA
e-mail: ayako.shimada@jefferson.edu

J. Francis
Information Services and Technology—Enterprise Analytics, Thomas Jefferson University Hospital, Philadelphia, PA, USA
e-mail: jude.francis@jefferson.edu

R. E. Myers (✉)
Medical Oncology, Thomas Jefferson University, Philadelphia, PA, USA
e-mail: Ronald.Myers@Jefferson.edu

It is well established that lung cancer screening (LCS) of high-risk individuals with low-dose computed tomography (LDCT) demonstrates a mortality benefit [2, 3]. However, despite recommendations, only a relatively small proportion of eligible individuals are currently being screened, as evidenced by low numbers of program enrollees relative to the estimated fewer than 2% of the eligible population (seven million) in the United States who would meet eligibility criteria [4]. While multiple interventions will be required to target this challenge, a solution currently being explored is the mass identification of high-risk individuals through population-based eligibility screening utilizing the electronic medical records (EMR) [5].

The widespread adoption of the EMR by primary care providers and health systems, and meaningful use incentives, which encourage using the EMR to document patients' tobacco status, create opportunities to implement EMR-based clinical decision support tools to promote appropriate LCS [6]. The eligible to have LDCT, who were 55 to 77 years old, had a ≥30 pack-year smoking history recorded at the time of the encounter, and had not quit smoking ≥15 years previously [7]. Pack-year cigarette smoking history is very important to determine eligibility of LCS. However, EMR data on pack-years of smoking exposure are currently limited and unreliably recorded due to incomplete, inaccurate, or underestimate true exposure [8–13]. Nevertheless, the accuracy of documentation of smoking history in the EMR has not been extensively examined [9, 10].

In this chapter, we explore the utilization of the EMR to improve efficiency in identifying patients who are eligible for LCS by comparing an EMR query to a patient self-report using Natural Language Processing (NLP) in a machine learning model.

Background

In 2019, we initiated the conduct of an institutional review board (IRB)-approved randomized controlled trial in Jefferson Health (Jefferson), a large health system in southeastern Pennsylvania [14]. Primary care physicians in this health system are encouraged to identify patients who are eligible for LCS for referral to a centralized LCS program, known as the Jefferson Lung Cancer Screening Program (JLCSP). To conduct the study, we identified four Jefferson primary care practices for inclusion in the study. Two of the practices were Family and Community Medicine practices and the other two were Internal Medicine practices.

The investigation involved using standard EMR methods to identify patients who were potentially eligible for LCS according to the existing guidelines based on age and having a history of cigarette smoking. Note, we did not attempt to assess pack-years of smoking exposure. The research team planned to randomize potentially eligible patients to one of three study groups: Outreach Contact plus Decision Counseling (OC-DC), Outreach Contact alone (OC), or usual care control group (UC). We also planned to contact patients allocated to the intervention groups to verify screening eligibility. The primary goal of the study was to determine the individual and combined effects of the OC-DC, and OC strategies on LCS rates compared to usual care. Over a seven-month period, we identified 4421 potentially eligible patients and randomized 2376 as follows: OC-DC group ($N = 314$), OC group ($N = 314$), and UC group (N-1748).

The research team did not attempt to contact patients in the UC group to assess screening eligibility, but did take steps to do so for patients in the OC-DC, and OC groups. Initially, we sent a study invitation letter to patients in the intervention groups, and, in response, a total of 29 patients refused further contact. We proceeded with the manual inspection of medical records followed by attempts to make telephone contact with the remaining 599 patients in order to assess screening eligibility. We were able to contact a total of 280 of these patients and were not able to contact 319 patients. A comparison of patients who were reached and those who were not reached showed that there were no statistically significant differences in age, gender, race, and self-reported smoking status, based on contact status. Among the patients who were contacted and who provided eligibility information, a total of 64 (23%) were found to eligible for LCS.

We used data collected for patients in the combined intervention group to conduct of a study that focused on determining whether the use of health system patients who are eligible for LCS. This effort aims to extend earlier reports in the literature on the use of alternative methods to ascertain LCS eligibility status from health system EMR data [15, 16].

Methods

Setting/Study Population To explore the potential for NLP and ML in identifying patients' eligible for LCS, we built an innovative model to identify which patients were most likely to be eligible. Since our training database was modest in size, we leveraged an existing rule-based system for extracting smoking history (SHAPES) [17]. Specifically, we combined the output from the rule-based system with a pre-trained language model (DistilBERT) [18] that we fine-tuned with the 2006 i2b2 NLP Shared Task smoking status dataset [19]. Finally, we used the combined feature set as the input for a random forest binary classifier that predicted a patient's probability of being eligible for lung cancer screening. Figure 9.1 provides a general overview of the NLP workflow's text preprocessing and model architecture.

Data Utilization For the randomized, controlled trial to test the effects of patient outreach and SDM contacts on LCS rates, 280 patients received a verified label of eligible or ineligible for lung cancer screening that we use as the target outcome. For each patient, we obtained clinical notes for any encounter present in the health system EMR, which resulted in 29,922 clinical notes for the 280 patients. We removed extra spaces, tabs, linebreaks, and stop words in each clinical note using the NLTK and pandas Python packages.

Rule-Based System The Smoking History And Pack-year Extraction System (SHAPES) is a rule-based pack-year extraction system that uses Python and regular expressions. These rules identify several indicators of explicit or implicit non-zero

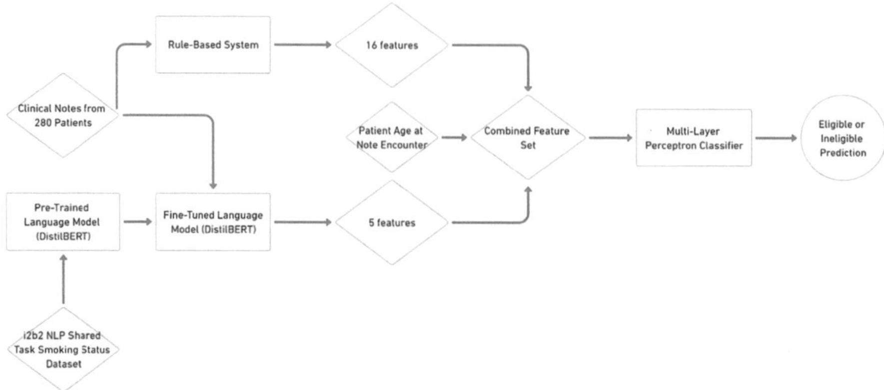

Fig. 9.1 Overview of the NLP workflow's text preprocessing and model architecture

pack-year history from clinical notes, including smoking history duration, smoking rate, current smoking status, quitting status, and others. We adapted SHAPES regular expression rules to create 16 features. In total, 7 of the 16 features are numeric and extract the year, age, or relative time difference since a subject started or quit smoking. The remaining nine features are boolean and indicate whether the notes mention the subject never smoking, ever smoking, attempts to quit, rates of cigarette consumption, or the duration of smoking history.

Fine-Tuned Language Model Transfer learning from large-scale pre-trained models has become commonly applied for NLP tasks. The latest generation of these language models, such as the Bidirectional Encoder Representations from Transformers (BERT) model [19], are deep learning models based on the transformer architecture, which are composed of encoder–decoder networks that use self-attention on the encoder side and attention on the decoder side. These transformer language models improve upon previous NLP techniques by learning context-based representations of text.

By training these language models on millions of sample texts, they can perform well on general-purpose NLP tasks. To apply these pre-trained language models on domain-specific tasks, we can fine-tune the pre-trained model on smaller, task-specific datasets. In our case, we fine-tuned the DistilBERT pre-trained model with clinical notes from the 2006 i2b2 NLP Shared Task smoking status dataset. DistilBERT is an adaptation of BERT that leverages knowledge distillation to reduce the model's size by 40% and increase the speed by 60% while retaining 97% of BERT's language understanding performance [20].

We used the 2006 i2b2 NLP Shared Task smoking status dataset, which consists of 502 clinical notes that annotators classified as one of five smoking status categories: "Smoker", "Current Smoker", "Past Smoker", "Non-Smoker", and "Unknown". Figure 9.2 shows the frequency of classes. We split the dataset to randomly select 30% as the test data and the remainder as the training data. After fine-tuning the

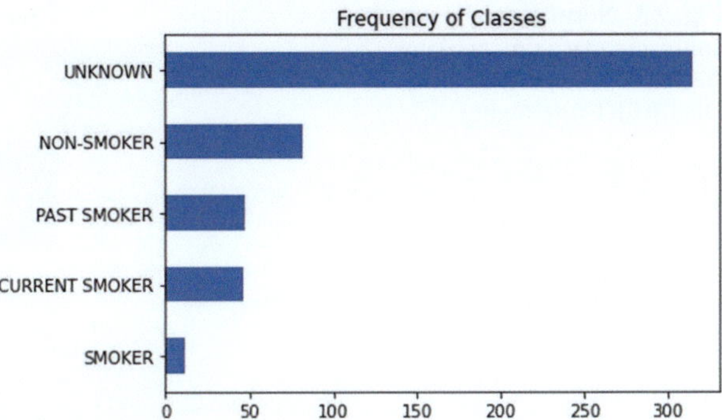

Fig. 9.2 Frequency of classes in the 2006 i2b2 Shared Task smoking status dataset

DistilBERT pre-trained model, the resulting F1 score and accuracy on the domain-specific test data were 0.70 and 0.71, respectively.

Results

In this study, we created a normalized confusion matrix for the test data prediction (see Fig. 9.3). We applied the fine-tuned DistilBERT model to produce probabilities for the five smoking status categories for each of the 29,922 clinical notes from our health system EMR for the 280 patients in our study. This effort allowed us to develop a final model that predicts the likelihood that a patient is eligible or ineligible for LCS.

The final model used a combined feature-set of the 16 features from the rule-based system, the five features from the fine-tuned language model, and the patient's age at the time of the note's encounter. Since patients have a variable number of notes, we aggregated the dataset from note-level to patient-level granularity by averaging features for each patient.

To find the best model architecture for our task, we leveraged the Tree-based Pipeline Optimization Tool (TPOT), a Python tool that uses genetic programming to automate feature selection, feature preprocessing, feature construction, model selection, and parameter optimization [21]. The TPOT classifier search optimized for the area under the receiver operating characteristic curve (ROC-AUC) and used a 5 × 2 repeated, stratified cross-validation (five repetitions of two folds per repetition) for 60 generations. The best-performing pipeline used a multi-layer perceptron classifier and achieved a cross-validation ROC-AUC and accuracy of 0.68 and 0.75, respectively. Figure 9.4 shows the ROC curve.

Determining the functional impact of the NLP/ML model on the efficiency of identifying eligible patients for LCS is a function of assessing the efficiency of identifying eligible patients and the cost of making contact to verify eligibility. Here, we assume that patients identified as "Eligible" by the model will be targeted for contact by screening personnel. Increased efficiency can be realized by allocating resources to contact a smaller proportion of ineligible patients (the number of patients identified as ineligible divided by the total number of patients), and the cost

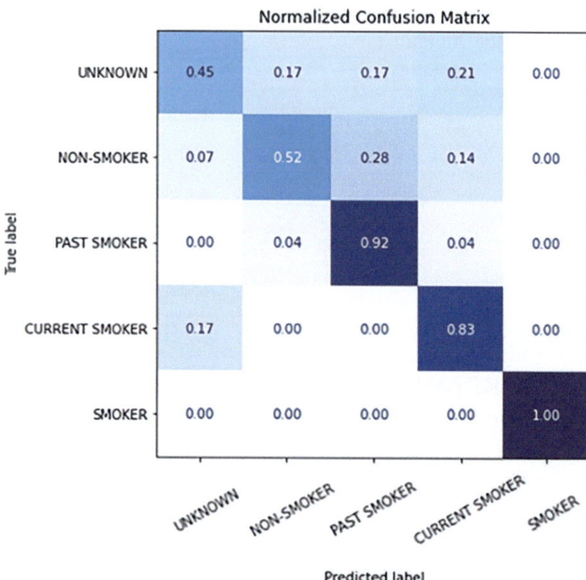

Fig. 9.3 Normalized confusion matrix of smoking status predictions after DistilBERT fine-tuning

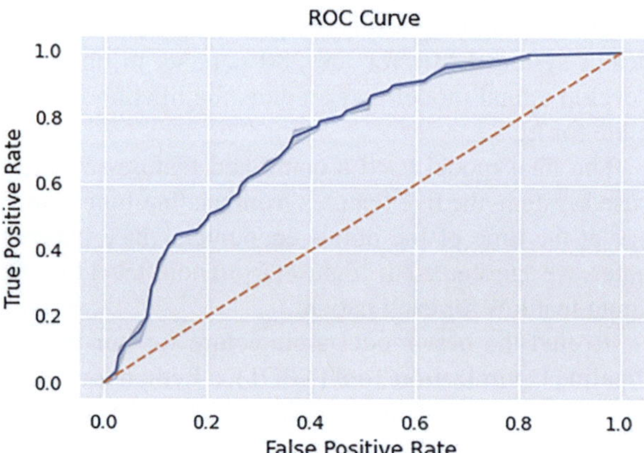

Fig. 9.4 ROC curve for lung cancer screening eligibility predictions from the final model

relates to the misidentification of eligible patients as ineligible (the number of false negatives divided by the sum of the true positives and the false negatives).

The output of the model is a continuous number between 0 and 1. To delineate between eligible and ineligible patients, health systems must decide on a threshold. For example, a threshold of 0.1 designates eligible patients as any patient with a model output higher than 0.1. However, the choice of threshold impacts the distribution of false positives (ineligible patients that are misidentified as eligible) and false negatives (eligible patients that are misidentified as ineligible). False positives reduce efficiency since resources are wasted to contact patients that are not eligible for screening. Conversely, there is a cost related to false negatives, since patients who are eligible for screening may not be contacted. One way to choose a threshold may be to find one that has the greatest difference between efficiency and cost, as defined previously. This solution is represented by the distance between the green and red curves in Fig. 9.5.

Figure 9.6 illustrates the efficiency gains from our model that corresponds to different levels of risk for eligible patient misidentification. At a threshold of 0.1, we can expect a 48% efficiency gain with a 20% chance of misidentifying eligible patients as ineligible. In practical terms, we would only need to contact 145 of the 280 patients using our model, and 35% of the contacted patients would be eligible for lung cancer screening. This result offers an improvement from the practice of contacting all 280 patients, as only 23% of the contacted patients were eligible for LCS.

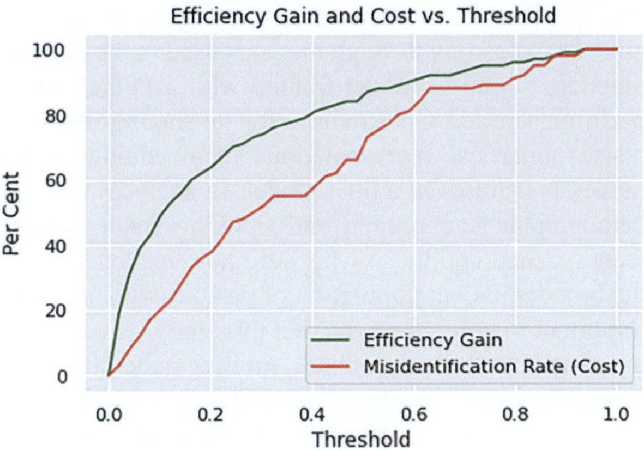

Fig. 9.5 A comparison of efficiency gain and misidentification rate with changing class threshold

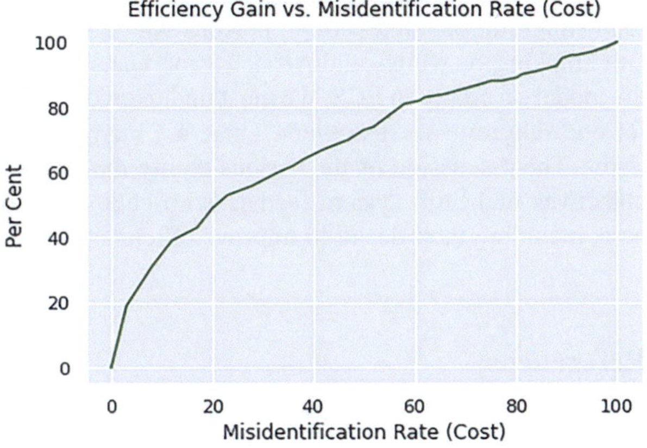

Fig. 9.6 Illustration of the trade-off between efficiency gain and misidentification rate

Conclusion

Applying a basic EMR data query strategy of identify primary care patients who are potentially eligible for screening using age and smoking status data is unfortunately inefficient. This observation has been well-documented in the literature on LCS and has been attributed largely to the incompleteness and inaccuracy of EMR smoking history data [22, 23]. In the study reported here, we found that in comparison of a standard approach to EMR data abstraction and a labor-intensive patient contact process to potentially eligible patients for LCS, our enhanced model was more efficient and is likely to substantially reduce the time and effort involved in LCS program operation.

The small training dataset available from the pilot study presented a considerable challenge to building and training an NLP model. However, we demonstrated that operationalizing such a model could substantially increase the likelihood that patients targeted for contact would actually be eligible for LCS. At a threshold of 0.1, we were able to determine the proportion of contacted patients who were eligible for screening through methods used in the original study from 23% to 35%. In practice, a similar model trained with a larger dataset would result in improved performance and would allow for leveraging other techniques, such as including dense numerical representations ("embeddings") from the fine-tuned language model as features in a final model. In analyses not shown here, we also found that demographic background and smoking status was comparable for patients who were reached and those who were not reached. Thus, results may be applicable to the broader patient population of persons who are potentially eligible for LCS. It is important to note, however, that this study was conducted in one health system and in a small number of practices, limiting generalizability.

Furthermore, it is important to pay special attention to algorithmic "fairness" in curating the training dataset and to examine model predictions. There are many ways to mitigate bias. One of the most straightforward strategies to reduce bias is to ensure that the training dataset includes an adequate number of samples to represent each subgroup of interest (e.g., persons who currently smoke and those who have quit smoking or whites and African Americans). To fully understand the effect of the model on equity in LCS, we must understand if the model is making more errors for one subgroup versus others. There are many ways to define equity in numeric terms. The discussion of the various equity metrics is dependent on the goals and objectives of health system leaders who choose to apply the methods described here, including their desire to improve efficiency and address equity in LCS.

References

1. American Cancer Society. Lung cancer statistics—how common is lung cancer?
2. National Lung Screening Trial Research Team, Aberle DR, Adams AM, et al. Reduced lung-cancer mortality with low-dose computed tomographic screening. N Engl J Med. 2011;365(5):395–409. https://doi.org/10.1056/NEJMoa1102873.

3. Humphrey LL, Deffebach M, Pappas M, et al. Screening for lung cancer with low-dose computed tomography: a systematic review to update the US preventive services task force recommendation. Ann Intern Med. 2013;159(6):411–20. https://doi.org/10.7326/0003-4819-159-6-201309170-00690.

4. GO2Foundation for lung cancer. Screening fact & figure. http://Go2foundation.org/risk-early-detection/screening-facts-figures/. Accessed 1 Mar 2022.

5. Fathi JT, White CS, Greenberg GM, Mazzone PJ, Smith RA, Thomson CC. The integral role of the electronic health record and tracking software in the implementation of lung cancer screening-a call to action to developers: a White paper from the National Lung Cancer Roundtable. Chest. 2020;157(6):1674–9. https://doi.org/10.1016/j.chest.2019.12.004. Epub 2019 Dec 23. PMID: 31877270.

6. Blumenthal D, Tavenner M. The "meaningful use" regulation for electronic health records. N Engl J Med. 2010;363(6):501–4. https://doi.org/10.1056/NEJMp1006114.

7. CMS. Medicare coverage of screening for lung cancer with low dose computed tomography (LDCT). 2015. https://www.cms.gov/Outreach-and-Education/Medicare-Learning-Network-MLN/MLNMattersArticles/Downloads/mm9246.pdf. Accessed 10 May 2018.

8. Kinsinger LS, Anderson C, Kim J, et al. Implementation of lung cancer screening in the veterans health administration. JAMA Intern Med. 2017;177(3):399–406. https://doi.org/10.1001/jamainternmed.2016.9022.

9. Modin HE, Fathi JT, Gilbert CR, Wilshire CL, Wilson AK, Aye RW, Farivar AS, Louie BE, Vallières E, Gorden JA. Pack-year cigarette smoking history for determination of lung cancer screening eligibility. Comparison of the electronic medical record versus a shared decision-making conversation. Ann Am Thorac Soc. 2017;14(8):1320–5. https://doi.org/10.1513/AnnalsATS.201612-984OC. PMID: 28406708.

10. Chen LH, Quinn V, Xu L, Gould MK, Jacobsen SJ, Koebnick C, Reynolds K, Hechter RC, Chao CR. The accuracy and trends of smoking history documentation in electronic medical records in a large managed care organization. Subst Use Misuse. 2013;48(9):731–42. https://doi.org/10.3109/10826084.2013.787095. Epub 2013 Apr 26. PMID: 23621678.

11. Cole AM, Pflugeisen B, Schwartz MR, Miller SC. Cross sectional study to assess the accuracy of electronic health record data to identify patients in need of lung cancer screening. BMC Res Notes. 2018;11(1):14. https://doi.org/10.1186/s13104-018-3124-0. PMID: 29321038; PMCID: PMC5763525.

12. Tarabichi Y, Kats DJ, Kaelber DC, Thornton JD. The impact of fluctuations in pack-year smoking history in the electronic health record on lung cancer screening practices. Chest. 2018;153(2):575–8. https://doi.org/10.1016/j.chest.2017.10.040.

13. Chan KS, Fowles JB, Weiner JP. Review: electronic health records and the reliability and validity of quality measures: a review of the literature. Med Care Res Rev. 2010;67(5):503–27. https://doi.org/10.1177/1077558709359007.

14. DiCarlo M, Myers P, Daskalakis C, Shimada A, Hegarty S, Zeigler-Johnson C, Juon HS, Barta J, Myers RE. Outreach to primary care patients in lung cancer screening: a randomized controlled trial. Prev Med. 2022;159:107069. https://doi.org/10.1016/j.ypmed.2022.107069. Epub 2022 Apr 22. PMID: 35469777.

15. Palmer EL, Higgins J, Hassanpour S, et al. Assessing data availability and quality within an electronic health record system through external validation against an external clinical data source. BMC Med Inform Decis Mak. 2019;19(1):143. https://doi.org/10.1186/s12911-019-0864-2.

16. Yang X, Yang H, Lyu T, et al. A natural language processing tool to extract quantitative smoking status from clinical narratives. IEEE Int Conf Healthc Inform. 2020;2020:10.1109/ICHI48887.2020.9374369. https://doi.org/10.1109/ICHI48887.2020.9374369.

17. Osterman TJ. Extracting detailed tobacco exposure from the electronic health record. Vanderbiltedu [Internet]. 2017 [cited 2022 Mar 11]. Available from: https://ir.vanderbilt.edu/handle/1803/13004.

18. Sanh V, Debut L, Chaumond J, Wolf T. DistilBERT, a distilled version of BERT: smaller, faster, cheaper and lighter. arXivorg [Internet]. 2019 [cited 2022 Mar 11]. Available from: https://arxiv.org/abs/1910.01108v4.

19. Uzuner Ö, Goldstein I, Luo Y, Kohane I. Identifying patient smoking status from medical discharge records. J Am Med Inform Assoc. 2008;15(1):14–24. https://doi.org/10.1197/jamia.M2408.
20. Devlin J, Chang M-W, Lee K, Google K, Language A. BERT: pre-training of deep bidirectional transformers for language understanding [Internet]. 2019. p. 4171–86. Available from: https://aclanthology.org/N19-1423.pdf.
21. Le TT, Fu W, Moore JH. Scaling tree-based automated machine learning to biomedical big data with a feature set selector. Kelso J, editor. Bioinformatics [Internet]. 2019 [cited 2022 Mar 11];36(1):250–6. Available from: https://academic.oup.com/bioinformatics/article/36/1/250/5511404?login=true.
22. Wilshire CL, Fuller CC, Gilbert CR, Handy JR, Costas KE, Louie BE, Aye RW, Farivar AS, Vallières E, Gorden JA. Electronic medical record inaccuracies: multicenter analysis of challenges with modified lung cancer screening criteria. Can Respir J. 2020;2020:7142568. https://doi.org/10.1155/2020/7142568.
23. Triplette M, Donovan LM, Crothers K, Madtes DK, Au DH. Prediction of lung cancer screening eligibility using simplified criteria. Ann Am Thorac Soc. 2019;16(10):1280–5. https://doi.org/10.1513/AnnalsATS.201903-239OC.

Chapter 10
Primary Care Provider Support and Patient Outreach in Lung Cancer Screening

Randa Sifri, William Curry, Heather Bittner Fagan, Beth Careyva, Brian Stello, and Ronald E. Myers

Background

Primary care is a fundamental component of healthcare and serves as a trusted channel of communication between health systems and diverse populations and communities. Operationalizing direct and indirect support for primary care providers

R. Sifri (✉)
Department of Family and Community Medicine, Thomas Jefferson University, Philadelphia, PA, USA
e-mail: randa.sifri@jefferson.edu

W. Curry
Department of Family and Community Medicine and Department of Public Health Sciences, Penn State Health, Hershey, PA, USA
e-mail: wjc8@psu.edu

H. B. Fagan
Department of Family and Community Medicine, Christiana Care Health System, Wilmington, DE, USA
e-mail: HBittner-Fagan@christianacare.org

B. Careyva · B. Stello
Department of Family Medicine, Lehigh Valley Health Network, Allentown, PA, USA
e-mail: Beth_A.Careyva@lvhn.org; Brian.Stello@lvhn.org

R. E. Myers
Department of Medical Oncology, Thomas Jefferson University, Philadelphia, PA, USA
e-mail: Ronald.Myers@Jefferson.edu

G. C. Kane et al. (eds.), *Lung Cancer Screening*,
https://doi.org/10.1007/978-3-031-33596-9_10

can promote positive health outcomes and health equity, such as in the case of lung cancer screening and follow-up [1–3]. To reduce lung cancer mortality and related disparities, health systems have an opportunity to help primary care providers increase both shared decision making (SDM) and lung cancer screening (LCS) rates in a manner that is patient centric and can reach diverse populations [4]. Unfortunately, there are few reports in the literature on successful health system efforts to develop, implement, evaluate, and sustain the use of evidence-based practices in preventive healthcare, including in cancer screening [5].

As described by Tabriz et al. [6], health systems offering LCS make this preventive health service available using a decentralized, centralized, or hybrid approach. In decentralized programs, "frontend providers," mostly primary care physicians, are encouraged to identify patients eligible for screening, educate eligible patients about screening, engage patients in counseling and SDM related to screening, refer/ schedule interested patients for screening, and follow patients who actually screen. Centralized LCS programs commonly rely on front-end practitioners to identify and refer LCS-eligible patients to a screening center. Center staff then seek to contact referred patients, verify screening eligibility, and schedule a screening visit with eligible patients. For those patients who are reached, found to be eligible, and present at a scheduled visit, center staff provide patient education, assess screening preference, guide interested patients through screening, and arrange follow-up care. Some health systems offer a hybrid approach that includes decentralized and centralized elements.

Irrespective of how screening services are made available, LCS rates are suboptimal. Health systems can change this reality by forming a lung cancer learning community of health system leaders, providers, patients, and other stakeholders committed to improving lung health [7]. In accordance with the Exploration, Preparation, Implementation, and Sustainment (EPIS) framework proposed by Moullin et al. [8], the health system learning community can analyze the health system's internal context and external environment to identify barriers to and facilitators of strategy implementation and then develop a strategy to support primary care providers and outreach to patients who are eligible for screening. This step is followed by an implementation phase, in which intervention processes are operationalized and evaluated as part of a process of continuous improvement [9]. Ultimately, this process can lead to the tailored integration of intervention strategies that can be sustained in routine care.

Supporting Primary Care Providers

Healthcare system and stakeholders have an opportunity to embrace the challenge of increasing LCS by supporting primary care provider efforts to identify eligible patients, engage patients in SDM, and facilitate the follow-up of patients, both those who complete screening and those who do not.

Supporting the Identification of Patients Eligible for Screening An initial step in increasing LCS is the identification of eligible patients. In accordance with current guidelines, the identification of eligible patients requires a current and accurate assessment of cigarette screening. Unfortunately, complete and accurate pack year-based smoking history data are not routinely captured in electronic medical records (EMRs) [10, 11].

Due to the stigma associated with smoking, patients may be reluctant to disclose accurately, and this along with varying cigarette use over the life span can introduce complexity and inconsistent in reporting of smoking history on the part of the patient. In terms of providers, these issues are exacerbated by time constraints experienced in busy outpatient practices, leading to inaccurate and longitudinally inconsistent documentation of smoking history. To address these issues, easy-to-use patient-facing tools could be made available for use outside of an office visit. Tools for patients and providers could include structured paper or digital templates that allow for the calculation of pack years.

A study by Dharod et al. [12] reported on the use of a patient portal interactive Website to assess screening eligibility and included a decision aid for LCS. Portal invitations were sent to 1000 patients, and while many (86%) read the invitation, the percentage of patients who visited the website (40%) and completed the decision aid (35%) was considerably lower. Ultimately, of the 99 patients who were confirmed screening eligible, 22 (22%) actually completed a LDCT scan. While it is encouraging that many patients read the invitation, the findings suggest that direct contact with a healthcare team member as part of the process may have increased the response rate. In this regard, pack-year assessment tools could be used by trained outreach personnel (e.g., care coordinators or patient navigators) prior to an office visit, with findings entered into the EMR, or by practice clinical staff at the time of an office visit.

Provider Education and Training in SDM Once patients and/or providers are aware of an individuals' eligibility for LCS, providers must be prepared with both knowledge, e.g., knowing the risks and benefits of screening, and skill to actively invite and engage a patient into a discussion to elicit patient values and beliefs. In a recent review, Müller et al. [13] found that a number of training programs have been developed to educate healthcare providers about SDM. These programs have aimed to increase provider knowledge and enhance provider skills and confidence in SDM across a spectrum of medical decisions [14]. There are a limited number of studies that have reported on the impact of SDM training related to LCS. SDM about LCS in primary care settings occurs infrequently and varies in quality [15]. Lack of time and/or training in SDM are likely contributors. Moreover, sub-optimal SDM for LCS is likely to contribute to low levels of LCS and to repeat screening.

In a study focused on training primary care physicians in SDM for LCS, Volk et al. [16] enrolled 49 primary care physicians in an online training course that used case-based learning that prepared participants to encourage patients to ask questions about screening, provide guidance to patients about decision making, tailor information about screening to patient needs, and establish a decision-making partnership. Using post-training data, the authors found that over 90% of providers correctly identified the steps in the SDM process, 65% said they felt very confident in their capacity to explore a patient's values related to screening, and more than 70% reported that they intended to engage their eligible patients in SDM about screening in the future.

To assess the effects of training providers in SDM about LCS on patient LCS rates, Olazagasti et al. [17] recruited 35 physicians and identified an initial cohort of consecutive patients who were eligible for LCS and had made a routine office visit. At baseline, only 26% of the patients were found to have had screening. Participating physicians attended a series of in-person training sessions on SDM and LCS. Subsequently, the research team identified a second cohort of patients who visited the provider after the training experience was completed. In the second cohort, 78% of screening-eligible patients underwent screening. This increase in the LCS rate was substantial and highly significant ($p < 0.001$).

Additional evidence on the impact of provider training in SDM about LCS has been provided by research on training practice staff to engage patients in SDM about LCS at the time of a primary care practice office visit [18]. The researchers recruited current smokers 55 to 77 years of age who were patients across five community health centers, and randomized participants to receive either an in-office patient navigation intervention or usual care. They also trained patient navigators to guide intervention group participants through an LCS eligibility assessment, educate participants about LCS, and cue participants to discuss LCS at an ensuing encounter with their primary care provider. Among 94 intervention group participants, 23 (24%) had LDCT screening, while among 69 control group participants, only 9% underwent screening ($p < 0.001$). In addition, Fagan et al. (2020) demonstrated that a telephone-based SDM intervention delivered by a trained care coordinator as an outreach contact before a scheduled primary care office visit promoted LCS.

A free, accredited online training program for providers has been developed to facilitate SDM training. This program, which can be accessed at https://www.chest-net.org/Store/Products/Standard-Products/eLearning/Shared-Decision-Making-in-Lung-Cancer-Screening, includes modules on assessing patient eligibility for screening, educating patients about LCS, performing SDM about LCS. Information about tobacco treatment resources is also included. The target audience for this program includes primary care physicians and other healthcare providers who are responsible for identifying and offering LCS to eligible patients. Healthcare systems could proactively disseminate information about this and other LCS training resources to their providers.

Facilitating Patient Referral and Appointment-Scheduling Once LCS eligibility is documented in the EMR, providers affiliated with health systems that offer decentralized screening can complete SDM, refer the patient for screening, and order an LDCT screening exam. Point-of-care alerts linked to a structured LDCT order set have been shown to help facilitate placing an order for LDCT [19]. Ideally, the order set would document SDM completion, treatment, and/or referrals for tobacco treatment, along with the LDCT order with scheduling logistics. In centralized screening programs, providers may choose to refer eligible patients to LCS program staff for appointment scheduling, SDM, initial screening and follow-up, and tobacco treatment. Support for the diagnostic follow-up of abnormal results and for the encouragement of repeat screening are also offered.

While it is imperative to improve LCS in patients who present at a primary care practice, health systems should devote resources to contacting patients who do not present for care at an office visit in order to assure inclusion and equity. Patient outreach methods can serve to augment provider capacity to identify and engage screening-eligible patients in LCS in decentralized, centralized, and hybrid screening programs.

Outreach to Primary Care Patients

LCS can be an important test of the increasingly common population focus of health systems; it is a case study of several outreach and navigation tools at play and the need to integrate these efforts into primary care. Patient outreach for LCS is particularly challenging as two main tenets of LCS must be met to be successful: (1) patients must be accurately identified as meeting eligibility for LCS and (2) a process for providing SDM must be documented to complete an order for testing.

These aspects of LCS necessitate a different level of interaction with the patient that theoretically could be facilitated through the use of EMR patient portals. Furthermore, outreach to patients to improve LCS must incorporate strategies that reach patients who do not typically or regularly access their primary care office. This is particularly important with LCS as tools for identifying eligible patients that lead PCPs to act at the time of the visit are not readily available. Due to poor tobacco history documentation in most EHRs, PCPs are not prompted to order screening at the point of care as they often are for colorectal cancer (CRC) or breast cancer screening.

Patient Contact Patient outreach and navigation to encourage different types of cancer screening are common and the more successful outreach approaches are via phone/text, mail, and the EMR portal. Historically, patient navigators have been nurses who are assigned to help patients diagnosed with cancer find their way through the complex and confusing diagnostic and treatment process; and numerous studies of such contacts have been shown to have positive effects on cancer prevention and control [20–24]. Patient navigation has had a positive impact on cancer screening and has been effective in increasing equity in screening utilization [25, 26]. It is important to note that SDM is not mandated in screening for breast, cervical, and colorectal cancer. In those instances, providers can generate and send orders or hand actual screening tests or prescriptions to patients directly (e.g., mammography scripts and FIT/FOBT kits), and patient navigation can be initiated immediately.

Patient Engagement at the Time of an Office Visit Patient navigation in the context of LCS has been reported in the clinic setting [27]. In the context of office-based efforts to engage patients in LCS, Reuland et al. [28] used EMR data to identify primary care patients who were potentially eligible for LCS. The research team contacted patients by telephone and arranged for them to visit their primary care practice to view an LCS educational video. In this study, patients were exposed to an educational video at the time of the office visit. Of 36 participants who visited the practice and viewed the video, 10 (28%) underwent LCS within 90 days after the visit. It is important to note that patients included in this study were not engaged in SDM about LCS prior to or at the time of the office visit. Research is needed on the design, delivery, and impact of health system patient outreach contacts via mail, telehealth, EMR based, and other communication channels to facilitate SDM and LCS.

Patient Engagement Prior to an Office Visit In an ongoing study being conducted in the Lehigh Valley Health Network in southeastern Pennsylvania, primary care patients in ten primary care practices who were currently smoking or formerly smoked and also had a scheduled primary care office visit were engaged to participate in a LCS study. In addition, the research team engaged a physician champion in each participating practice. Project staff identified 993 patients as potentially eligible for LCS through EMR queries and sent these individuals a screening invitation letter and a copy of an LCS decision aid. As a result of outreach contacts, a project care coordinator succeeded in enrolling 253 screening-eligible participants in the study, reviewed the decision aid with each participant, assessed participant interest in screening, and encouraged the participant to discuss screening with a provider at their scheduled office visit. Furthermore, the care coordinator entered the results of the contact into the EMR prior to the visit. The research team found that 174 (69%) participants completed LCS.

In a patient outreach study that involved primary care patients from a health system in Delaware, Bittner-Fagan et al. [29] used EMR data to identify patients who were potentially eligible for LCS. A research assistant contacted identified individuals, assessed eligibility for LCS, obtained consent, scheduled a telephone call with a study care coordinator, and mailed a copy of a 1-page LCS decision aid to each participant. During the ensuing call, a care coordinator trained in SDM reviewed information in the decision aid and used an online software application (the Decision Counseling Program©, or DCP), to guide the participant through a decision counseling exercise that served to clarify the participant's screening preference (to be screened, unsure about being screened, not to be screened). This project identified 419 patients who were potentially eligible for LCS and enrolled 55 eligible participants in the study. Of this number, 36 participants completed a decision counseling session, and 13 (36%) underwent LCS.

An additional ongoing 3-arm randomized controlled trial was conducted in four primary care practices of a metropolitan health system [30]. Practice patients identified through medical records who were aged 50–80 years and who currently smoked heavily or had a history of heavy smoking were randomized to receive Outreach Contact plus Decision Counseling (OC-DC, $n = 314$), Outreach Contact alone (OC, $n = 314$), or usual care (UC, $n = 1748$). OC-DC involved mailing a 1-page decision aid to the participant and a care coordinator telephone call. The care coordinator verified LCS eligibility, guided eligible participants through the LCS decision aid, completed a screening decision counseling exercise, and developed an action plan based on participant preference. The OC involved mailing the 1-page decision aid, determining eligibility, and delivery of care coordinator telephone call to verify screening LCS eligibility and record participant interest in screening. LCS was significantly higher in the combined OC/OC-DC group versus usual care controls ($p = 0.001$). Among screening-eligible patients, screening was higher in the OC-DC group than in the OC group (40% and 28%, respectively).

Elsewhere, Tanner et al. [31] reported that outreach contacts which included SDM before a primary care office visit and an SDM encounter that took place at the time of an office had comparable effects on LCS rates. Findings from the studies described here strongly suggest that the use of patient outreach strategies should be explored.

Conclusion

Primary care faces ongoing tension between priorities of acute care, chronic illness, and prevention. Even prior to the COVID-19 pandemic, patient-initiated visits in a fee-for-service structure prioritize acute care over prevention. The COVID-19 pandemic further deprioritized prevention and cancer screening [32]. Until COVID-19 becomes endemic, practice strain is likely to continue, both in terms of access demands for acute illness care as well as staffing shortages which may limit practice capacity to engage in population health management. Health systems should reimagine quality improvement in LCS, consider using incentives in a creative manner, promote the reimbursement of value-based care, and broaden support for team-based care in the management of competing demands.

Reimagine Quality Improvement Structured quality improvement in LCS requires the ability to accurately capture the denominator of eligible patients and will require more accurate data collection especially related to smoking history. Depending on in-person visits to capture this information will likely miss many eligible patients and underestimate the true denominator of those who are eligible for screening. Current practices of monitoring the number of screening tests ordered and completed are also likely to exclude patients in vulnerable populations experiencing disparities and those who do not make routine office visits. The strategies presented above for documentation of smoking history will help to mitigate this challenge.

Most quality improvement initiatives in cancer screening are based on patient completion of screening, a binary measurement that does not support the more subtle act of engaging in SDM where sometimes choosing not to screen is aligned with the patient values and their comorbidities. While healthcare team can facilitate adherence through motivational interviewing and navigation, there may be patient-level factors that are not easily addressed that prevent a patient from screening completion. Assessing the number of eligible patients who have participated in SDM in addition to completion of LDCT would provide a patient-centered view of quality improvement. Proceeding with the choice made by an informed patient would be considered successful SDM in LCS, even if this activity does not result in testing. Creating systems and practices to support patients to operationalize their decisions after the primary care encounter, including via navigation, may also aid in supporting patient goals.

Reconsider Incentives Aligning incentives may help to facilitate improvement in rates of shared decision making and LCS. Most traditional quality programs incentivize via bonuses and/or linkage to salary, most often for clinicians. Programs that only incentivize clinicians have not been found to consistently improve patient-related outcomes [33]. Another possibility for health systems to consider is to also incentivize staff, who play a pivotal role in ensuring documentation of smoking history needed for effective screening, in order to promote further alignment of efforts.

Health systems may also consider implementing alternative incentives that may be even more important to clinicians and teams, such as using quality incentive payments to add staff and/or community health workers in lieu of a traditional bonus structure. This approach would allow clinicians and practices to be rewarded with the capacity to develop the teams needed to deliver more effective patient care. For some, this may be more motivating than an incremental payment. It has also been acknowledged that there is not a single incentive model most likely to be effective and that a combination of financial and non-financial incentives may be best able to influence change [34].

Our recommendations align with the literature and Wernli et al. [35] to identify several steps that health systems can take in order to increase SDM and LCS. These steps include training both care coordinators and clinicians in SDM about LCS and using care coordination as a means of supporting primary care and specialty care efforts to provide high-quality preventive care to patients. We recommend that health systems train and support primary care providers and care coordinators to identify patients who are eligible for screening, guide patients through SDM about screening, and facilitating the referral and follow-up of patients who make an informed decision to screen. This effort should involve enhancing the use of the EMR to identify patients who are eligible for screening, providing providers with tools and training needed to integrate SDM in routine care, and supporting patient outreach.

Managing Competing Demands In response to competing demands, practices have adopted multiple strategies to address prevention outside of the patient visit. However, LCS is only one of many quality measures and needs that clinicians and teams are asked to address. Values-based reimbursement (VBR) contracts and other incentive payments currently emphasize other more easily measured screening tests, e.g., breast and colon cancer screening, in part because of limitations with determining the true denominator for LCS, yet the financial reality is of particular concern given that lung cancer is the number one cause of cancer deaths worldwide.

To achieve and sustain LCS, healthcare systems need the capability to engage in data-driven population health, moving beyond our current system of reactive and transactional care for those who schedule appointments and reaching out to the greater communities we serve. This requires a pivot to increased reimbursement for value-based care. In addition to restructuring payment for primary care, an optimal practice context includes both a team-based approach and a functional EMR infrastructure.

The team-based approach includes clinical staff ensuring the documentation of smoking history and notating those who are eligible, followed by SDM with a provider and support for the patient after the encounter. While point-of-care reminders have been found to be effective for patients who have scheduled appointments, population health management via registry review is needed to engage those with barriers to accessing routine primary care. Health systems should support registry review and outreach to capture those individuals who may meet screening criteria but are not regularly accessing healthcare. Moreover, the health system EMR infrastructure should include tools to facilitate the capture of smoking history, tailored order sets with decision tools, and health maintenance alerts to provide cues for both initial and annual screening for the appropriate age ranges.

Finally, a "one size fits all" approach is unlikely to be effective given the unique contexts of healthcare systems and individual primary care practices. Workflows and infrastructure that can be tailored to best meet the needs of patients and healthcare teams and can utilize multi-modal approaches are needed to accelerate LCS across patient populations and fully leverage the power of primary care.

References

1. Lawn JE, Rohde J, Rifkin S, Were M, Paul VK, Chopra M. Alma-Ata 30 years on: revolutionary, relevant, and time to revitalise. Lancet. 2008;372(9642):917–27.
2. World Health Organization. Primary health care: now more than ever. The World Health Organization; 2008.
3. Shi L. The impact of primary care: a focused review. Scientifica (Cairo). 2012;2012:432892.
4. Myers RE. Health organizations have an opportunity to improve shared decision-making and raise lung cancer screening rates. Chest. 2021;159(1):23–4.
5. Allen C, Coleman K, Mettert K, Lewis C, Westbrook E, Lozano P. A roadmap to operationalize and evaluate impact in a learning health system. Learn Health Sys. 2021;5(4):e10258.
6. Alishahi Tabriz A, Neslund-Dudas C, Turner K, Rivera MP, Reuland DS, Elston Lafata J. How health-care organizations implement shared decision-making when it is required for reimbursement: the case of lung cancer screening. Chest. 2021;159(1):413–25.
7. Man LC, DiCarlo M, Lambert E, Sifri R, Romney M, Fleisher L, et al. A learning community approach to identifying interventions in health systems to reduce colorectal cancer screening disparities. Prev Med Rep. 2018;12:227–32.

8. Moullin JC, Dickson KS, Stadnick NA, Rabin B, Aarons GA. Systematic review of the Exploration, Preparation, Implementation, Sustainment (EPIS) framework. Implement Sci. 2019;14(1):1.

9. Deming WE. Out of the crisis. Reprint. The MIT Press; 2000.

10. Polubriaginof F, Salmasian H, Albert DA, Vawdrey DK. Challenges with collecting smoking status in electronic health records. AMIA Annu Symp Proc. 2017;2017:1392–400.

11. Modin HE, Fathi JT, Gilbert CR, Wilshire CL, Wilson AK, Aye RW, et al. Pack-year cigarette smoking history for determination of lung cancer screening eligibility. comparison of the electronic medical record versus a shared decision-making conversation. Ann Am Thorac Soc. 2017;14(8):1320–5.

12. Dharod A, Bellinger C, Foley K, Case LD, Miller D. The reach and feasibility of an interactive lung cancer screening decision aid delivered by patient portal. Appl Clin Inform. 2019;10(1):19–27.

13. Müller E, Strukava A, Scholl I, Härter M, Diouf NT, Légaré F, et al. Strategies to evaluate healthcare provider trainings in shared decision-making (SDM): a systematic review of evaluation studies. BMJ Open. 2019;9(6):e026488.

14. Légaré F, Adekpedjou R, Stacey D, Turcotte S, Kryworuchko J, Graham ID, et al. Interventions for increasing the use of shared decision making by healthcare professionals. Cochrane Database Syst Rev. 2018;7:CD006732.

15. Brenner AT, Malo TL, Margolis M, Elston Lafata J, James S, Vu MB, et al. Evaluating shared decision making for lung cancer screening. JAMA Intern Med. 2018;178(10):1311–6.

16. Volk RJ, Shokar NK, Leal VB, Bulik RJ, Linder SK, Mullen PD, et al. Development and pilot testing of an online case-based approach to shared decision making skills training for clinicians. BMC Med Inform Decis Mak. 2014;14:95.

17. Olazagasti C, Sampat D, Rothman A, Seetharamu N, Steiger D. Implementing physician education to increase lung cancer screening compliance. J Clin Oncol. 2019;37(15_suppl):e18282.

18. Percac-Lima S, Ashburner JM, Rigotti NA, Park ER, Chang Y, Kuchukhidze S, et al. Patient navigation for lung cancer screening among current smokers in community health centers a randomized controlled trial. Cancer Med. 2018;7(3):894–902.

19. Coma E, Medina M, Méndez L, Hermosilla E, Iglesias M, Olmos C, et al. Effectiveness of electronic point-of-care reminders versus monthly feedback to improve adherence to 10 clinical recommendations in primary care: a cluster randomized clinical trial. BMC Med Inform Decis Mak. 2019;19(1):245.

20. Freeman HP, Muth BJ, Kerner JF. Expanding access to cancer screening and clinical follow-up among the medically underserved. Cancer Pract. 1995;3(1):19–30.

21. Till JE. Evaluation of support groups for women with breast cancer: importance of the navigator role. Health Qual Life Outcomes. 2003;1:16.

22. Oluwole SF, Ali AO, Adu A, Blane BP, Barlow B, Oropeza R, et al. Impact of a cancer screening program on breast cancer stage at diagnosis in a medically underserved urban community. J Am Coll Surg. 2003;196(2):180–8.

23. Guadagnolo BA, Dohan D, Raich P. Metrics for evaluating during cancer diagnosis and treatment: crafting a policy-relevant research agenda for in cancer care. Cancer. 2011;117(15 Suppl):3565–74.

24. Myers RE, Sifri R, Daskalakis C, DiCarlo M, Geethakumari PR, Cocroft J, et al. Increasing colon cancer screening in primary care among African Americans. J Natl Cancer Inst. 2014;106(12):dju344.

25. Ali-Faisal SF, Colella TJF, Medina-Jaudes N, Benz Scott L. The effectiveness of to improve healthcare utilization outcomes: a meta-analysis of randomized controlled trials. Patient Educ Couns. 2017;100(3):436–48.

26. Shusted CS, Barta JA, Lake M, Brawer R, Ruane B, Giamboy TE, et al. The case for in lung cancer screening in vulnerable populations: a systematic review. Popul Health Manag. 2019;22(4):347–61.

27. Lowenstein LM, Godoy MCB, Erasmus JJ, Zirari Z, Bennett A, Leal VB, et al. Implementing decision coaching for lung cancer screening in the low-dose computed tomography setting. JCO Oncol Pract. 2020;16(8):e703–25.
28. Reuland DS, Cubillos L, Brenner AT, Harris RP, Minish B, Pignone MP. A pre-post study testing a lung cancer screening decision aid in primary care. BMC Med Inform Decis Mak. 2018;18(1):5.
29. Fagan HB, Fournakis NA, Jurkovitz C, Petrich AM, Zhang Z, Katurakes N, et al. Telephone-based shared decision-making for lung cancer screening in primary care. J Cancer Educ. 2020;35(4):766–73.
30. DiCarlo M, Myers P, Daskalakis C, Shimada A, Hegarty S, Zeigler-Johnson C, Juon HS, Barta J, Myers RE. Outreach to primary care patients in lung cancer screening: a randomized controlled trial. Prev Med. 2022;159:107069. https://doi.org/10.1016/j.ypmed.2022.107069. Epub 2022 Apr 22. PMID: 35469777.
31. Tanner NT, Silvestri GA. Shared decision-making and lung cancer screening: let's get the conversation started. Chest. 2019;155(1):21–4.
32. Alkatout I, Biebl M, Momenimovahed Z, Giovannucci E, Hadavandsiri F, Salehiniya H, et al. Has COVID-19 affected cancer screening programs? A systematic review. Front Oncol. 2021;11:675038.
33. Doran T, Maurer KA, Ryan AM. Impact of provider incentives on quality and value of health care. Annu Rev Public Health. 2017;38:449–65.
34. Custers T, Hurley J, Klazinga NS, Brown AD. Selecting effective incentive structures in health care: a decision framework to support health care purchasers in finding the right incentives to drive performance. BMC Health Serv Res. 2008;8:66.
35. Wernli KJ, Tuzzio L, Brush S, Ehrlich K, Gao H, Anderson ML, et al. Understanding patient and clinical stakeholder perspectives to improve adherence to lung cancer screening. Permanent J. 2021;25:20.295.

Chapter 11
Shared Decision Making in the Lung Cancer Screening Context

Jamie L. Studts, Erin A. Hirsch, Nina A. Thomas, Channing E. Tate, Amy G. Huebschmann, Melissa DiCarlo, and Ronald E. Myers

Background

In response to the landmark results of the National Lung Screening Trial (NLST), the US Preventive Services Task Force (USPSTF) updated their lung cancer screening (LCS) guideline at the end of 2013, recommending annual low-dose computed tomography (LDCT) for individuals at elevated risk of developing lung cancer [1],

J. L. Studts (✉)
Division of Medical Oncology, Department of Medicine, University of Colorado School of Medicine, Aurora, CO, USA
e-mail: jamie.studts@cuanschutz.edu

E. A. Hirsch
Division of Medical Oncology, Department of Medicine, University of Colorado School of Medicine, Aurora, CO, USA
e-mail: erin.hirsch@cuanschutz.edu

N. A. Thomas
Division of Pulmonary Sciences and Critical Care, Department of Medicine, University of Colorado School of Medicine, Aurora, CO, USA
e-mail: nina.thomas@cuanschutz.edu

C. E. Tate · A. G. Huebschmann
Division of General Internal Medicine, Department of Medicine, University of Colorado School of Medicine, Aurora, CO, USA
e-mail: channing.tate@cuanschutz.edu; amy.huebschmann@cuanschutz.edu

M. DiCarlo
Department of Medical Oncology, Thomas Jefferson University, Philadelphia, PA, USA
e-mail: Melissa.DiCarlo@Jefferson.edu

R. E. Myers
Department of Medical Oncology, Thomas Jefferson University, Philadelphia, PA, USA
e-mail: Ronald.Myers@Jefferson.edu

G. C. Kane et al. (eds.), *Lung Cancer Screening*,
https://doi.org/10.1007/978-3-031-33596-9_11

and there was little surprise that the guideline also favored shared decision making (SDM) as the preferred approach to discussing the LCS opportunity with potentially eligible candidates. This recommendation was not surprising, because the USPSTF has favored a SDM approach to virtually all preventive health service options and recommendations since 2004 [2], and has recently updated and reaffirmed a commitment to SDM [3]. Nearly all relevant authoritative professional and community organizations have developed recommendations favoring LCS implementation following the publication of the NLST primary results, which showed a favorable benefit-to-risk ratio for LDCT and both a lung cancer specific and overall mortality reduction compared to standard chest radiographs [4].

When the Centers for Medicare and Medicaid Services (CMS) offered their National Coverage Determination on LCS in 2015 [5, 6], the organization mandated delivery and documentation of SDM as a *requirement* for LDCT reimbursement for a Medicare beneficiary and allocated payment for SDM performance. Furthermore, CMS stipulated several key points that must be addressed during the SDM consultation with patients who are determined to be eligible for LCS, including patient education about the benefits and harms of screening, follow-up diagnostic testing, and the importance of adhering to annual screening. In addition to outlining key considerations, CMS took an additional step. Specifically, CMS required the use of at least one decision aid or decision support tool as part of the SDM consultation [5].

The decision support stipulation may have been premature, given the lack of widely available evidence-based decision aids to support the SDM consultation at the time [7]. Importantly, however, this requirement signaled a clear focus on helping eligible candidates make informed and collaborative choices that are based not only on the evidence but also based on candidate's personal values and preferences. Subsequent guidance from CMS regarding interventions for other health conditions, including implantable cardioverter-defibrillators and for left atrial appendage closure (LAAC) for stroke prophylaxis in atrial fibrillation, has also required documentation of SDM and decision aids as part of the care delivery and reimbursement process [8, 9].

Based on evidence provided by the publication of the NELSON Trial results [10], as well as additional accumulating evidence [11], the USPSTF revisited their LCS guidelines. This effort led to the presentation of updated guidance in 2021 [12], which again included a recommendation for clinicians to employ SDM as the preferred approach to addressing the LCS opportunity with potentially eligible patients. Subsequently, CMS initiated a coverage analysis that led to a revised determination that retained the SDM requirement for LCS reimbursement, but relaxed requirements on who could deliver the SDM consultation and also modified the required content to be covered in the consultation [13]. The required content now includes (1) determination of beneficiary eligibility, (2) SDM using a decision aid, (3) counseling on the importance of adherence, impact of comorbidities, and/or ability/willingness to undergo treatment, and (4) counseling on the importance of smoking cessation or sustained abstinence.

To summarize, LCS has been consistently recommended by professional guidelines and by the USPSTF since 2013 and by CMS since 2015, and virtually all guidelines have recommended or required the use of SDM to support clinician and candidate consideration of the LCS opportunity. However, few of these guidelines have specifically defined best practices for how to implement SDM into clinical workflows. Despite recommendations and mandates, data have unfortunately shown a combination of limited implementation of SDM [14] and poor quality implementation when attempted [15].

What Is Shared Decision Making?

As defined by Elwyn and colleagues, SDM refers to "…an approach where clinicians and patients share the best available evidence when faced with the task of making decisions, and where patients are supported to consider options, to achieve informed preferences" [16]. Beyond the fundamental principle of respecting the autonomy of individuals to make decisions regarding their own health, what does SDM seek to achieve? One way to think of this is that in a SDM process, the goal is for patients to reflect on the best available evidence in light of their own personal values, preferences, and health goals—thus, some have also termed SDM as a "meeting of two experts"—where the patient is an expert in their own values, preferences, and goals, and the clinician is the expert in the data regarding the benefits and risks of the intervention. In the LCS context, an additional goal would be to enhance engagement and personal commitment to achieving an informed choice, and, for those who choose to screen, participation in the full screening algorithm (i.e., initial screening, diagnostic follow-up, and repeat screening). The fundamental value proposition of LCS, as demonstrated in the literature (e.g., NLST, the NELSON Trial, etc.) [4, 10], is that to achieve the individual and population health benefits offered by LCS, adherence to the screening algorithm is essential.

Studies have demonstrated that SDM can play a central role—helping screening candidates develop a thorough understanding of the LCS opportunity (e.g., potential benefits, potential harms, and unknowns) and make an informed choice that is consistent with their values, preferences, and health goals [17, 18], and is built on a foundation of commitment to the algorithm of screening that will give them the best chance of benefitting from periodic LCS. A recent report demonstrated that Medicare beneficiaries who have an SDM consultation documented via billing records are more likely to be adherent to repeat screening in comparison to those individuals who don't have a documented SDM consultation [19]. Recognizing both the benefits and challenges of implementing SDM for LCS, the American Thoracic Society and the U.S. Department of Veterans Affairs have developed stakeholder research priorities to identify best practices, prioritize research questions, and select preferred outcomes for this line of inquiry.

Shared Decision-Making Frameworks

There are several available SDM frameworks to help guide skill-building for clinicians and SDM implementation in clinical and community settings to support optimal decision making in the context of complex medical decisions [20, 21]. While each framework may integrate variations around the SDM process, two of the key principles relevant to all models include the notion described above that any SDM consultation includes two experts—the *clinician expert*, who is the authority on the potential risks and benefits for the choices under consideration, and the *patient expert*, who is the authority on their personal beliefs, values, and preferences that need to be integrated into the decision-making process. The second key principle recognizes that the SDM consultation is a collaborative process. Responsibility and power are shared by the participants in a conversation that takes place in the context of the clinician–patient relationship, one that is focused on delivering patient-centered care with respect for patient autonomy in decisions that will impact their health [22].

To support the implementation of SDM in the LCS context, two common models of SDM are briefly presented. First, developed by the Agency for Healthcare Research and Quality, the SHARE approach offers a five-step process from *Seek* (S) to *Evaluation (E)* [21]. Second, the Elwyn Model proposes three key phases of SDM, including choice talk, option talk, and decision talk, simplifying the process of achieving SDM [20].

The SHARE Approach The SHARE Approach to SDM includes five steps, representing each letter in the SHARE acronym [21]. The portal on the Agency for Healthcare Research and Quality (AHRQ) website provides a set of training modules, support materials, and other resources to facilitate implementation. Within this approach to SDM, clinicians first *Seek* the participant's active participation in the specific decision through an invitation to consider the option under consideration and a clear description of the choice to be made. Next, the clinician *Helps* the individual explore and compare each of the available options by reviewing the potential benefits, harms, and unknowns associated with each. Third, the clinician *Assesses* the individual's values and preferences by eliciting them through discussion and connecting them with the choice under consideration. In the fourth step, the clinician collaborates with the individual to *Reach* a decision and develop a plan of action. While many SDM approaches may stop at that point, the SHARE Approach adds a final step, *Evaluation*, that emphasizes the importance of evaluating the individual's decision, including the process and the outcomes from the decision, whether the plan was implemented or not, and sorting through any challenges that may have altered the plan. This SHARE approach outlines a step-by-step process that clinicians can use to implement SDM into their clinical practice, including SDM about LCS. The model has been integrated into primary clinician training regarding LCS with favorable preliminary outcomes [23].

Elwyn Talk Model Elwyn and colleagues have introduced a model of SDM implementation that highlights three essential steps [20]. The model emphasizes three types of discussion that should occur within the clinician–patient exchange to fulfill the principles of SDM. The first step involves *choice talk*, which introduces the choice to be discussed and considered, including the range of available options. The second step covers *option talk*, and it involves a description of the available options, including potential benefits, harms, and unknowns about each option. This component may integrate the use of a decision aid to support the accurate and efficient delivery of information about each option. The final step, *decision talk*, aims to elicit patient values and integrate them with the evidence to achieve an informed preference. Ideally, reaching an informed preference is followed by planning a course of action, which may include the choice to defer definitive action.

The fundamental elements of these two models are quite similar and capture the principles and spirit of SDM. Early data from primary care clinicians suggest that they support the principles of SDM as it applies to LCS. However, neither model is very informative about how to elicit patient values nor to clarify patient preference. Rather they assume an implicit understanding of candidate values and beliefs [24].

To facilitate the full collaborative process, ensuring all elements of the SDM process are addressed, patient decision aids (PtDAs) may be used. Although many different types of PtDAs have been developed, tools that are used directly in the clinician–patient visit are called encounter or consultation-style PtDAs. Also called decision support tools, PtDAs are designed to facilitate the efficient, accurate, and unbiased presentation of options and support consideration of personal values, beliefs, and preferences into the decision-making process.

Decision Aids or Decision Support Tools

Consistent with guidance to support the implementation of SDM as a key element of the LCS trajectory, PtDAs have been recommended or required [6, 13] as tools to facilitate high-quality SDM that can help clinicians and candidates/participants navigate the screening decision. As defined by the International Patient Decision Aid Standards (IPDAS) Collaboration, "Patient decision aids are tools designed to help people participate in decision making about healthcare options. They provide information on the options and help candidates clarify and communicate the personal value they associate with different features of the options" [25].

It is important to recognize what decision aids are not—they are not designed to advise, persuade, or direct individuals to a certain choice. Rather they are tools that invite participants to play an active role in managing their care, by clearly articulating the choice to be made, carefully presenting available evidence regarding available options, supporting elicitation of patient values and clarification of personal preference related to the decision, and helping the clinician and participant arrive at an optimal choice.

Updated most recently in 2017, a series of systematic literature reviews conducted as part of the Cochrane Collaboration have consistently identified a number of reliable benefits of implementing PtDAs for use in health decision making [26]. Specifically, the use of PtDAs improves patient understanding of attributes related to the choices to be made (e.g., increased knowledge, accuracy of risk perceptions, and congruence between values and choices) and a high-quality decision-making process (e.g., reduced decisional conflict, elicitation of personal values and preference, and increased active engagement in decision making). In addition, using PtDAs is associated with improvements in clinician–patient communication, preparation for action, and decision satisfaction [26].

Implementing SDM as a central component of the LCS process has received nearly universal support from all authoritative organizations and has even been mandated in the process of screening Medicare beneficiaries. In tandem with this support and based on substantial historical evidence, there has been an encouragement to integrate PtDAs to help structure the LCS dialogue between clinicians and candidates/participants. Yet, data evaluating application of SDM for LCS has identified a range of implementation barriers and threats to realizing the value of SDM [15, 27].

Challenges to Implementing Shared Decision Making in the Lung Cancer Screening Context

The established literature regarding barriers to implementing SDM in broader clinical settings identifies three principal challenges to provider performance: (1) perceived time constraints (additional time burden), (2) perceived relevance to patients, and (3) concerns regarding the value of SDM in the specific context [28]. Conversely, the literature has also demonstrated that clinician motivation, and the perceived favorable impact on clinical processes and patient outcomes constitute the three primary facilitators of implementing SDM [29]. In addition to these constraints and supports, there are important challenges, including a lack of training and skill development in this new application of SDM [30, 31], and deeply embedded negative sociocultural perspectives related to lung cancer and persons who smoke (e.g., nihilism and fatalism) [32].

Time Burden/Constraints As with implementing SDM generally [28], the time burden for clinicians stands as one of the most commonly sited challenges to integrating SDM into the LCS process [7, 33]. Given the responsibility for encouraging preventive healthcare that is embraced by primary care clinicians, adding any time to the patient consultation constitutes a significant challenge. The broader literature suggests that integrating SDM using PtDAs may extend clinic visits by 2.5 min on average [34], but objective data regarding the extended time burden of SDM for LCS remains scarce. One study showed no difference between usual care and implementation of a PtDA [35], but additional data are needed to build efficient and effective workflows and processes. Furthermore, the perceived time burden [7] related to SDM and the need to address SDM in the context of the cultural stigma and nihilism associated with lung cancer need to be addressed [32]. As with the implementation of any new evidence-based practice, growing pains are inevitable. However, progress is being made in the development of efficient, person-centered care approaches that utilize technology as well as build relationships to support the quality implementation of SDM and LCS.

Skills/Training Another threat to optimally implementing SDM, many clinicians lack appropriate LCS knowledge [36–38] and do not have sufficient skills to engage patients in SDM and to integrate SDM in routine practice [31]. Overestimating provider knowledge of LCS and overstating SDM skills have the combined functional effect of missing the opportunities to learn about LCS and pursue training in SDM. Novel approaches to circumnavigate this challenge are needed.

SDM Misunderstanding An interesting challenge to implementing SDM in LCS is that there is a widespread belief that clinicians are already doing SDM and that training is not needed [39]. Compelling data presented by Brenner and colleagues provides important insights into the reality of SDM performance in clinical care related to LCS [15]. In this study, investigators reviewed transcribed consultations between a clinician and an LCS candidate. Using a rigorous coding algorithm, the data showed that none of the consultations met the minimum criteria for SDM, and the overall mean SDM score was 6 on a scale of 0–100 for the essential elements of SDM. It is not clear if clinicians would have indicated that they were conducting SDM in these consultations, yet, it was very clear that SDM was not being conducted as required or recommended in these consultations. Furthermore, there was no evidence of PtDA use.

Lack of Patient Decision Aids (PtDAs) When CMS initially adopted the SDM requirement for reimbursement of LCS services, it may have been premature to require utilization of decision tools [7]. While a robust literature has developed supporting the utility of PtDAs to improve a range of important outcomes [26], no LCS-focused tools were available at the time the policy was adopted. Since that time, there has been substantial development of decision preparation aids and consultation-style decision support tools to facilitate SDM for LCS [40, 41], but implementation remains suboptimal [42] despite the potential of these tools to help clinicians and candidates achieve a structured, efficient, and collaborative consideration of LCS.

Inadequate Staff and Technology Support In addition to a lack of clinician education and training regarding SDM for LCS, additional clinical staff also have limited experience and knowledge to facilitate high-quality LCS and SDM [7]. Some clinical settings have reported challenges or resistance to developing new workflows that integrate LCS and SDM [33]. Similarly, technological platforms have been slow to adapt to the new clinical service pathways, creating challenges to identifying potential screening candidates and delivering efficient SDM procedures in the primary care setting [43].

Incompatibility with Clinical Practice Guidelines In the broader SDM literature, there has been concern that SDM can be in conflict with clinical practice guidelines that dictate strong recommendations for patient behavior [39]. This concern has also been raised in the LCS context, suggesting that SDM is unnecessary given the strengths of the evidence supporting LCS [44], but this concern is commonly based on a misunderstanding of SDM and lack of familiarity with the extensive data reported in the literature that support the short-term and long-term benefits of SDM. Furthermore, patients have reported favorable responses to SDM and the use of PtDAs, expressing a preference for more information and more communication and involvement in the decision-making process [45].

Combining the anticipated complexity of a new evidence-based cancer screening, the novel SDM mandate adopted by CMS, and the unique aspects of populations and communities that will be served by LCS, it is in many ways understandable that implementation of SDM for LCS has faced a slow start. However, when reflecting on the quality of the data supporting LCS and the consistent policies recommending and/or mandating SDM as a vital component of the LCS process, we realize that there is an urgent need to expedite the implementation. Without such efforts to accelerate implementation, we will continue to fall far short of realizing the full individual and population health benefits of LCS. Identifying effective and innovative approaches to facilitating the adoption and implementation of sustainable high-quality SDM have been underway and will play a central role in reducing lung cancer death through early detection.

Supporting Implementation of Shared Decision Making in the Lung Cancer Screening Context

To support quality implementation of SDM, a number of approaches and materials have been developed to achieve optimal SDM and LCS outcomes. These approaches include a combination of implementation strategies [46] that improve how SDM is delivered and may be considered as ways to "package" the core components of SDM into discrete decision coaching and counseling approaches [4]. Packages of core SDM components are ways to operationalize discrete decision coaching and counseling approaches, such as the Share model or the Elwyn 3-step model, in terms of the PtDAs and other decision support tools that can guide clinicians and patients through the SDM process.

Some key implementation strategies for delivering these packages of SDM core components include: (1) training and skill development, (2) expanding the clinical staff roles trained to deliver SDM, and (3) expanding the modes/ways that SDM may be delivered to promote better overall uptake by patients, as well as improving the equitable reach to patients. Some ways to improve overall reach as well as equitable reach include the use of telehealth delivery methods to deliver the core SDM components with attention to the literacy levels and visuals used in patient decision aids (PtDAs). Fundamentally, each of these approaches seeks to expand the high-quality implementation of SDM for LCS that considers efficiency and appropriateness in ways that support clinician and candidate consideration of LCS.

Training and Skill Development One of the most substantial barriers to integrating high-quality SDM in any clinical setting involves a lack of appropriate training and skill development, including both the necessary knowledge regarding the key principles and research on LCS but also the development of the skills to elicit patient values and clarify preferences [31]. Légaré has led international efforts to train a broad array of clinicians in SDM and has identified core competencies, including listening skills, language skills, nonverbal skills, contextual appropriateness, and attitudinal skills [47]. Unfortunately, outcomes data related to SDM skills training is limited and has not substantially improved outcomes according to a Cochrane Review [48]. Despite the limited literature, there is a persistent need to expand clinical training in LCS and SDM to support implementation and expedite the realization of the benefits of LDCT.

Recognizing the acute need for SDM training for clinicians regarding the LCS context, Myers and colleagues collaborated with the American College of Chest Physicians (ACCP) to develop a brief, no-cost, accredited online training program to help clinicians learn the principles and practices of SDM. Importantly, the 45–60 minute training program integrates key contextual factors related to LCS [49]. The program integrates content regarding LCS eligibility criteria, documentation requirements, LCS benefits and harms, brief efforts to address tobacco treatment, SDM steps, examples of candidate motivations to screen/not screen, and support for helping candidates make high-quality choices. Built by a transdisciplinary team, early testing and feedback of the program have been favorable, and broader evaluation efforts are ongoing. However, additional training efforts using diverse platforms (e.g., in-person, online, integrated into graduate medical education) remain necessary to facilitate broader implementation of SDM, particularly regarding LCS. Other training resources developed by our team and others include online training with prompts to develop a clinical workflow for a specific clinic, and other implementation resources like PtDAs.

Expanding Clinician Delivery Options The initial CMS criteria required that licensed clinicians (e.g., physicians, advanced practice nurses, or physician assistants) conduct SDM and perform the patient counseling session [6], potentially constraining delivery options and hampering efficiency. There does not appear to be sufficient data showing the superiority of licensed clinician delivery of SDM or the use of decision aids. Furthermore, observational data suggest that busy clinicians may not be able to allocate sufficient effort to engage patients in high-quality SDM [15]. Thus, the most recent CMS coverage statement has withdrawn the requirement that SDM be delivered by a licensed clinician, creating a wider range training and implementation options. However, while this flexibility permits broader implementation, SDM consultation provided by non-licensed clinicians may not be reimbursable or reimbursable at a lower rate. Hoffman and colleagues [7] have advocated for the use of trained decision coaches in LCS based on data collected in other settings [50]. Other research has successfully explored the use of patient navigators or community health workers to conduct engagement activities and SDM to expand delivery options [51, 52].

Decision Coaching and Counseling Decision coaching involves a decision counselor or coach that offers a "…individualized, nondirective facilitation of patient preparation for shared decision making" [50]. The approach commonly seeks to prepare candidates/participants to finalize their healthcare choice with the responsible clinician but offers a more efficient and less time-constrained delivery of information, elicitation of values and preferences, and supports readiness to make the choice in question. This approach combined with telehealth or the use of PtDAs can fulfill the SDM consultation requirement but may not be reimbursable in certain situations.

Decision counseling commonly employs a trained clinician, whose credentials would not meet the licensure requirements as a physician, advanced practice nurse, or physician assistant, but would have ample training in SDM and LCS to communicate appropriate information about LCS, elicit personal values, beliefs, and preferences, and integrate those sources of information into an informed choice about becoming engaged in screening. While decision counseling may not be reimbursable by some health insurers, it offers a unique and efficient opportunity to achieve an informed choice for screening candidates and build engagement with the LCS program for those who chose to pursue screening.

Lowenstein and colleagues conducted a cohort comparison study examining outcomes comparing a decision coaching intervention with a decision aid against a standard of care condition [35]. Results showed that candidates reported greater LCS knowledge and a better SDM process in the decision coaching cohort than in the usual care condition. Additionally, the decision coaching intervention did not increase visit time, and decision coaches fulfilled the CMS-required elements of SDM in nearly all consultations. Fagan and colleagues have also demonstrated the utility of a decision counseling approach to achieving high-quality SDM and enhanced uptake of LCS, providing additional support for the feasibility and effectiveness of decision coaching and counseling in real-world settings [53]. These data support the feasibility and potential efficacy of the decision coaching approach, and additional research is warranted to explore the potential of this approach to implementing SDM without expanding consultation time.

Patient Decision Aids/Decision Support Tools Patient decision aids (PtDAs) constitute one of the fundamental approaches to supporting participant engagement by facilitating a structured conversation about the LCS opportunity. As noted previously, PtDAs provide support to achieve a structured conversation between two experts, a clinician expert, and a patient expert, that enhances the likelihood of a quality decision process and a quality decision. Systematic literature reviews have consistently demonstrated a broad range of benefits associated with the implementation of PtDAs [34]. There have been substantial efforts to develop tools to support LCS consideration in advance of meeting with a clinician, including video-based approaches [54, 55] and web-based approaches [56, 57].

While these approaches have demonstrated feasibility and efficacy in helping prepare individuals for an SDM consultation, encounter-style PtDAs are meant to be used during the consultation and play a more proximal role in supporting SDM for LCS. Led by Volk and colleagues as part of the Eisenberg Center for Clinical

Decisions and Communications Science, AHRQ has developed a suite of tools to support SDM regarding LCS, including a robust encounter PtDA, "A Decisionmaking Tool for You and Your Health Care Professional" [58]. Additional encounter tools have been developed and evaluated [59], but there is a need for more tools that target specific communities and take additional factors (e.g., health literacy, unique backgrounds) into consideration [60].

Fukunaga and colleagues reported an early systematic review of tools to promote SDM for LCS that reviewed a relatively modest set of instruments. The review concluded that the tools improved knowledge, reduced decisional conflict, and were acceptable to both clinicians and candidates/participants [40]. More recently, Jallow and colleagues have reported a scoping review examining the content and presentation styles used in LCS PtDAs [41], concluding that there was notable heterogeneity in content coverage and design. The authors suggested efforts to achieve greater consistency and the application of consensus guidelines regarding PtDA design.

Specifically, PtDAs create a unique opportunity to guarantee coverage of all the essential points outlined regarding the LCS opportunity, consistent with the initial CMS guidelines [6]. While CMS no longer mandates specific content regarding potential benefits and harms, to achieve a quality decision within the SDM framework, PtDAs should continue to include several essential elements. These elements include: (1) a clear description of the LCS opportunity and process and an invitation to engage the decision, (2) the potential benefits, the potential harms, and the unknowns of each screening option (i.e., only LDCT), (3) the importance of adherence and tobacco cessation services, if appropriate, and (4) a form of values elicitation and preference elicitation that allows candidates to align the information with their individual perspectives, values, and health goals in order to achieve an optimal decision and plan.

Telehealth Delivery Patient counseling and SDM (procedural code G0296) were not initially allowed for use in billing for services delivered via telehealth [6]. However, in 2018 CMS added G0296 to the list of telehealth services that could be delivered by a licensed clinician and reimbursed. CMS further expanded support for telehealth delivery of G0296 and many other services to help address challenges presented by the SARS-COV2 pandemic that emerged in 2020. Importantly, telehealth does not require an in-person visit in advance of the LDCT scan, can focus attention on individuals who are eligible for screening, and can minimize transportation costs.

Clinician–researchers have recently explored the use of telehealth delivery of the patient counseling and SDM session using a decision aid, comparing it against the face-to-face visiting using the same decision aid [61]. Results were comparable across setting on outcomes related to screening uptake, decision satisfaction, and decisional conflict. All outcomes were favorable for both groups, including 88% uptake, very high levels of decision satisfaction, and minimal residual decisional conflict post-intervention [61]. These results provide early support for the use of telephone-delivered SDM for LCS and open the door for other platforms (e.g., secure Zoom or MS Teams) approaches to conducting SDM and reducing access barriers and clinical burden.

Supporting Health Equity In addition to respecting patient autonomy, implementing SDM has been proposed as a key strategy to reduce health inequity [7, 60, 62], and systematic reviews of the SDM literature have supported the value of SDM in supporting socially disadvantaged populations [63, 64]. One of the motivating factors for expanding the eligibility criteria for LCS was to address the burden of lung cancer that emerges earlier and with less tobacco exposure in underserved communities. The warranted historical mistrust of healthcare by individuals among underserved communities (including individuals with diverse racial and ethnic backgrounds, individuals who reside in rural areas, those who are facing socioeconomic challenges, or other vulnerable communities that are likely to experience challenges to engaging high-quality healthcare (e.g., LGBTQIA+, seriously mentally ill)) undoubtedly impedes the process of making LCS widely available.

As SDM for LCS respects individual autonomy and supports person-centered care principles, implementing LCS may help build and restore trusting relationships [65] that can not only enhance opportunities for initiating LCS but also sustaining adherence to the LCS algorithm that will help tilt the benefit-risk equation toward benefit. It is important to consider factors that may improve the equitable reach to patients as part of the implementation planning process, including the use of PtDAs designed with ample consideration of health literacy and numeracy, use of appropriate imagery, and cultural adaptations appropriate for unique communities.

Conclusions

While there have been notable challenges to implementing SDM in the LCS context (as well as challenges to implementing a host of other aspects of high-quality LCS) [66], there have been substantial efforts to develop tools and approaches to overcome these challenges. Ongoing and expanding development and research efforts continue to design and revise more effective tools and approaches to continue to support quality decision making and LCS implementation. While the pace of translation from the clinical trials and supportive policy stances to community uptake remains slow, it is vital to sustain person-centered efforts like SDM to build trust with at-risk persons, populations, and communities that often operate at the fringes of the healthcare system. Changing this situation will require substantial targeted and compassionate efforts to support uptake and adherence to achieve the promise offered by LCS. It is essential that the next phase of efforts to implement high-quality SDM and LCS begin with a fundamental understanding of the community to be served and their unique and sometimes complicated relationships that exist with and within healthcare systems. By placing the people to be served at the center of the process, we will have a better chance to reduce the burdens associated with lung cancer morbidity and mortality.

References

1. Moyer VA. US Preventive Services Task Force. Screening for lung cancer: U.S. Preventive Services Task Force recommendation statement. Ann Intern Med. 2014;160(5):330–8.
2. Sheridan SL, Harris RP, Woolf SH, Shared Decision-Making Workgroup of the U.S. Preventive Services Task Force. Shared decision making about screening and chemoprevention. A suggested approach from the U.S. Preventive Services Task Force. Am J Prev Med. 2004;26(1):56–66.
3. Davidson KW, Mangione CM, Barry MJ, Nicholson WK, Cabana MD, Caughey AB, et al. Collaboration and shared decisionmaking between patients and clinicians in preventive health care decisions and US preventive services task Force recommendations. JAMA. 2022;327(12):1171–6.
4. Aberle DR, Adams AM, Berg CD, Black WC, Clapp JD, Fagerstrom RM, et al. Reduced lung-cancer mortality with low-dose computed tomographic screening. N Engl J Med. 2011;365(5):395–409.
5. Centers for Medicare & Medicaid Services. National coverage determination (NCD) for lung cancer screening with low dose computed tomography (LDCT (210.14). 2015.
6. Centers for Medicare & Medicaid Services. Decision memo for screening for lung cancer with low dose computed tomography (LDCT) (cag-00439n). 2015.
7. Hoffman RM, Reuland DS, Volk RJ. The centers for Medicare & Medicaid services requirement for shared decision-making for lung cancer screening. JAMA. 2021;325(10):933–4.
8. Merchant FM, Dickert NW, Howard DH. Mandatory shared decision making by the centers for Medicare & Medicaid services for cardiovascular procedures and other tests. JAMA. 2018;320(7):641–2.
9. Knoepke CE, Allen LA, Kramer DB, Matlock DD. Medicare mandates for shared decision making in cardiovascular device placement. Circ Cardiovasc Qual Outcomes. 2019;12(7):e004899.
10. de Koning HJ, van der Aalst CM, de Jong PA, Scholten ET, Nackaerts K, Heuvelmans MA, et al. Reduced lung-cancer mortality with volume CT screening in a randomized trial. N Engl J Med. 2020;382(6):503–13.
11. Pastorino U, Sverzellati N, Sestini S, Silva M, Sabia F, Boeri M, et al. Ten-year results of the multicentric Italian lung detection trial demonstrate the safety and efficacy of biennial lung cancer screening. Eur J Cancer. 2019;118:142–8.
12. Krist AH, Davidson KW, Mangione CM, Barry MJ, Cabana M, Caughey AB, et al. Screening for lung cancer: US preventive services task force recommendation statement. JAMA. 2021;325(10):962–70.
13. Centers for Medicare & Medicaid Services. Decision memo for screening for lung cancer with low dose computed tomography (LDCT) (CAG-00439R). 2022.
14. Goodwin JS, Nishi S, Zhou J, Kuo YF. Use of the shared decision-making visit for lung cancer screening among Medicare enrollees. JAMA Intern Med. 2019;179(5):716–8.
15. Brenner AT, Malo TL, Margolis M, Elston Lafata J, James S, Vu MB, et al. Evaluating shared decision making for lung cancer screening. JAMA Intern Med. 2018;178(10):1311–6.
16. Elwyn G, Laitner S, Coulter A, Walker E, Watson P, Thomson R. Implementing shared decision making in the NHS. BMJ. 2010;341:c5146.
17. Tan NQP, Nishi SPE, Lowenstein LM, Mendoza TR, Lopez-Olivo MA, Crocker LC, et al. Impact of the shared decision-making process on lung cancer screening decisions. Cancer Med. 2022;11(3):790–7.
18. Mazzone PJ, Tenenbaum A, Seeley M, Petersen H, Lyon C, Han X, et al. Impact of a lung cancer screening counseling and shared decision-making visit. Chest. 2017;151(3):572–8.
19. Hirsch EA, Studts JL. Significance of a shared decision-making consultation on lung cancer screening efficacy. American society of preventive oncology 46th annual conference, Tucson, AZ; 2022.
20. Elwyn G, Frosch D, Thomson R, Joseph-Williams N, Lloyd A, Kinnersley P, et al. Shared decision making: a model for clinical practice. J Gen Intern Med. 2012;27:1361–7.

21. Agency for Healthcare Quality and Research. The SHARE approach, Rockville, MD; 2020.
22. Barry MJ, Edgman-Levitan S. Shared decision making--pinnacle of patient-centered care. N Engl J Med. 2012;366(9):780–1.
23. Mejia MG, Hinchey MC, Byrne MM, Han P, Studts JL. Lung cancer screening: evaluation of a pilot continuing education program for primary care providers. 35th annual meeting and scientific sessions of the society of behavioral medicine, Philadelphia, PA; 2014.
24. Melzer AC, Golden SE, Ono SS, Datta S, Crothers K, Slatore CG. What exactly is shared decision-making? A qualitative study of shared decision-making in lung cancer screening. J Gen Intern Med. 2020;35(2):546–53.
25. International Patient Decision Aid Standards (IPDAS) Collaboration. What are patient decision aids? 2017. Available from: http://ipdas.ohri.ca/what.html.
26. Stacey D, Légaré F, Lewis K, Barry MJ, Bennett CL, Eden KB, et al. Decision aids for people facing health treatment or screening decisions. Cochrane Database Syst Rev. 2017;4:CD001431.
27. Kinsinger LS, Anderson C, Kim J, Larson M, Chan SH, King HA, et al. Implementation of lung cancer screening in the veterans health administration. JAMA Intern Med. 2017;177(3):399.
28. Légaré F, Ratté S, Gravel K, Graham ID. Barriers and facilitators to implementing shared decision-making in clinical practice: update of a systematic review of health professionals' perceptions. Patient Educ Couns. 2008;73(3):526–35.
29. Légaré F, Witteman HO. Shared decision making: examining key elements and barriers to adoption into routine clinical practice. Health Aff (Millwood). 2013;32(2):276–84.
30. Myers RE. Health organizations have an opportunity to improve shared decision-making and raise lung cancer screening rates. Chest. 2021;159(1):23–4.
31. Alishahi Tabriz A, Neslund-Dudas C, Turner K, Rivera MP, Reuland DS, Elston Lafata J. How health-care organizations implement shared decision-making when it is required for reimbursement: the case of lung cancer screening. Chest. 2021;159(1):413–25.
32. Hamann HA, Ver Hoeve ES, Carter-Harris L, Studts JL, Ostroff JS. Multilevel opportunities to address lung cancer stigma across the cancer control continuum. J Thorac Oncol. 2018;13:1062–75.
33. Allen CG, Cotter MM, Smith RA, Watson L. Successes and challenges of implementing a lung cancer screening program in federally qualified health centers: a qualitative analysis using the consolidated framework for implementation research. Transl Behav Med. 2021;11(5):1088–98.
34. Stacey D, Légaré F, Lewis K, Barry MJ, Bennett CL, Eden KB, et al. Decision aids for people facing health treatment or screening decisions. Cochrane Database Syst Rev. 2017;2017(4):CD001431.
35. Lowenstein LM, Godoy MCB, Erasmus JJ, Zirari Z, Bennett A, Leal VB, et al. Implementing decision coaching for lung cancer screening in the low-dose computed tomography setting. JCO Oncol Pract. 2020;16(8):e703–e25.
36. Kanodra NM, Pope C, Halbert CH, Silvestri GA, Rice LJ, Tanner NT. Primary care provider and patient perspectives on lung cancer screening. A qualitative study. Ann Am Thorac Soc. 2016;13(11):1977–82.
37. Raz DJ, Wu GX, Consunji M, Nelson RA, Kim H, Sun CL, et al. The effect of primary care physician knowledge of lung cancer screening guidelines on perceptions and utilization of low-dose computed tomography. Clin Lung Cancer. 2018;19(1):51–7.
38. Raz DJ, Wu GX, Consunji M, Nelson R, Sun C, Erhunmwunsee L, et al. Perceptions and utilization of lung cancer screening among primary care physicians. J Thorac Oncol. 2016;11(11):1856–62.
39. Légaré F, Thompson-Leduc P. Twelve myths about shared decision making. Patient Educ Couns. 2014;96(3):281–6.
40. Fukunaga MI, Halligan K, Kodela J, Toomey S, Furtado VF, Luckmann R, et al. Tools to promote shared decision-making in lung cancer screening using low-dose CT scanning: a systematic review. Chest. 2020;158(6):2646–57.
41. Jallow M, Bonfield S, Kurtidu C, Baldwin DR, Black G, Brain KE, et al. Decision support tools for low-dose CT scan lung cancer screening: a scoping review of information content, format, and presentation methods. Chest. 2021;162:930.

42. Lopez-Olivo MA, Minnix JA, Fox JG, Nishi SPE, Lowenstein LM, Maki KG, et al. Smoking cessation and shared decision-making practices about lung cancer screening among primary care providers. Cancer Med. 2021;10(4):1357–65.
43. Brenner AT, Cubillos L, Birchard K, Doyle-Burr C, Eick J, Henderson L, et al. Improving the implementation of lung cancer screening guidelines at an academic primary care practice. J Healthc Qual. 2018;40(1):27–35.
44. Mulshine JL, Yankelevitz DF, Pyenson B. Concerns related to benefits and harms of real-world shared decision-making for lung cancer screening. American Health & Drug Benefits. 2021. https://www.ahdbonline.com/issues/2021/september-2021/3148-concerns-related-to-benefits-and-harms-of-real-world-shared-decision-making-for-lung-cancer-screening.
45. Crothers K, Kross EK, Reisch LM, Shahrir S, Slatore C, Zeliadt SB, et al. Patients' attitudes regarding lung cancer screening and decision aids. A survey and focus group study. Ann Am Thorac Soc. 2016;13(11):1992–2001.
46. Powell BJ, Waltz TJ, Chinman MJ, Damschroder LJ, Smith JL, Matthieu MM, et al. A refined compilation of implementation strategies: results from the Expert Recommendations for Implementing Change (ERIC) project. Implement Sci. 2015;10(1):21.
47. Légaré F, Moumjid-Ferdjaoui N, Drolet R, Stacey D, Härter M, Bastian H, et al. Core competencies for shared decision making training programs: insights from an international, interdisciplinary working group. J Contin Educ Heal Prof. 2013;33(4):267–73.
48. Légaré F, Adekpedjou R, Stacey D, Turcotte S, Kryworuchko J, Graham ID, et al. Interventions for increasing the use of shared decision making by healthcare professionals. Cochrane Database Syst Rev. 2018;2018(7):CD006732.
49. Myers RE, Volk RJ, Studts JL, Tanner N, Sederstrom N, Giamboy T, et al. Shared decision making in lung cancer screening. American College of Chest Physicians. 2021. Available from: https://www.chestnet.org/Store/Products/Standard-Products/eLearning/Shared-Decision-Making-in-Lung-Cancer-Screening.
50. Stacey D, Kryworuchko J, Bennett C, Murray MA, Mullan S, Légaré F. Decision coaching to prepare patients for making health decisions: a systematic review of decision coaching in trials of patient decision AIDS. Med Decis Mak. 2012;32(3):E22–33.
51. Williams LB, Shelton BJ, Gomez ML, Al-Mrayat YD, Studts JL. Using implementation science to disseminate a lung cancer screening education intervention through community health workers. J Community Health. 2020;46:165.
52. Percac-Lima S, Ashburner JM, Rigotti NA, Park ER, Chang Y, Kuchukhidze S, et al. Patient navigation for lung cancer screening among current smokers in community health centers a randomized controlled trial. Cancer Med. 2018;7(3):894–902.
53. Fagan HB, Fournakis NA, Jurkovitz C, Petrich AM, Zhang Z, Katurakes N, et al. Telephone-based shared decision-making for lung cancer screening in primary care. J Cancer Educ. 2020;35(4):766–73.
54. Volk RJ, Lowenstein LM, Leal VB, Escoto KH, Cantor SB, Munden RF, et al. Effect of a patient decision aid on lung cancer screening decision-making by persons who smoke: a randomized clinical trial. JAMA Netw Open. 2020;3(1):e1920362.
55. Reuland DS, Cubillos L, Brenner AT, Harris RP, Minish B, Pignone MP. A pre-post study testing a lung cancer screening decision aid in primary care. BMC Med Inform Decis Mak. 2018;18(1):5.
56. Carter-Harris L, Comer RS, Slaven Ii JE, Monahan PO, Vode E, Hanna NH, et al. Computer-tailored decision support tool for lung cancer screening: community-based pilot randomized controlled trial. J Med Internet Res. 2020;22(11):e17050.
57. Studts JL, Thurer RJ, Brinker K, Lillie SE, Byrne MM. Brief education and a conjoint valuation survey may reduce decisional conflict regarding lung cancer screening. MDM Policy Pract. 2020;5(1):2381468319891452.
58. Agency for Healthcare Research and Quality. Overview: is lung cancer screening right for me? Rockville, MD: Effective Health Care Program, Agency for Healthcare Research and Quality; 2016.

59. Ito Fukunaga M, Balwan A, Janis JA, Gutheil C, Yahwak J, Han PKJ. Pilot study of an encounter decision aid for lung cancer screening. J Cancer Educ. 2021;37:1161.
60. Haddad DN, Sandler KL, Henderson LM, Rivera MP, Aldrich MC. Disparities in lung cancer screening: a review. Ann Am Thorac Soc. 2020;17(4):399–405.
61. Tanner NT, Banas E, Yeager D, Dai L, Hughes Halbert C, Silvestri GA. In-person and telephonic shared decision-making visits for people considering lung cancer screening: an assessment of decision quality. Chest. 2019;155(1):236–8.
62. Rivera MP, Katki HA, Tanner NT, Triplette M, Sakoda LC, Wiener RS, et al. Addressing disparities in lung cancer screening eligibility and healthcare access. an official American Thoracic Society statement. Am J Respir Crit Care Med. 2020;202(7):e95–e112.
63. Yen RW, Smith J, Engel J, Muscat DM, Smith SK, Mancini J, et al. A systematic review and meta-analysis of patient decision aids for socially disadvantaged populations: update from the International Patient Decision Aid Standards (IDPAS). Med Decis Mak. 2021;41(7):870–96.
64. Durand MA, Carpenter L, Dolan H, Bravo P, Mann M, Bunn F, et al. Do interventions designed to support shared decision-making reduce health inequalities? A systematic review and meta-analysis. PLoS One. 2014;9(4):e94670.
65. Golden SE, Ono SS, Thakurta SG, Wiener RS, Iaccarino JM, Melzer AC, et al. "I'm putting my trust in their hands": a qualitative study of patients' views on clinician initial communication about lung cancer screening. Chest. 2020;158(3):1260–7.
66. National Academies of Sciences Engineering, and Medicine, Health and Medicine Division, Board of Health Care Services, National Cancer Policy Forum. Implementation of lung cancer screening: proceedings of a workshop. 2016.

Chapter 12
Advances in Tobacco Treatment

Sung Whang

Smoking continues to be one of the most modifiable risk factors of morbidity and mortality. Despite decades of ongoing efforts in smoking cessation, tobacco products continue to be the leading cause of preventable death worldwide [1]. Cigarette smoke contains an estimated 70 different chemicals that are suspected human carcinogens and are responsible for half a million American deaths each year [2]. Deaths from tobacco smoke can be attributed to cancers and pulmonary disease for persons who smoke or have smoked, and among persons who have been exposed to secondhand smoke [2]. An estimated 70% of smokers visit a clinician each year, making each appointment an opportunity for the provider to assess tobacco use and potentially intervene. No matter how brief, advice given face-to-face about quitting has been shown to increase cessation rates [1]. The United States Public Health Service outlines the 5-As (ask, advise, assess, assist, and arrange) as a framework that guides a proactive approach to tobacco treatment, regardless of a smoker's readiness to quit [1]. Identifying patients who use tobacco, assessing readiness to quit, providing practical counseling and treatment options, and ensuring follow-up have been the mainstay in evidence-based tobacco treatment.

In contrast to tobacco treatment options in decades past, numerous advances have been made in effective smoking cessation interventions [1]. Tobacco treatment must be individualized according to the severity of nicotine dependence and likelihood of developing withdrawal symptoms, medical comorbidities or potential contraindications to pharmacotherapy, financial resources, compliance, and patient preference [3]. This approach and the use of combination therapies, both behavioral interventions and pharmacotherapy, provide optimal tobacco treatment. Behavioral interventions may be comprised of various platforms such as in-person meeting,

S. Whang (✉)
Division of Thoracic and Esophageal Surgery, Department of Surgery, Philadelphia, PA, USA
e-mail: Sung.Whang@Jefferson.edu

© The Author(s), under exclusive license to Springer Nature Switzerland AG 2023   117
G. C. Kane et al. (eds.), *Lung Cancer Screening*,
https://doi.org/10.1007/978-3-031-33596-9_12

support groups, and text messaging and are held by specialists who are certified in tobacco treatment [3].

Motivational interviewing has come to the fore, providing a more intense counseling intervention intended to increase motivation among persons who smoke and may not be interested in quitting, encourage agency over smoking behaviors, and assist in creating a plan or implementing techniques to control urges and triggers [3]. This approach uses techniques that include exploring personal feelings and discovering ambivalence regarding smoking. In this regard, motivational interviewing involves using *change talk* about smoking cessation and *commitment language* related to intentions to practice specific actions to change smoking-related behaviors [1]. Rather than lecturing a tobacco user, this approach encourages clinician to help patients use their own words to commit to change [1]. To strengthen future quit attempts during motivational interviewing, the clinician can address relevance, risk, rewards, roadblocks, and repetition [1].

Another counseling intervention shown to be effective is problem-solving and skills training. Using problem-solving in practical counseling may include: (1) recognizing potentially risky situations by identifying circumstances that increase the threat of smoking or relapse, (2) developing coping skills to manage those threats, and (3) providing information about the harms of smoking and the benefits of successful cessation. An additional element of practical counseling is a supportive treatment which includes encouraging cessation attempts, communicating concerns, and encouraging the patient to discuss quitting [1].

Nicotine is the primary addictive substance in tobacco products and sustains tobacco use [2]. When quitting, patients experience symptoms of nicotine withdrawal such as cravings, mood changes, insomnia, and increased appetite [4]. Nicotine replacement therapy (NRT) supplies a controlled amount of nicotine to help gradually wean the patient away from smoking with decreased withdrawal symptoms and without the additional harmful chemicals of tobacco products. Assessing nicotine dependence can determine smoking behavior and guide patient therapy.

The Cutting Down, Annoyance by Criticism, Guilty Feelings, and Eye Openers (CAGE) questionnaire is a tool clinicians can use for screening patients for addictive behaviors and has been modified for smoking behavior. As a simple acronym, CAGE is amended to four questions where two affirming responses constitute a positive screen [5]. CAGE can be broken down into feeling a need to *Control* or *Cut down*, getting *Annoyed* or *Angry* with criticism, feeling *Guilty*, and needing an *Eye-Opener* [5]. Similarly, the "Four Cs" Test, known to mental health clinicians, may also be applied to nicotine dependence—compulsion, control, cutting down, and consequences [5]. The Heaviness of Smoking Index is another simple and quick tool to determine the severity of nicotine dependence using two questions: (1) How many cigarettes do you smoke a day? and (2) How soon after waking up do you smoke your first cigarette? [3]. Finally, the Fagerstrom Test for Nicotine Dependence is a standard instrument used to determine the intensity of nicotine addiction and guide prescribing medications to alleviate nicotine withdrawal [5]. Although this tool may take longer to administer, it has proven to be an important reference in nicotine dependence and can help dictate NRT dosing and frequency [5].

The United States Food and Drug Administration (FDA) has approved seven first-line medications for tobacco treatment shown to be more effective in increasing the chances of cessation, and in recent years have largely been covered by most insurance companies [4]. When deciding on initial pharmaco-therapeutics, the choice will be determined by patient preference. Guidelines will recommend either varenicline or a nicotine replacement therapy (NRT) combination of two products, the nicotine patch and a short-acting nicotine product [3]. NRT is most effective when using the nicotine patch, delivering a basal dose of nicotine throughout the day, along with a more rapid-acting NRT as needed to relieve withdrawal symptoms [3]. NRT is used to replace nicotine in lieu of combustible tobacco products to aid in reducing urges and during trigger situations [3]. Fortunately, several NRT are commercially available over the counter without a need for prescription, including the long-acting transdermal patch and rapid-acting chewing gum or lozenges.

Additional short-acting NRT is available with a prescription, such as an oral inhaler as well as a nasal spray under the brand Nicotrol [4]. It is recommended NRT be used at least 8 weeks after smoking cessation or as needed during a high risk of relapse, however, there are no reported findings that are definitive in clarifying whether gradual or abrupt withdrawal is more favorable. NRT is generally well-tolerated. However, specific side effects typically pertain to the delivery method and may be mitigated by titrating doses or changing delivery methods. There are no clear contraindications to initiating NRT. Notably, long-term use of NRT has been deemed safe and not associated with harmful effects and the risk of dependence on NRT products is low [3].

Varenicline tartrate (brand name Chantix) and bupropion hydrochloride (brand names Zyban, Wellbutrin) are two FDA-approved oral prescription cessation medications that do not contain nicotine. Varenicline is a partial agonist on nicotinic receptors that mediate the release of dopamine, the neurotransmitter that perpetuates addiction, effectively reducing the rewarding effects of nicotine [3]. Because smokers enjoy cigarettes less on varenicline, some may even reduce their consumption prior to an established quit date. The partial agonist action helps to decrease the intensity of withdrawal symptoms as well [3]. Varenicline can begin when the person who smokes is currently smoking and chooses a flexible quit date within a month of beginning the medication or choosing to gradually reduce their amount of smoking before quitting completely. Varenicline can be used for up to 6 months to aid in continued abstinence [3]. In clinical trials, varenicline alone has proved more effective in promoting smoking cessation than the nicotine patch or bupropion and is comparable to combining multiple NRT modalities [2].

Bupropion and the nicotine patch have been found to be comparable to one another and performed significantly superior to placebo. Bupropion was initially marketed as an antidepressant, blocking the reuptake of dopamine and norepinephrine and allowing increased levels in the brain, effectively simulating the effects of nicotine. Bupropion additionally has antagonist activity on nicotinic receptors. It can be used alone as a second-line therapy after varenicline and combination NRT, or in combination with NRT which increases cessation rates than with either alone [2]. Bupropion can be used for as little as 12 weeks, however, continued use for a year has been shown to enhance abstinence rates [2]. General practices using pharmacotherapy are described in Table 12.1. However, prescribers are recommended to refer to specific manufacturers' recommendations far as dosing information, adverse effects, and contraindications.

Table 12.1 FDA-approved first-line pharmacotherapy for tobacco cessation

Drug	Dosing	Administration	Common side effects
Nicotine patch • 7 mg • 14 mg • 21 mg	• Less dependence start with nicotine patch 14 mg/day • High dependence start with nicotine patch 21 mg/day	Apply one patch to hairless, clean, dry skin for 24 h rotate the site daily to avoid skin irritation	• Skin irritation • Insomnia • Vivid dreams
Nicotine gum • 2 mg • 4 mg	• Less dependence, use 2 mg pieces • High dependence, use 4 mg pieces	"Chew and park": Chew until tingling sensations occurs, then "park" between gum and cheek until tingling disappears. Then chew again to repeat, parking in the opposite cheek. Chew one piece of gum whenever there is an urge to smoke. Use up to 24 pieces per day	• Mouth soreness • Oral irritation • GI irritation • Hiccups • Jaw pain • Excess salivation • Headache • Heart palpitations
Nicotine lozenge • 2 mg • 4 mg	• Less dependence, use 2 mg • High dependence, use 4 mg	Place lozenge in the mouth and allow to dissolve for 30 min. Maximum 20 lozenges per day	• Oral irritation • Mouth ulcers • Abdominal pain • Hiccups • Heartburn • Nausea/vomiting • Diarrhea • Headache • Palpitations
[a]Nicotine inhaler (10 mg/cartridge)	Puff into mouth as needed; use 6–16 cartridges per day. Each cartridge is about 20 min of continuous use	Puff into mouth to back of throat or in short breaths for mucosal absorption (not inhaling into chest). Maximum 16 cartridges per day	• Oral irritation • Throat irritation • Cough
[a]Nicotine nasal spray (10 mg/mL)	Use 1 spray in each nostril 1–2 times per hour	Maximum of 10 sprays per hour or 80 spray per day	• Nasal irritation • Throat irritation • Cough • Rhinitis • Headache
[a]Bupropion SR (sustained release) 150 mg	150 mg once daily for the first 3 days, then increase to 150 mg twice daily	Begin at least 1–2 weeks before target quit date	• Insomnia • Headache • Dizziness • Diaphoresis • Weight loss • Xerostomia • Nausea/vomiting

(continued)

Table 12.1 (continued)

Drug	Dosing	Administration	Common side effects
[a]Varenicline • Starting month pack • 0.5 mg • 1 mg	Starting month pack: Days 1–3: 0.5 mg once daily Days 4–7: 0.5 mg twice daily Day 8 and later: 1 mg twice daily	Treatment should be continued for at least 12 weeks; consider dose reduction if 1 mg doses twice daily is not tolerated	• Insomnia • Nausea/vomiting • Vivid dreams • Headache • Nasopharyngitis • Xerostomia

[a]Requires prescription

Earlier in the chapter, it was noted that pharmacotherapy should typically be based on patient preferences and, although few, contraindications need to be considered with patient comorbidities. Fortunately, recent studies have dispelled historical fears regarding particular adverse reactions. For example, large studies have found treatment with varenicline or bupropion did not increase neuropsychiatric adverse effects and now suggest the use of varenicline as more efficacious than NRT in patients with psychiatric illnesses [6]. Tobacco cessation medications have now been shown to probably be safe to use in patients in the setting of acute coronary syndrome [6]. Bupropion reduces seizure threshold and is still contraindicated in patients with seizure disorder [6].

With today's advances in tobacco treatment and control, the prevalence of current cigarette smokers has significantly declined and now there are more persons who formerly smoked than there are persons who currently smoke [7]. National use of the tobacco quitline 1–800-QUIT-NOW has made it possible for persons who smoke to access intensive interventions including counseling and pharmacotherapy more than ever [1]. Tobacco control measures have also been helpful in decreasing tobacco use including restrictions on advertising and sponsorship, increased prices, indoor smoke-free policies, warning labels, and additional government campaigns and community tobacco control programs have reduced the prevalence of tobacco use [7].

Although much progress has been made, disease and death attributed to tobacco use have remained a significant public health concern. Visions of a tobacco-free society have spurred additional strategies to complement ongoing efforts such as reducing nicotine content and even greater restrictions on sales for categories of tobacco products. For example, electronic cigarettes (e-cigarettes) have not been shown to be beneficial in smoking cessation, due to their potential for nicotine addiction and various risks of respiratory complications [3]. Although studies demonstrate e-cigarettes may be beneficial in achieving abstinence of cigarettes, individuals continued to use these products found to have carcinogens and toxins [3]. Because long-term health consequences are unknown, clinicians should advise complete cessation of e-cigarettes when the patient can do so without threatening their abstinence from conventional tobacco products [7].

It is important for healthcare providers to remember nicotine dependence is an addiction—a chronic disease prone to relapse. In order to become a tobacco-free society, clinicians must continue to develop, implement, and disseminate evidence-based clinical practice guidelines for smoking interventions. Smoke-free policies and increasing the price of cigarettes continue to reduce smoking prevalence, reduce cigarette consumption, and increase smoking cessation [7]. Mass media campaigns, pictorial health warnings, and local tobacco control programs also reduce the prevalence of smoking and increase quit attempts and must therefore be optimized [7]. In the future, a push for comprehensive insurance coverage for tobacco treatment including counseling and pharmacotherapy, as well as reimbursement for clinician tobacco treatment, should help to create an environment that is more supportive of cessation. Combining both clinical and public health tobacco strategies will continue to reinforce smoking cessation interventions for individuals, populations, and communities [7].

References

1. Clinical Practice Guideline Treating Tobacco Use and Dependence 2008 Update Panel, Liaisons, and Staff. A clinical practice guideline for treating tobacco use and dependence: 2008 update. A U.S. public health service report. Am J Prev Med. 2008;35(2):158; https://www.ncbi.nlm.nih.gov/pmc/articles/PMC4465757/#:~:text=These%20steps%20are%3A%20(1),up%20contact%20to%20prevent%20relapse.
2. Prochaska JJ, Benowitz NL. Current advances in research in treatment and recovery: nicotine addiction. Sci Adv. 2019;5:eaay9763; https://www.ncbi.nlm.nih.gov/pmc/articles/PMC6795520/.
3. Choi HK, Ataucuri-Vargas J, Lin C, Singrey A. The current state of tobacco cessation treatment. Cleve Clin J Med. 2021;88(7):393; https://www.ccjm.org/content/88/7/393.
4. Office of the Commissioner. Want to quit smoking? FDA-approved products can help. Silver Spring, MD: US Food and Drug Administration; 2017; https://www.fda.gov/consumers/consumer-updates/want-quit-smoking-fda-approved-products-can-help.
5. Rustin TA. Assessing nicotine dependence. Leawood, KS: American Family Physician; 2000; https://www.aafp.org/afp/2000/0801/p579.html.
6. Rigotta NA. Pharmacotherapy for smoking cessation in adults. UpToDate; 2021; https://www.uptodate.com/contents/pharmacotherapy-for-smoking-cessation-in-adults.
7. US Department of Health and Human Services. Smoking cessation: a report of the surgeon general; 2020; https://www.hhs.gov/sites/default/files/2020-cessation-sgr-full-report.pdf.

Part III
Organizing a Quality Program

Chapter 13
Organizational Workflow for Lung Cancer Screening

Teresa Giamboy and Julie A. Barta

Background

Lung cancer screening with low-dose CT (LDCT) imaging has been proven to be an effective tool in recognizing those at risk for developing lung cancer and offering this preventative measure in an effort to detect the disease earlier, when more treatment options are available and ultimately when more lives can be saved. There are many aspects to offering this service, which requires coordination and organization across several disciplines. Implementing LDCT screening for lung cancer is a highly complex process that requires substantial upfront planning and investment among leadership and staff, as well as ongoing communication to help troubleshoot challenges that arise throughout the implementation process [1]. Organizing a high-quality lung cancer screening (LCS) program will be discussed throughout this chapter, outlining the numerous components that are necessary to offer individuals seamless preventative care and "top box" patient experience.

T. Giamboy
Jefferson Health Northeast, Sidney Kimmel Cancer Center at Torresdale, Thomas Jefferson University, Philadelphia, PA, USA
e-mail: Teresa.Giamboy@jefferson.edu

J. A. Barta (✉)
Department of Medicine, Thomas Jefferson University, Philadelphia, PA, USA
e-mail: Julie.Barta@jefferson.edu

G. C. Kane et al. (eds.), *Lung Cancer Screening*,
https://doi.org/10.1007/978-3-031-33596-9_13

Planning for Implementation of a Lung Cancer Screening Program

When organizing a lung cancer screening program, the first undertaking is to determine the goals of the organization in which you are structuring this program and to engage relevant stakeholders [2]. There are various models of programmatic structure for such an offering, however, the more centralized and comprehensive a program is designed to be, the more resources and coordination it takes to organize and oversee this operationally. It is our opinion that a centralized model of lung cancer screening, hosted by a dedicated clinical team with multidisciplinary and interdepartmental support, is critical to the program's success and most beneficial to the individuals the program serves. We know that adherence to annual lung cancer screening is higher among individuals who were screened through a centralized program, demonstrating the value of centralization and the need to further implement strategies that improve adherence to annual screening for lung cancer [3, 4].

Selecting a motivated leader and team of multidisciplinary specialists to drive the program forward is important. Establishing a program steering committee that meets regularly to plan, and then frequently to assess outcomes once the program is implemented, is a sound approach to accomplishing this task. Quality improvement should be a continuous process, ensuring the screening program remains competitive in a rapidly changing healthcare environment [5]. Pinpointing key stakeholders and ensuring their teams and departments have the capability to execute their portion of the screening process is vital; the bones need to be there. That includes a CT scanner with low-dose capability and calibration, reading radiologists who are well acquainted with CT chest imaging and appropriate reading protocols, and a CT technologist team accustomed to providing this service in a safe way to patients, ensuring radiation dosage is delivered in the appropriate manner. The multidisciplinary team members may vary based on who is available at the institution. However, remote support and connectivity, which are better established now secondary to widespread familiarity wtih telemedicine, may allow for specialty collaboration at a distance in order to be comprehensive. Most commonly, those stakeholders include primary care providers, pulmonologists, thoracic surgeons, and oncologists, among others. Once the team is assembled, the discussion of how the patients will make their way through the program can be generated.

It is essential to determine the scope and subsequent workflow of the program. Given the potential for such a large number of lives to be positively affected by a timely diagnosis of early stage treatable disease, the initiation of lung cancer screening programs should be given the highest priority by healthcare institutions and providers [6]. It is important to have a strong understanding of any challenges that may exist in the current state, and to anticipate issues that may arise once a program is implemented. A realistic timeline should be created based on these factors, particularly if modifications and/or additions are required. There needs to be a clear goal and vision to help direct program development that encompasses all of these relevant variables, to be most effective to the population you serve. There is a need to understand how best to coordinate care with and engage referring providers, as well as how to educate providers about requirements and patient eligibility [7].

Understanding guidelines and recommendations of eligibility for lung cancer screening is critical to program intake and patient throughput. Governmental and private payors will dictate which of their patients should receive preventative cancer screening based on evidence-based research and publications. Programmatic structure must align to screen appropriately within these guidelines and recommendations, in order to achieve maximum financial return while ensuring all patients receive equitable care. Finally, it is important to recognize that this is cancer screening, and in order for patients to be attracted to preventative care, it should be easy, accessible, covered, and relatively painless to complete. The centralized program model assists in providing this service in a concierge-type approach, as the team assists in coordinating the screening continuum for each patient. Centralized programs can even access potential charitable sources with greater ease to cover screenings for patients who lack insurance.

The Centralized Model

Investing in a centralized program model will require the support of multiple clinical positions, including a dedicated clinician, most often an advanced practice provider (nurse practitioner or physician assistant), as well as a navigator and program coordinator (Fig. 13.1). Finally, there are other logistical considerations when determining the feasibility of building a lung cancer screening program, inclusive of collaboration and planning with other teams, most importantly scheduling and radiology, and ensuring that there is enough support within those departments to take on an additional volume of significant work. Finally, recognizing the financial components to hosting this type of program is key in justifying and advocating for centralization, understanding that downstream revenue will ultimately flow from this investment.

With a dedicated team, program coordinators begin the process by managing all referred patients to screening, as well as individuals who self-refer. The role of the program coordinator is to handle all intake (calls/electronic referrals, work queues, etc.), confirm eligibility based on age, smoking status, risk, and insurance coverage, and to schedule patients for shared decision making and then, if the opt in, a LDCT. Based on the structure of the program, these appointments may occur in one visit or can be in two separate encounters. Patient encounters may occur via telephone, telehealth, or in-person. The coordinator, ensuring that the patient's entrance into the program is simple and efficient, also manages referrals, authorizations, and all communication at this stage of the process. A crucial component to program coordination is strong and consistent customer service, as this is a patient's initial touch point with the program, and first impressions are long lasting. Documentation of calls and updates should be recorded in the electronic medical record, and any issues or barriers brought to the attention of the team to address and/or prepare for prior to the patient's appointment. Maintaining referral queues and pending authorizations must

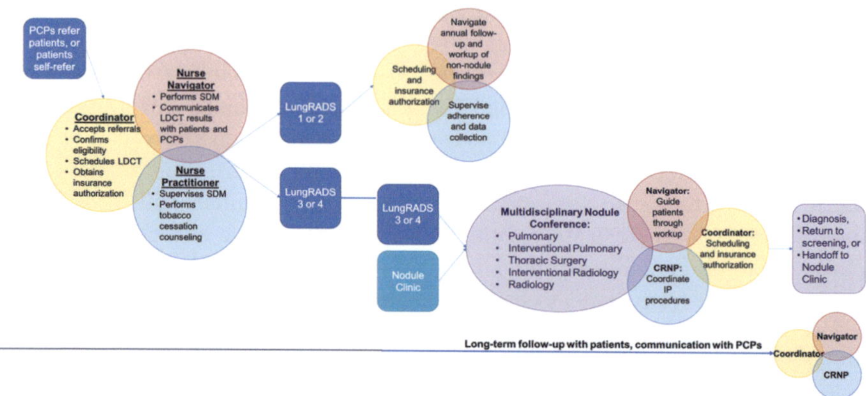

Fig. 13.1 Workflow for a Nursing-Driven, Centralized LCS Program Supported by a Multidisciplinary Team. A clinical trial comprised of a Nurse Practitioner, Nurse Navigator, and Coordinator with well-defined roles can guide patients through the LCS process in a comprehensive fashion. All individuals with positive LDCT scans are reviewed at a weekly Multidisciplinary Nodule Conference, receiving critical collaborative guidance from Pulmonary, Thoracic Surgery, and Radiology. The core team maintains relationships and communication with referring primary care providers throughout the LCS process

be kept up to date daily, and always supported. In a program with significant volume, additional coordinators may be required to support these efforts.

The navigator role is flexible in the sense that this can be filled by a non-clinical or clinical person. However, the benefit of having a nurse navigator in this position is significantly positive, as they have a strong educational background in healthcare and can field more complex questions and concerns from patients as well as provide patient education. Centralization allows the nurse navigator to become involved at the time of shared decision making, which is a critical component of the lung cancer screening process that is considered best practice, and an opportunity for the navigator and provider to work together to care for the patient comprehensively. Shared decision making (SDM) consists of communication, collaboration, aspects of evidence-based medicine, and relationship building—all based on the principle of the autonomy of the patient. It is a complex process, with each consultation unique [8]. Nurse navigators also assist in counseling patients on tobacco addiction and cessation opportunities, during shared decision making and while following the patient through the screening process. They will often be involved in calling patients with screening results to review pulmonary and/or incidental findings found on LDCT, and continuing cessation follow-up and treatment recommendations in coordination with the provider's prescribed treatment plan. Having navigators who are certified tobacco treatment specialists further boosts strong support for patients who commit to cessation.

When suspicious findings are detected and individuals require additional testing or diagnostic intervention, nurse navigators assist in collaborating with the multidisciplinary team to ensure patients travel through the care continuum successfully, helping to identify and overcome any barriers along the way. Involvement in nodule conferences or tumor boards with the comprehensive team allows for the navigator to practice at the top of their clinical scope, remaining involved in the care of the patients and tracking the status of pending work-up. Communication with the patient and the team is key throughout this process, and navigators are typically the glue that holds it all together. This work helps to support more robust screening program rates, adherence to annual and follow-up screening, shortening time to treatment, increased patient satisfaction, and improved quality of life for the patient [9]. Data keeping, tracking, and reporting are often responsibilities supported by the nurse navigator, allowing them to remain abreast of any shifts or trends that may be occurring or to identify efficiencies or improvements that could be implemented.

Finally, the provider who is dedicated to a lung cancer screening program has the task to complete the shared decision-making discussion, in collaboration with the patient and the nurse navigator, and to make final recommendations for tobacco cessation treatment. LDCT orders and tobacco cessation treatments are prescribed by this provider, who is ultimately responsible for the results and continuation of medications when appropriate. Advanced practitioners are uniquely positioned to provide lung cancer screening within a formal screening program [10]. Those with a background in pulmonology or thoracic surgery are strong candidates for this role, given their clinical expertise. In fact, many practices will embed a lung cancer screening program into these groups, which harbors immediate and continued support by a team of physicians and other providers. The benefit of this model is that those APPs have the knowledge and proficiency to read CT imaging and are able to make recommendations as licensed providers who can also bill for their services. A background, and ideally certification, in tobacco treatment is ideal for this role as a large portion of patients will require tobacco addiction counseling and cessation treatment planning.

Other APP involvement includes follow-up with those who are discovered to have suspicious findings, educating patients, and referring providers about potential disease differentials and appropriate next steps. Presenting these cases at multidisciplinary tumor boards and communicating those recommendations to patients ensures that diagnosis is never delayed. Coordinating care with other specialists to ensure timely work-up is critical when malignancy is a concern. Very importantly, continual and consistent documentation in the patient's electronic medical record is necessary so that the care team can stay informed. Direct messaging through the medical record is a preferred method of communication so that other members of the care team can easily access additional details of the patient's case if needed. The APP can also communicate with the patient directly through the electronic medical record, if the functionality exists and the patient is adept.

Multidisciplinary Teams in Lung Cancer Screening

A multidisciplinary team serves both operational and clinical care aims in a centralized LCS program. Foundational partnerships must be built among a core team of physicians and APPs in Pulmonary Medicine and Interventional Pulmonology, Thoracic Surgery, and Radiology and Interventional Radiology. Additional critical members of the multidisciplinary steering committee include Primary Care champions, Pathology and Cytology specialists with expertise in lung cancer, Thoracic Medical Oncology and Radiation Oncology providers, research coordinators and data analysts from the Clinical Trials Office, medical administrators representing each of the core specialties, and marketing specialists [2]. From an operational standpoint, the multidisciplinary steering committee's objective is to develop an integrated workflow and high-quality screening process for eligible individuals [11]. This includes a multitude of logistical challenges ranging from scheduling and coordinating appointments, to streamlining referral processes in the electronic health record, to the governance of LDCT results, and setting standard protocols for screen-detected nodules and other findings.

From a clinical standpoint, the multidisciplinary team frequently reflects existing Lung Cancer Tumor Board or Lung Nodule Clinic membership and can leverage clinical partnerships that are already in place. Processes for multidisciplinary teams have been described for the management of both incidental and screen-detected nodules [12, 13]. Goals for multidisciplinary Lung Nodule teams include an emphasis on standardized, guideline-concordant care (or clear reasons for guideline deviation) and reliable follow-up, as well as the reduction in diagnostic delay for cancers and also reduction of unnecessary procedures for low-risk nodules. A common theme across such interdisciplinary collaborations is a time-intensive commitment to this process, which may be a barrier for some healthcare systems.

Tracking Data and Quality Metrics

Beginning in the planning phase of LCS implementation, developing mechanisms for tracking data and quality metrics are critically important. At the patient level, LCS programs must know when screened patients are due to return for ongoing annual LDCT or short-interval scans following a positive LDCT [14]. At the program level, basic quality metrics for LCS may include the percentage of individuals completing screening who are eligible by the United States Preventive Services Task Force Criteria and documentation of tobacco treatment counseling for individuals who currently smoke [15, 16]. Additional quality metrics proposed by the National Lung Cancer Roundtable focus on screening adherence by the American College of Radiology Lung-RADS category and require detailed data entry for calculation of adherence rates at annual and short-interval time points [15]. These and other metrics have clinical, programmatic, and financial implications for LCS programs. Administrators and healthcare organization leadership may use such outcomes to drive resource allocation across health systems, making accurate and standardized patient tracking imperative for the success of LCS programs.

Conclusions

A well-organized workflow will lead to improved performance for the lung cancer screening program with a mechanism to address timely referrals for suspected cancers, quality improvement to achieve timely patient follow-up, and standardized approaches for addressing incidental findings. Coupled with a multi-disciplinary steering committee; highly organized workflow will yield benefits through identifying early stage lung cancers and substantially impacting the mortality of lung cancer in the community served (Fig. 13.1).

References

1. Allen CG, Cotter MM, Smith RA, Watson L. Successes and challenges of implementing a lung cancer screening program in federally qualified health centers: a qualitative analysis using the consolidated framework for implementation research. Transl Behav Med. 2021;11(5):1088–98.
2. Wiener RS, Gould MK, Arenberg DA, Au DH, Fennig K, Lamb CR, et al. An official American Thoracic Society/American College of Chest Physicians policy statement: implementation of low-dose computed tomography lung cancer screening programs in clinical practice. Am J Respir Crit Care Med. 2015;192(7):881–91.
3. Sakoda LC, Rivera MP, Zhang J, Perera P, Laurent CA, Durham D, et al. Patterns and factors associated with adherence to lung cancer screening in diverse practice settings. JAMA Netw Open. 2021;4(4):e218559.
4. Smith HB, Ward R, Frazier C, Angotti J, Tanner NT. Guideline-recommended lung cancer screening adherence is superior with a centralized approach. Chest. 2022;161(3):818–25.
5. Batile JC, Maroules CD, Latif MA, Cury RC. A five-step strategy for building an LDCT lung cancer screening program. Appl Radiol. 2018;47(1):12–8.
6. Sands J, Tammemägi MC, Couraud S, Baldwin DR, Borondy-Kitts A, Yankelevitz D, et al. Lung screening benefits and challenges: a review of the data and outline for implementation. J Thorac Oncol. 2021;16(1):37–53.
7. Copeland A, Criswell A, Ciupek A, King JC. Effectiveness of lung cancer screening implementation in the community setting in the United States. J Oncol Pract. 2019;15(7):e607–e15.
8. Matthys J. Shared decision making: an ideal and an art. BMJ. 2021;374:n2033.
9. Shusted CS, Barta JA, Lake M, Brawer R, Ruane B, Giamboy TE, et al. The case for patient navigation in lung cancer screening in vulnerable populations: a systematic review. Popul Health Manag. 2019;22(4):347–61.
10. Strong A. A nurse practitioner's experience in the development and implementation of a lung cancer screening program. J Adv Pract Oncol. 2018;9(5):524–9.
11. Mazzone P, Powell CA, Arenberg D, Bach P, Detterbeck F, Gould MK, et al. Components necessary for high-quality lung cancer screening: American College of Chest Physicians and American Thoracic Society Policy Statement. Chest. 2015;147(2):295–303.

12. Madariaga ML, Lennes IT, Best T, Shepard J-AO, Fintelmann FJ, Mathisen DJ, et al. Multidisciplinary selection of pulmonary nodules for surgical resection: diagnostic results and long-term outcomes. J Thorac Cardiovasc Surg. 2020;159(4):1558–66.e3.
13. Verdial FC, Madtes DK, Cheng G-S, Pipavath S, Kim R, Hubbard JJ, et al. Multidisciplinary team-based management of incidentally detected lung nodules. Chest. 2020;157(4):985–93.
14. Mazzone PJ, Silvestri GA, Souter LH, Caverly TJ, Kanne JP, Katki HA, et al. Screening for lung cancer: CHEST guideline and expert panel report. Chest. 2021;160:e427.
15. Mazzone PJ, White CS, Kazerooni EA, Smith RA, Thomson CC. Proposed quality metrics for lung cancer screening programs: a national lung cancer roundtable project. Chest. 2021;160:368.
16. Force UPST. Screening for lung cancer: US preventive services task force recommendation statement. JAMA. 2021;325(10):962–70.

Chapter 14
Lung-RADS® and Radiology Reporting Requirements

Cole Miller and Baskaran Sundaram

Background

Lung cancer is the leading cause of cancer-related mortality in the United States. The US Preventative Services Task Force (USPSTF) recommends lung cancer screening for current high-risk smokers with low-dose computed tomography (LDCT) or those that have quit within the past 15 years. High risk is defined as adults aged 50–80 with at least a 20-pack-year history of smoking. This recommendation was mainly based on the National Lung Screening Trial (NLST) data. The NLST enrolled 53,454 randomly assigned participants and found a 20% reduction in mortality from lung cancer in the LDCT group compared to chest radiography [1]. Chest radiography and alternative methods of screening such as sputum cytology have previously failed to show survival benefits [2]. LDCT provides many advantages over plain chest radiography, including increased resolution and contrast in the lung tissue and cross-sectional data acquisition, eliminating overlying structures obscuring pulmonary nodules. LDCT scanning produces high-resolution volumetric imaging of the thoracic cavity performed in a single breath-hold, which reduces artifacts from respiratory motion and low levels of radiation exposure [3, 4], without compromising image quality [5]. The major disadvantage of LDCT for lung cancer screening is the high false-positive rate, leading to over-testing, additional radiation exposure, patient anxiety, invasive

C. Miller
Sidney Kimmel Medical College, Thomas Jefferson University, Philadelphia, PA, USA
e-mail: CJM039@students.jefferson.edu

B. Sundaram (✉)
Department of Radiology, Thomas Jefferson University Hospital, Philadelphia, PA, USA
e-mail: Baskaran.Sundaram@jefferson.edu

G. C. Kane et al. (eds.), *Lung Cancer Screening*,
https://doi.org/10.1007/978-3-031-33596-9_14

procedures, and high cost of care [1, 6]. Despite the proven benefit of lung cancer screening, recent data suggest that implementation of lung cancer screening remains low in the United States [7].

Lung-RADS®

One of the essential aspects of the lung cancer screening process is interpreting and outputting screening test findings accurately in a practical and reliable manner. Hence, it is critical to have a simple, meaningful, reproducible, and universally applicable system that allows data collection. It is comprehensively accomplished by Lung-Reporting And Data Systems (Lung-RADS®) developed by the American College of Radiology (ACR). There are other ACR reporting systems for different organs and diseases, such as coronary artery disease (CAD-RADS®), liver imaging (LI-RADS®), prostate imaging (PI-RADS®), and thyroid imaging (TI-RADS®). ACR modeled Lung-RADS® after the Breast Imaging RADS (BI-RADS®) for breast cancer screening, the most successful and longest-standing reporting system in any cancer screening. BI-RADS®, currently in its fifth edition, was initiated in the 1980s to address heterogeneity in mammography reporting and management recommendations. It includes a lexicon of image descriptors, a reporting structure with assessment categories, corresponding management recommendations, and a data collection and quality assurance implementation framework. Further editions continued to enhance its performance, reducing the interobserver variability in reporting breast mammograms and sonograms [8–12]. Therefore, ACR introduced Lung-RADS® version 1.0 in 2014 with the hope of finding similar success and updated it in 2019 with version 1.1. Currently, version 2.0 is in coming out in mid-late 2022.

The ACR has licensed Lung-RADS® under a Creative Commons Attribution-No Derivatives 4.0 International License. Lung-RADS® is a quality assurance tool used to standardize lung cancer screening CT reporting and management recommendations, reduce confusion in CT interpretations, and facilitate outcome monitoring. Lung-RADS® helps determine an accurate categorization of CT scan results to maximize the lung cancer screening potential for lowering lung cancer-specific morbidity and mortality while minimizing false-positive results. Moreover, it facilitates improvement in screening performance by compiling data such as positive screening rates in individual practices and comparing them with regional and national benchmarks.

Comparison of Fleischner and NLST Criteria

It is essential to differentiate Lung-RADS® from Fleischner Society Criteria for lung nodule management, which refers to the management of pulmonary nodules incidentally detected on CT examinations performed for purposes other than lung cancer screening [13]. They apply to the general population in patients over 35 years without new or growing pulmonary nodules. The Fleischner criteria apply to the lung nodules in immunocompetent individuals without a known malignancy or who do not meet the lung cancer screening eligibility [13]. Lung-RADS® guidelines apply to patients with a high risk for developing lung cancer.

Understanding the similarities and differences between Lung-RADS® and NLST parameters is also essential. In the NLST, researchers determined a positive screen as any lung nodule equal to or greater than 4 mm in size in its greatest dimension regardless of consistency or other characteristics. This cutoff significantly reduced lung cancer mortality by 20%, but the positive screening rate was over 27% on initial screening, while lung cancer was only diagnosed in 1.1% of the CT screening group [1]. Later, the International Early Lung Cancer Action Program (I-ELCAP) studied the effect of using alternative thresholds for defining a positive screen. They found that increasing the size threshold to 6 mm reduced the positive screening rate to 10.2% while also reducing additional diagnostic testing by 36%. This 2 mm increase in size threshold found that no patients experienced a 9 months or longer delay in their cancer diagnosis [14]. The researchers then introduced new size thresholds to NLST data and found that 64% of positive screens were 7 mm or smaller. If the threshold was raised to 8 mm, they found that false-positive rates were reduced to only 10.5%, however, missed or delayed cancer diagnoses increased to 15.8% [15]. Hence, the Lung-RADS® determined that the optimal lung nodule size threshold can be raised to 6 mm, balancing the benefits and harms.

Additionally, nodule characteristics were incorporated into Lung-RADS®, including calcifications, solid or non-solid components, ground-glass appearance, and changes over time. NLST did not specify a different threshold for non-solid nodules. NLST considered a nodule larger than 4 mm nodule benign only if it remained stable in size for 2 years [4]. To further decrease false-positive screening, Lung-RADS® set the positive screening threshold to 20 mm for ground-glass nodules (later increased to 30 mm in Lung-RADS® V1.1) and the duration of nodule stability required to qualify as benign to 3 months [16].

Lung-RADS® Version 1.0

The initial 2014 Lung-RADS® version 1.0 includes a set of assessment categories ranging from zero to 4X. They specify different parameters for solid nodules, part-solid (PS) nodules, and non-solid ground-glass nodules (GGN). Category zero indicates an incomplete screen, which warrants additional imaging. Other designations include the modifier "S," indicating clinically significant non-lung cancer-related findings, and modifier, "C" indicating prior lung cancer to append to each Lung-RADS® assessment category and their corresponding management recommendations. A Category 1 (negative) screen indicates a scan with no lung nodules and solid nodules with a benign pattern of calcifications (complete, central, popcorn, or concentric rings) and fat-containing (hamartoma) nodules (Fig. 14.1). Category 2 nodules (benign appearance or display benign behavior) include solid or PS nodules smaller than 6 mm, non-solid nodules under 20 mm, or the Lung-RADS® category 3 and 4 nodules that have remained stable for three or more months. These nodules (Fig. 14.2) also carry a very low risk of malignancy and are

Fig. 14.1 LDCT shows a smoothly marginated 15 mm left upper lobe lung nodule (arrow) with internal adipose contents (ACR-Lung RADS category 1)

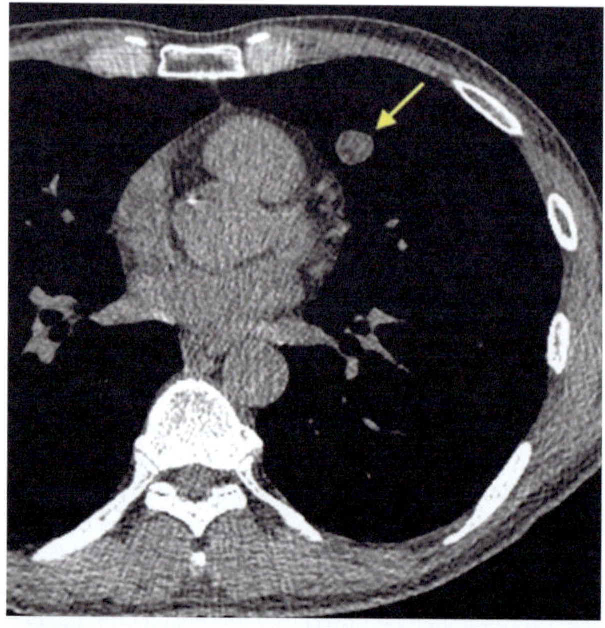

Fig. 14.2 LDCT shows a stable (for 5 years) 3 mm middle lobe solid lung nodule (arrow) without internal calcifications or adipose contents (ACR-Lung RADS category 2)

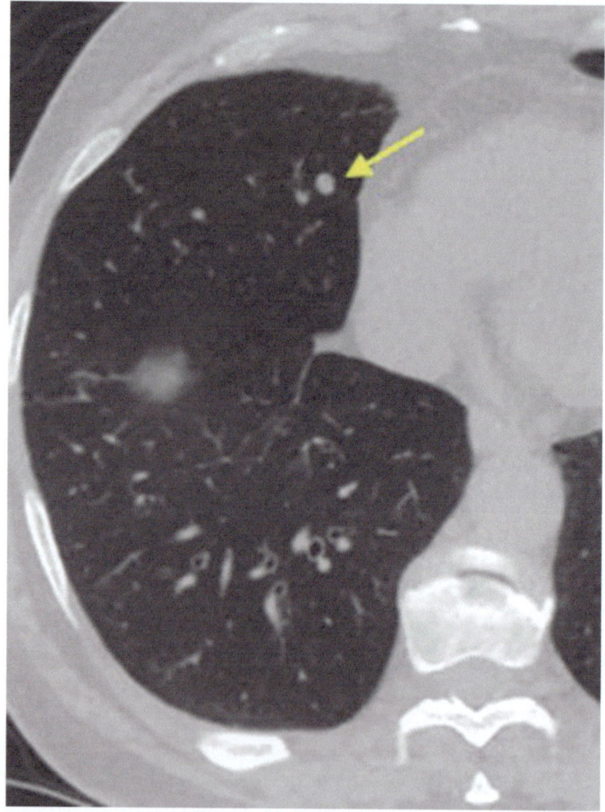

Fig. 14.3 LDCT shows a right upper lobe solid 7 mm lung nodule (arrow) without internal calcifications (ACR-Lung Rads category 3) that was downgraded later to a ACR-Lung Rads category 2 nodule due to its stability for more than 3 months

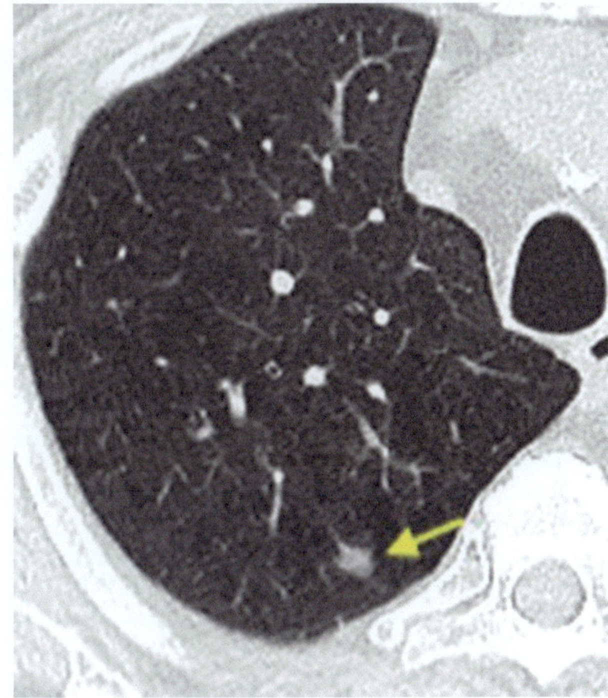

returned to annual LDCT screenings [16]. Category 3 nodules (probably benign) include 6 mm or larger to under 8 mm sized solid nodules at baseline (or new 4 and 5 mm), ≥ 6 mm PS nodules with solid component <6 mm (or new 1–5 mm nodules), or GGN nodules ≥20 mm (baseline or new). These nodules (Fig. 14.3) have a 1–2% risk of malignancy and are recommended to get a 6-month follow-up LDCT [16]. Category 4A nodules are (suspicious) characterized by solid nodules 8–14 mm at baseline (or growing <8 mm or new 6 and 7 mm nodules), PS nodules that are 6 mm or larger with the solid component 6–7 mm (or new or increasing by <4 mm solid part), or an endobronchial nodule. These nodules (Fig. 14.4) have a 5–15% risk of malignancy and are recommended to get a 3-month follow-up with LDCT. PET/CT may be used if the solid component is 8 mm or larger [16]. Category 4B nodules (suspicious) include solid nodules (Fig. 14.5) 15 mm or larger (or new/growing 8 mm or larger) and PS nodules with a solid component 8 mm or larger (or new/growing 4 mm or larger solid part). The category 4X refers to any category o three or four nodules (Fig. 14.6) with additional features or imaging findings that increase the suspicion of malignancy. These category 4B and 4X nodules carry a risk of malignancy of more than 15% and require prompt evaluation with a diagnostic standard radiation dose CT with or without contrast, PET/CT, or tissue sampling depending on the probability of malignancy and comorbidities. Category 1 and 2 LDCTs are considered screen negatives, and 3 and 4 LDCTs are considered screen positives [16]. The estimated population

Fig. 14.4 LDCT shows a left upper lobe part-solid nodule (arrow) with a 6 mm to 8 mm solid component (ACR-Lung RADS category 4A)

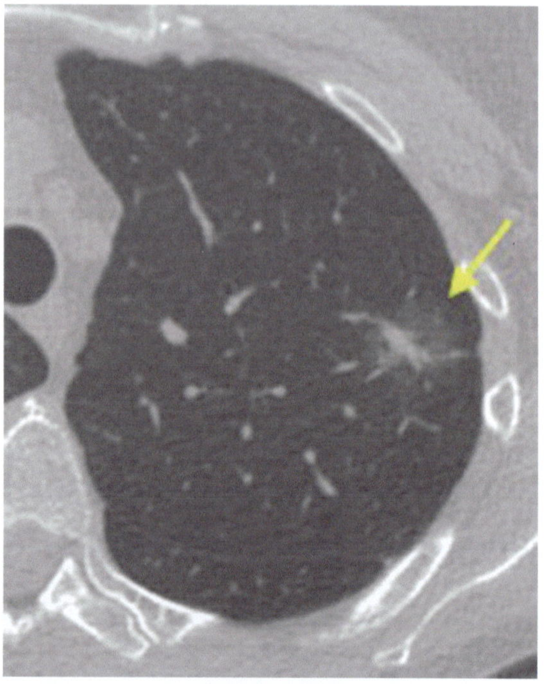

Fig. 14.5 LDCT shows a right upper lobe solid 12 mm lung nodule (arrow) that grew from 7 to 8 mm to 12 months previously (ACR-Lung RADS category 4B). The patient underwent surgical resection and the final diagnosis was determined to be squamous cell carcinoma pathologic stage 1A2 (pT1b, pN0, cM0)

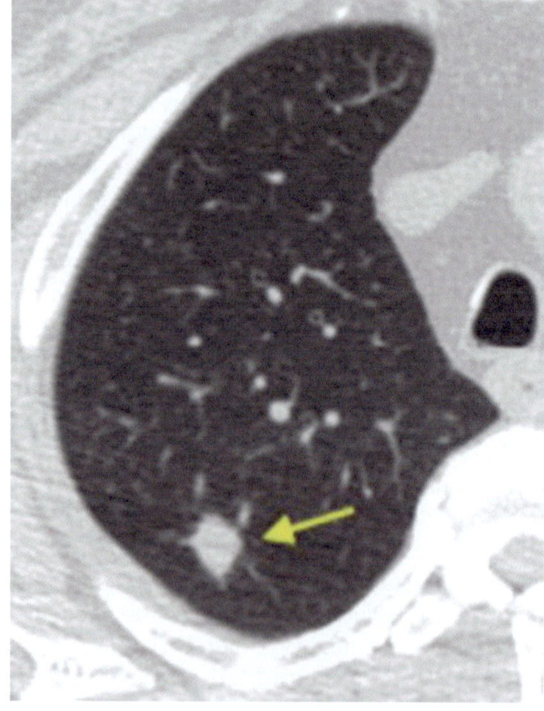

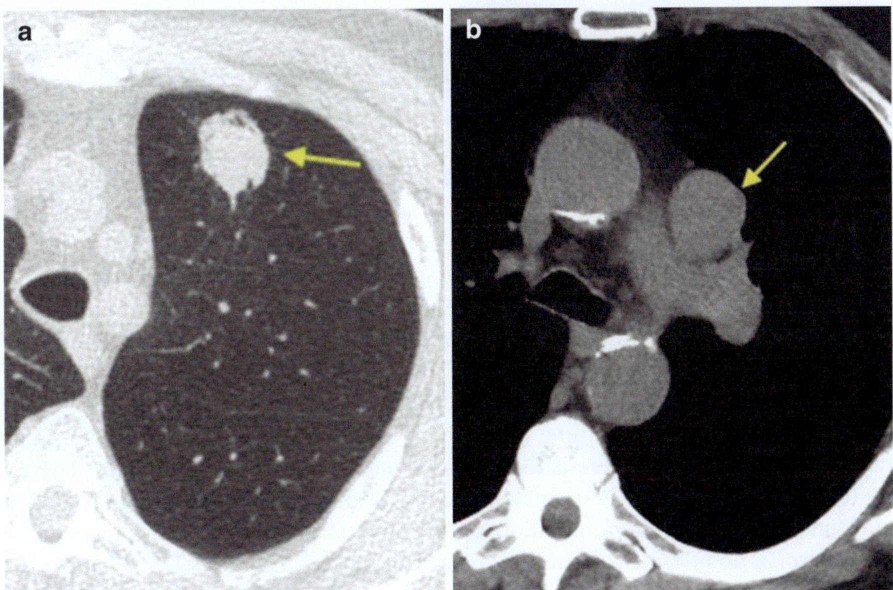

Fig. 14.6 LDCT shows a 30 mm left upper lobe lung nodule (arrow in 6A) with a 50 mm left AP window lymph node (arrow in 6B) indicating ACR-Lung RADS 4X. The patient underwent surgical resection and the final diagnosis was determined to be small cell carcinoma

prevalence for category 2 nodules is 90%, 3 is 5%, and 4 is 2%. Similarly, the estimated prevalence for the clinically significant non-lung cancer findings is 10% [16].

Lung-RADS® Versions

In 2019, ACR introduced Lung-RADS® version 1.1 with several significant updates to the categorizing and managing of pulmonary nodule subtypes. The first update addressed the perifissural nodules, and the intrapulmonary lymph nodes near or contiguous with pleural layers and fissures. They are typically oval, lentiform, or triangular solid nodules with smooth margins and a maximum diameter of under 10 mm. Lung-RADS® 1.1 classified these nodules as category 2 (benign), while previously, any 6–10 mm solid nodules were in category 3 or 4A. Xu et al. found that perifissural nodules comprised 83% of the intermediate solid pulmonary nodules in the NELSON trial, and at 1 year follow-up, no cancer was found [17]. Additionally, McWilliams et al. found that in the pooled data from Canada's PANCAN and BCCA trials, the probability of developing lung cancer from a perifissural nodule was 0% [18]. In addition, a secondary analysis of NLST data revealed that none of the 216 perifissural nodules out of 1092 solid nodules in the 6–10 mm size range later became malignancy [19]. ACR implemented this change based on data on perifissural nodules that make up a significant percentage of detected nodules yet are invariably benign. Although, in clinical practice, the subjective variations of perifissural nodules may pose management challenges.

Another major update in Lung-RADS® 1.1 was increasing GGN's positive screen size threshold from 20 to 30 mm. In the baseline CT, the GGN under 20 mm is classified as category 2 with lung RADS- version 1.0, and a GGN of 20 mm or larger is classified as category 3. With Lung-RADS® version 1.1, a GGN of up to 30 mm is classified as category 2. Another addition to Lung-RADS® 1.1 addresses the management of new large 4B category nodules that develop on annual repeat screening. Lung-RADS® 1.1 recommends a 1-month follow-up LDCT to identify infectious or inflammatory nodules rather than proceeding with immediate diagnostic testing or tissue sampling [16]. The fourth update for improving the accuracy of the nodule diameters is the mean diameter to one decimal point (derived by the long and short axis diameter measurements to one decimal point). They may not round the individual short and long-axis measurements, allowing for more precise nodule measurements [16]. Additionally, Lung-RADS 1.1 included the nodule volumetry with diameter measurements [16]. The lung nodule volumetry has the potential to improve the inter-reader agreement for nodule size and Lung-RADS® categorization [20]. Although, the lung nodule volumetric measurements are not possible or reliable for every lung nodule due to their non-spherical nature. Lung nodule contouring for volumetric analysis is time-consuming and with a significant measurement threshold variation between software programs.

Based on Nelson trial data, Lung-RADS® version two published in mid-late 2022 addresses additional items such as atypical lung cysts, endobronchial nodules, and costal pleural nodules and update management recommendations for some of the clinical scenarios [6]. Future studies need to demonstrate the performance and outcome of the current version of Lung-RADS.

Lung-RADS® Performance

Researchers retrospectively assessed the impact of the Lung-RADS 1.0 on a real-world clinical lung cancer program [21]. Their initial categorization of positive and negative screen results was based on National Comprehensive Cancer Network (NCCN), which was in alignment with the NLST study data. In their analysis, the screen negatives per NCCN criteria was 72.4% (1579 of 2180 patients) versus 89.4% (1949 of 2180 patients) with Lung-RADS®. They found the same number of (1.8%) lung cancers diagnosed in both methods. Lung-RADS® reduced the overall positive rate from 27.6% to 10.6%. No false negatives were present in the 152 patients with longer than 12-month follow-up reclassified as benign. Applying ACR Lung-RADS increased the positive predictive value for diagnosed malignancy in 1603 patients with follow-up from 6.9% to 17.3% [21].

Similarly, Pinsky et al. retrospectively researched the performance of Lung-RADS® 1.0 on NLST study data [22]. In their study, Lung-RADS® 1.0 would potentially miss 13% of 649 lung cancers that NLST found (86 total cancers; 25 at baseline and 61 at subsequent screenings). Although, potentially missed and the not-missed cancers had similar characteristics in stage (two-thirds were stage one), cell type (similar small-cell and adenocarcinoma proportions), and 5-year survival (71.7% vs. 64.2%; $p = 0.22$). They also found that Lung-RADS® would potentially avoid 66.6% overall false-positive screening (52% at baseline and 76% at subsequent screenings) with NLST. As a result, Lung-RADS® would potentially avoid 23.4% of invasive procedures and 48.5% of follow-up chest CT examinations (50.5% at baseline and 45.5% at subsequent screenings) due to false-positive tests [22].

Chung et al. explored if Lung-RADS ® category 4X improves malignancy prediction in subsolid nodules [23]. It is important to remember that the definition for category 4X is the category 3 or 4 lesions with suspicious features such as spiculation, GGN that doubles in size in 1 year, and enlarged lymph nodes. These features may be subjective, and upgrading a nodule from the lower category may trigger an immediate intensive diagnostic work-up. Their analysis included 374 subsolid nodules, and 56 were considered malignant nodules. They found that 15–24% of subsolid nodules were upgraded to 4X, and they successfully increased the malignancy rate in category 4X to approximately 50%. They also found that they falsely upstaged an average of 27% of lesions from benign to malignant lesions [23]. The findings indicate that the 4X category may be cautiously assigned to category 3 and 4 nodules by experienced radiologists. Although, a short-term follow-up could avoid unnecessary invasive management.

Kastner et al. studied the impact of reclassifying nodules in Lung RARS® version 1.1 compared to version 1.0 using secondary analysis of the NLST study data [19]. It is important to note that the introduction of perifissural nodules and 30 mm instead of 20 mm size threshold change for ground-glass nodules between Lung RADS® 1.1 and Lung-RARS® 1.0 [19]. They found that 1092 nodules between 6 and 10 mm. 216 (19.8%) were perifissural nodules, and none turned malignant. New size-based reclassification of the ground glass nodules did not reach statistical significance [19]. Their results support the idea that the perifissural nodules measuring under 10 mm can be safely categorized as benign category two lesions. These results validated the safety of Lung-RADS® use and indicated that Lung-RADS® application increases the accuracy and cost-effectiveness of lung cancer screening with LDCT.

Lung-RADS® Limitations

Lung-RADS®, while effective in decreasing false-positive rates in lung cancer screening and standardizing reporting and managing pulmonary nodules, has limitations. Lung-RADS® does not explicitly address definitions for identification, documentation, characterization, and management of common co-existing abnormalities such as pneumonia, vascular aneurysm, coronary calcifications, enlarged lymph nodes, findings in the upper abdominal organs, and chest wall findings, including osseous abnormalities in this high-risk population [16, 24]. We typically assign an "S" modifier; however, referring physicians need to recognize and manage these findings appropriately. There are other scenarios that Lung-RADS® does not explicitly address. Many of these limitations are nicely discussed in a review article by Martin et al. [24]. For example, it is unclear how best to manage a newly found category 3 (probably benign) solid lung nodule in patients exiting the screening eligibility age range [24]. Also, unclear guidance for nodules with prolonged growth rates, nodules that reduce in size and increase in attenuation (such as primary adenocarcinoma), the best methodology to measure complex nodules such as part-solid nodules, the optimal time to reenroll patients in the screening pathway after a stable abnormality, patients with a lung infection, and categorizing cavitary nodules [24].

Imaging Facility and Physician Requirements

Radiology imaging facilities interested in providing lung cancer screening must meet the Centers for Medicare and Medicaid Services (CMS) requirements that allow LDCT examinations for reimbursement as a preventative service under Medicare. Per these guidelines, radiology imaging facilities must perform LDCT with a volumetric CT dose index (CTDIvol) of 3.0 mGy or less for standard-sized patients (defined as 5′7″ and approximately 155 lbs) with appropriate adjustments in CTDIvol for smaller or larger patients [25]. The facilities must also use a standardized lung nodule identification, classification, and reporting system [25]. They are also highly encouraged to submit data to a CMS-approved registry (ACR Lung Cancer Screening Registry) for each LDCT examination performed. Submission data includes details about the facility, ordering physician, radiologist, patient identifiers, screening date, CT scanner, radiation dose, indication for the examination, lung nodules, reporting system used, patient smoking status, and smoking cessation interventions [25]. Also, there are expectations for the interpreting radiologist such as American Board of Radiology certification or board eligibility, diagnostic radiology and radiation safety training, involvement in the supervision and interpretation of at least 300 chest CTs in the past 3 years, CME participation, and perform lung cancer screening with LDCT in a radiology imaging facility that meets the requirements discussed above [25]. The CMS selected slightly different beneficiary eligibility criteria compared to the guidelines set forth by the USPSTF. The CMS now agreed to cover asymptomatic patients aged 50–77 with a 20-pack-year or more smoking history who is currently smoking or quitting within the last 15 years. Additionally, the beneficiary must receive an order for their LDCT lung cancer screening after lung cancer screening education and shared decision making with their physician. This visit must include counseling on eligibility, risks and benefits of screening, adherence to the annual screening protocols, and adherence to smoking abstinence and cessation interventions [25].

Conclusion

In conclusion, Lung-RADS® provides an effective tool for defining, classifying, and reporting findings of LDCT examinations for lung cancer screening. Lung-RADS® successfully identifies and risk-stratifies positive lung cancer screens and standardizes follow-up management. The implementation of Lung-RADS® has decreased the rate of false-positive findings without reducing sensitivity for detecting malignancy. Reporting data to organizations such as the ACR lung cancer screening registry has allowed for continued improvement of the Lung-RADS® classification schema. The updates included in Lung-RADS® 1.1 have proven to benefit the rates of false-positive examinations further. As imaging-related technology improves tools for segmentation, volumetric analysis, and AI integration, the Lung-RADS® system will continue to enhance the early detection of lung cancer while minimizing the deleterious effects of false-positive screens. While there are a few limitations to the current Lung-RADS® version, it will continue to improve at regular intervals based on updated knowledge and understanding.

References

1. National Lung Screening Trial Research Team. Reduced lung-cancer mortality with low-dose computed tomographic screening. N Engl J Med. 2011;365(5):395–409.
2. Early lung cancer detection: summary and conclusions. Am Rev Respir Dis. 1984;130(4):565–70.
3. Naidich DP, Marshall CH, Gribbin C, Arams RS, McCauley DI. Low-dose CT of the lungs: preliminary observations. Radiology. 1990;175:729–31.
4. National Lung Screening Trial Research Team. The national lung screening trial: overview and study design. Radiology. 2011;258(1):243–53.
5. Kubo T, Ohno Y, Takenaka D, Nishino M, Gautam S, Sugimura K, Kauczor HU, Hatabu H, iLEAD Study Group. Standard-dose vs. low-dose CT protocols in the evaluation of localized lung lesions: capability for lesion characterization-iLEAD study. Eur J Radiol Open. 2016;3:67–73.
6. de Koning HJ, van der Aalst CM, de Jong PA, Scholten ET, Nackaerts K, Heuvelmans MA, Lammers JJ, Weenink C, Yousaf-Khan U, Horeweg N, Van't Westeinde S, Prokop M, Mali WP, FAA MH, van PMA O, JGJV A, den Bakker MA, Thunnissen E, Verschakelen J, Vliegenthart R, Walter JE, Ten Haaf K, HJM G, Oudkerk M. Reduced lung-cancer mortality with volume CT screening in a randomized trial. N Engl J Med. 2020;382(6):503–13.
7. Zahnd WE, Eberth JM. Lung cancer screening utilization: a behavioral risk factor surveillance system analysis. Am J Prev Med. 2019;57(2):250–5.
8. Ciccone G, Vineis P, Frigerio A, Segnan N. Inter-observer and intra-observer variability of mammogram interpretation: a field study. Eur J Cancer. 1992;28(6–7):1054–8.
9. Elmore JG, Wells CK, Lee CH, Howard DH, Feinstein AR. Variability in radiologists' interpretations of mammograms. N Engl J Med. 1994;331(22):1493–9.
10. Lazarus E, Mainiero MB, Schepps B, Koelliker SL, Livingston LS. BI-RADS lexicon for US and mammography: interobserver variability and positive predictive value. Radiology. 2006;239(2):385–91.
11. Baker JA, Kornguth PJ, Floyd CE Jr. Breast imaging reporting and data system standardized mammography lexicon: observer variability in lesion description. AJR Am J Roentgenol. 1996;166(4):773–8.

12. Abdullah N, Mesurolle B, El-Khoury M, Kao E. Breast imaging reporting and data system lexicon for US: interobserver agreement for assessment of breast masses. Radiology. 2009;252(3):665–72.
13. Bueno J, Landeras L, Chung JH. Updated fleischner society guidelines for managing incidental pulmonary nodules: common questions and challenging scenarios. Radiographics. 2018;38(5):1337–50.
14. Henschke CI, Yip R, Yankelevitz DF, Smith JP, I-ELCAP Investigators. CT screening for lung cancer: update of the definition of positive test result and its implications. Ann Intern Med. 2013;158:246–52.
15. Gierada DS, Pinsky P, Nath H, Chiles C, Duan F, Aberle DR. Projected outcomes using different nodule sizes to define a positive CT lung cancer screening examination. J Natl Cancer Inst. 2014;106(11):dju284. https://doi.org/10.1093/jnci/dju284.
16. American College of Radiology. Lung CT screening reporting and data system (Lung-RADS); http://www.acr.org/Quality-Safety/Resources/LungRADS. Accessed 31 Jul 2014.
17. Xu DM, van der Zaag-Loonen HJ, Oudkerk M, Wang Y, Vliegenthart R, Scholten ET, Verschakelen J, Prokop M, de Koning HJ, van Klaveren RJ. Smooth or attached solid indeterminate nodules detected at baseline CT screening in the NELSON study: cancer risk during 1 year of follow-up. Radiology. 2009;250(1):264–72.
18. McWilliams A, Tammemagi MC, Mayo JR, Roberts H, Liu G, Soghrati K, Yasufuku K, Martel S, Laberge F, Gingras M, Atkar-Khattra S, Berg CD, Evans K, Finley R, Yee J, English J, Nasute P, Goffin J, Puksa S, Stewart L, Tsai S, Johnston MR, Manos D, Nicholas G, Goss GD, Seely JM, Amjadi K, Tremblay A, Burrowes P, MacEachern P, Bhatia R, Tsao MS, Lam S. Probability of cancer in pulmonary nodules detected on first screening CT. N Engl J Med. 2013;369(10):910–9.
19. Kastner J, Hossain R, Jeudy J, Dako F, Mehta V, Dalal S, Dharaiya E, White C. Lung-RADS version 1.0 versus lung-RADS version 1.1: Comparison of categories using nodules from the national lung screening trial. Radiology. 2021;300(1):199–206.
20. Gierada DS, Rydzak CE, Zei M, Rhea L. Improved interobserver agreement on lung-RADS classification of solid nodules using semiautomated CT volumetry. Radiology. 2020;297(3):675–84.
21. McKee BJ, Regis SM, McKee AB, Flacke S, Wald C. Performance of ACR lung-RADS in a clinical CT lung screening program. J Am Coll Radiol. 2015;12(3):273–6.
22. Pinsky PF, Gierada DS, Black W, Munden R, Nath H, Aberle D, Kazerooni E. Performance of lung-RADS in the national lung screening trial: a retrospective assessment. Ann Intern Med. 2015;162(7):485–91.
23. Chung K, Jacobs C, Scholten ET, Goo JM, Prosch H, Sverzellati N, Ciompi F, Mets OM, Gerke PK, Prokop M, van Ginneken B, Schaefer-Prokop CM. Lung-RADS category 4X: does it improve prediction of malignancy in subsolid nodules? Radiology. 2017;284(1):264–71.
24. Martin MD, Kanne JP, Broderick LS, Kazerooni EA, Meyer CA. Lung-RADS: pushing the limits. Radiographics. 2017;37(7):1975–93.
25. National coverage determination: lung cancer screening with low dose computed tomography (LDCT). Centers for Medicare & Medicaid Services; 2016. https://www.cms.gov/medicare-coverage-database/view/ncd.aspx?ncdid=364&ncdver=1.

Chapter 15
Managing Incidental Findings

Brooke Ruane and Debra Dyer

Background

Lung cancer is the leading cause of cancer-related mortality among men and women. There were 235,760 new cases of lung cancer and 131,880 deaths in 2021, more than breast, colon, and prostate cancer combined [1]. Preventative healthcare with screenings is an essential strategy in the early detection and/or prevention of various medical conditions, including cancers. Screening with low-dose chest computed tomography (LDCT) can identify early stage lung cancer and also provides an opportunity to identify significant incidental findings (IFs) unrelated to lung cancer. IFs are common in lung cancer screening CT (LCS CT). Some are considered significant or potentially significant and actionable while others are considered insignificant and not actionable. It is important that the actionable IFs receive appropriate attention as they may have a significant impact on patient care and outcomes. This chapter will examine IFs commonly detected during lung cancer screening, review pathways to report findings, and discuss the management of clinically significant IFs.

B. Ruane (✉)
Department of Medicine, Jane and Leonard Korman Respiratory Institute, Thomas Jefferson University, Philadelphia, PA, USA
e-mail: Brooke.Ruane@Jefferson.edu

D. Dyer
Department of Radiology, National Jewish Health, University of Colorado Denver, Denver, CO, USA
e-mail: DyerD@NJHealth.org

G. C. Kane et al. (eds.), *Lung Cancer Screening*,
https://doi.org/10.1007/978-3-031-33596-9_15

Lung Cancer Screening

The National Lung Screening Trial (NLST) demonstrated the benefit of screening high-risk individuals for lung cancer using an LDCT scan to decrease lung cancer death and all-cause mortality. The NLST demonstrated a 20% relative reduction in lung cancer mortality and a 6.7% reduction in all-cause mortality with LDCT compared to standard chest radiography [2].

The United States Preventive Services Taskforce (USPSTF) guidelines recommend annual screening with LDCT for eligible patients. The eligibility criteria, which were recently expanded in 2021, include individuals aged 50–80, with at least a 20-pack-year smoking history, and who continue to smoke or have quit within the last 15 years [3, 4]. Individuals must be asymptomatic for lung cancer or infection. Eligible individuals are at high risk for smoking-related comorbidities and also age-related competing causes of death, which may be a contributing factor to the reduction in all-cause mortality [5]. While lung cancer screening (LCS) is aimed at the early detection of lung cancer, there may be an additional benefit in the identification of incidental findings in this population.

Incidental Findings

IFs are defined as unexpected findings discovered on imaging studies unrelated to the intent, diagnosis, or symptoms that led to the imaging [6]. Many times, these findings have been present for years but go undetected, and they may have minimal impact on patient outcomes. It is not uncommon for patients to have abnormalities without ever having any symptoms [6, 7].

By definition, the LDCT is performed at a lower radiation dose than a routine chest CT. The low-dose technique for LCS is designed to optimize the visualization of the lung parenchyma but does not optimally visualize the soft tissues in the chest. In addition, since the CT extends from the lower neck into the upper abdomen, some solid organs may be only partially imaged such as the thyroid or kidney. An abnormality may be recognized and identified as an IF but not well demonstrated or incompletely visualized. Follow-up imaging may be needed to better characterize or fully image the abnormality.

IFs may be located in any of the following anatomic locations: abdominal, musculoskeletal, cardiovascular, breast, chest wall, esophagus, lung/pleura, mediastinum, and thyroid [8]. The identification of IFs has been reported as a cause of increased anxiety in patients [7]. Given the frequency of their discovery, a discussion about IFs should be included in the shared decision-making conversations with patients about lung cancer screening [9].

Individuals eligible for LCS are inherently at higher risk for other comorbidities, such as cardiovascular disease (heart disease and stroke), diabetes mellitus, and osteoporosis [10]. Cigarette smoking is attributed to one of every four cardiovascular deaths, and early signs of cardiovascular disease (CVD) have been seen in light smokers, who smoke less than five cigarettes a day [10]. Therefore, screening has the additional benefit of allowing us to identify other health issues that need to be addressed.

Types of Incidental Findings

A retrospective review of the LDCT cohort in the NLST trial found that 58.7% of participants had "minor" IFs and 19.6% had "potentially significant" findings [11]. The IFs were divided into five organ groupings: cardiovascular, thyroid, adrenal, renal, and hepatobiliary [11]. At least one in five patients undergoing LDCT for LCS may be expected to have potentially actionable incidental findings on imaging. The prevalence of potentially significant abnormalities was highest for cardiovascular (8.5%), renal (2.4%), hepatobiliary (2.1%), adrenal (1.2%), and thyroid (0.6%). However, it was rare (0.39%) for individuals to be diagnosed with an extrathoracic malignancy on a LDCT scan. The most common cancers were kidney (0.26%), thyroid (0.08%), and liver (0.05%) [11].

Not all IFs are considered clinically significant or actionable. For example, renal findings such as a non-obstructing calculus or simple or hyperdense/hemorrhagic cyst <4 cm requires no additional workup. However, an MRI or CT with or without contrast is recommended for a soft tissue density (or mixed) density renal mass [8].

Other clinically significant findings may include mediastinal lymphadenopathy (>15 mm in short axis), thyroid nodule >15 mm, ascending aortic aneurysm >42 mm, and interstitial lung disease [8]. All masses should have dedicated imaging of that specific area [8].

Incidental Findings and Follow-up Testing

As the adoption of LDCT has grown, the need for guidance on the management of IFs has become recognized. In response to this need, the American College of Radiology (ACR) LCS Steering Committee created the ACR Lung Cancer Screening CT Incidental Findings Quick Reference Guide to assist providers in identifying appropriate next steps (Fig. 15.1). The Quick Guide defines the most common IFs and outlines which are significant and which are "OK," or typically insignificant or benign. The Guide provides recommended actions for common IFs involving seven anatomic regions including 15 discrete organs. The recommendations are based on the references in the medical literature including multiple White Papers developed by the ACR for managing IFs [12–20]. For IFs not addressed in the White Papers, recommendations were based on content from other peer-reviewed publications and input from subspecialty experts. The Guide is intended to be used by LCS Program coordinators or nurse navigators as they assist in care coordination in collaboration with referring providers.

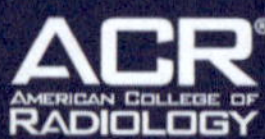

ACR® Lung Cancer Screening CT Incidental Findings
Quick Reference Guide

This Quick Guide is intended for use by Lung Cancer Screening (LCS) program coordinators and nurse navigators as they assist in the care coordination of LCS patients in collaboration with the referring providers.

- The Quick Guide lists common incidental findings on LCS CT and the typical management and/or appropriate follow–up recommendations.

- Comparison to prior exams is important to assess for stability or change.

- The guidance provided is intended to serve as a simple reference tool and does not replace the more comprehensive White Paper, ACR Appropriateness Criteria® and reference documents listed on the third page.

- The interpreting radiologist should include significant incidental findings that need attention, with recommended follow-up, in the "Impression" section of the report.

- Questions about the findings in a radiology report are best answered by the radiologist who interpreted the exam.

Legend/Abbreviations:

ASCVD = atherosclerotic cardiovascular disease
CAC = coronary artery calcification
CE = contrast enhanced
CT = computed tomography
→ = action recommended, text in **Bold** type

MR = magnetic resonance imaging
OK = typically, but not always, insignificant or benign
US = ultrasound
w/u: = work up with follow-up imaging
PCP = primary care provider

Anatomic Region	Findings/Recommendations
Abdominal	
Adrenal[1]	• Adrenal calcification – OK. • Nodule < 10 HU (fat density), likely adenoma – OK. • Soft tissue density nodule < 1 cm – OK. • Adrenal nodule stable ≥ 1 year – OK. → **Any other nodule or mass → w/u: CE Adrenal CT or MRI.**
Kidney[2]	• Non-obstructing renal calculi – OK. • Simple or hyperdense/hemorrhagic cyst ("Bosniak 1 or 2") < 4 cm – OK. → **Soft tissue density (or mixed density) renal mass → w/u: CT or MRI of the Kidneys without and with IV contrast.**
Liver[3]	• Simple cyst – OK. • Nodule < 1 cm – OK, likely benign. → **Soft tissue nodule/mass ≥ 1cm → w/u: CE Abdomen CT or MRI.** → **Fatty liver/hepatic steatosis or cirrhosis → PCP evaluation.**
Pancreas[4]	• Coarse calcifications – OK. → **Cyst/mass → w/u: CE Abdomen CT or MRI.**
Musculoskeletal	
Bone Density[13,14,15]	• > 130 HU at L1 – OK. → **100 – 130 HU at L1 (Osteopenia) → consider PCP evaluation.** → **< 100 HU at L1 (Osteoporosis) → PCP evaluation and consider DEXA.**
Other	• Degenerative disc disease – OK.

a

Fig. 15.1 (**a**) ACR lung cancer screening incidental findings quick reference guide (Page 1). (**b**) ACR lung cancer screening incidental findings quick reference guide (Page 2)

Cardiovascular	
Aorta[6]	• "Ectasia of the thoracic aorta" – OK. • Mural calcification – OK. • Ascending Aorta < 42mm – OK. → **Ascending Aorta ≥ 42 mm → PCP surveillance or cardiology consult for aneurysm surveillance.**
Cardiac/pericardium	• Trace/small pericardial effusion – OK. → **Moderate or large pericardial effusion → discuss with PCP.** → **Other Abnormalities (such as moderate or greater aortic valve calcification) → PCP evaluation.**
Coronary arteries[7,8]	• Coronary artery calcifications (CAC) typically reported as none, mild, moderate, or severe. → **CAC present → PCP evaluation for ASCVD risk assessment.**
Main PA measurement[9,10]	• < 31 mm – OK. • **→ 31 mm → PCP evaluation, consider Cardiology or Pulmonary consult.**
Breast	
	• Coarse calcifications – OK. • Cyst with no associated solid component – OK. → **Any other nodule/mass or asymmetric density → w/u: diagnostic mammogram +/- US.**
Esophagus	
	→ **Large hiatal hernia or dilated esophagus → PCP evaluation.** → **Focal wall thickening or mass → PCP evaluation, consider GI consult.**
Lung/Pleura	
Lung[11]	• Atelectasis – mild/subsegmental – OK. • Emphysema/bronchial wall thickening (Expected findings) – consider PCP evaluation; may benefit from Pulmonary consult. → **Fibrotic interstitial lung disease (ILD) → recommend pulmonary consultation.** → **Bronchiectasis/ground glass opacity/cystic lung disease/diffuse nodular disease → PCP evaluation, consider pulmonary consultation.**
Pleura	→ **New disease – effusion, thickening, mass → PCP evaluation, consider pulmonary consultation.**
Mediastinum	
Lymph nodes (Short axis measurement)[12]	• < 15 mm – OK. → **≥ 15 mm & no explainable cause → PCP evaluation; consider pulmonary consultation. Consider follow-up CE Chest CT in 3–6 months.**
Other[12]	• Cyst – OK. → **Mass (soft tissue or mixed density) → CE Chest MRI or CT.**
Thyroid[16]	
Features	• Large and heterogeneous, likely goiter – probably OK; consider thyroid function testing. • Nodule < 15 mm – OK. → **Nodule ≥ 15 mm or with suspicious features → w/u: thyroid US and clinical evaluation.**

b   Link to the ACR white papers on incidental findings:
https://publish.smartsheet.com/42d18e874a164318a0f702481f2fbb70

Fig. 15.1 (continued)

Unnecessary additional testing following LDCT is a significant concern among providers and patients. To minimize the risk of additional testing, the ACR Quick Guide clearly outlines the most common incidental findings, which need follow-up and which are considered insignificant. Additional testing related to IFs may include a dedicated CT with or without contrast, MRI, or Ultrasound of that specific organ. Others may include primary care evaluation, cardiology, pulmonary, or gastrointestinal referrals [8].

While the ACR Quick Guide advises appropriate next steps, it is important to evaluate any IF within the clinical context of each individual patient. Patients should be screened for any potential symptoms or family history related to IF. At our urban academic medical center's centralized screening program, we review patient charts for previous workup of IFs and confirm patients are on appropriate medications for findings. It is critical to review all prior imaging, if available, to evaluate for stability or change [8].

The findings should be discussed in detail with the patient's primary care physician (PCP) and/or referring provider. While the LCS program may determine an IF does not require further intervention, the PCP may feel differently based on prior interactions with the patient and additional findings that are unknown to the screening program.

Reporting Incidental Findings on LCS, "S" Modifier

Ideally, the radiologist interpreting the LCS CT provides clear guidance regarding recommended follow-up in the CT report. This can be optimized if the LCS report contains a section dedicated to "significant incidental findings" or "other actionable findings." Studies have shown that appropriate follow-up is improved if actionable items are listed in the Impression section of the report [21]. It is also important that the CT report indicate when an IF does not need follow-up to avoid unnecessary cost and resource utilization and any potential complications of unneeded work-up.

Radiologists typically use the ACR Lung CT Screening Reporting and Data System (Lung-RADS) to report LCS CT. The Lung-RADS classifies the CT findings into categories 0,1,2,3,4A,4B, and 4X based on the size, characteristics, and behavior of lung nodules [22, 23].

Lung-RADS includes an "S" modifier for IFs. The radiologist should add the modifier to the Lung-RADS category when there is a significant or potentially significant IF. The modifier flags the report indicating an IF is present that needs further attention. It is to be used when there is a new or previously unknown finding. The modifier does not need to be used if the finding is already known such as CAC which was described on a previous LCS CT. The S modifier can be particularly useful on the baseline CT such as identifying interstitial lung disease (ILD) in a patient with no prior diagnosis of ILD.

Repeated use of the modifier is however not needed unless there is a new IF or significant change in a pre-existing IF such as increased size of an aortic aneurysm. The "S" modifier is unfortunately used inconsistently [5]. An IF is deemed "clinically significant" at the discretion of the reading radiologist. As a result, there is much variability in the reported prevalence and associated costs of IFs [5, 9, 11].

If the CT report does not contain clear recommendations for follow-up, the interpreting radiologist can be contacted for further information. The Quick Guide can be a useful resource for the navigators and referring providers to clarify the next steps and to discuss the rationale for follow-up with the LCS patients.

Common IFs on LDCT

The reported frequency of IFs in LCS varies considerably with studies reporting a wide range from 4 to 94% [11, 24–26]. The variability likely relates to having no consistent definition of what constitutes an IF and which are considered significant. The Quick Guide helps address this issue.

The most common IFs in LCS are pulmonary and cardiovascular abnormalities [2, 5, 9, 27]. A study by Morgan et al. found respiratory IFs in 69% of cases and cardiovascular IFs in 67.5% of cases [9]. In their review, nearly all patients had at least one reported IF but only 15% were actionable.

Most pulmonary IFs are related to emphysema, airways disease, or ILD. Emphysema is the most commonly reported IF, accounting for up to 75% of the pulmonary IFs. Since it is not unexpected, some argue it may not be appropriate to consider emphysema an "incidental" finding. However, most agree on the presence of emphysema can be significant and has prognostic value [28]. The extent (trace, mild, moderate, and severe) and type of emphysema (centrilobular, confluent, paraseptal, and advanced destructive) can be assessed on LCS CT (Fig. 15.2).

Interstitial lung disease is observed in 5–25% of patients receiving LCS CT [29–31]. Although not as common as emphysema and airways disease, it can be very significant and carry prognostic ramifications. Respiratory Bronchiolitis (RB) is the most common smoking-related ILD and typically appears as upper lung predominant hazy ground glass nodules (Fig. 15.3). Other smoking-related ILDs include Desquamative Interstitial Pneumonia (DIP) and Pulmonary Langerhans cell histiocytosis (LCH). RB-associated ILD, DIP, and Pulmonary LCH are considered

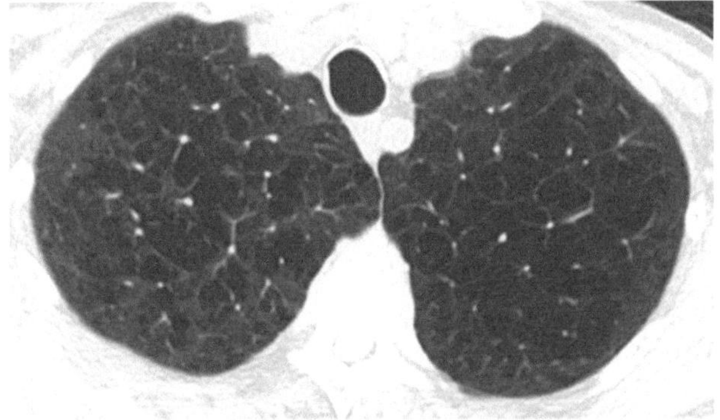

Fig. 15.2 72-year-old LCS patient with severe upper lung confluent emphysema

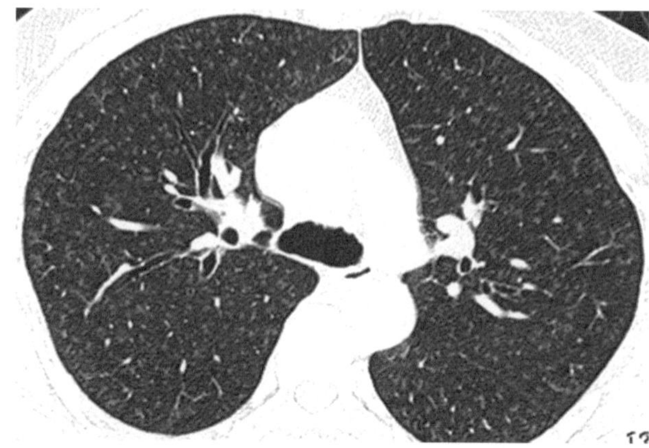

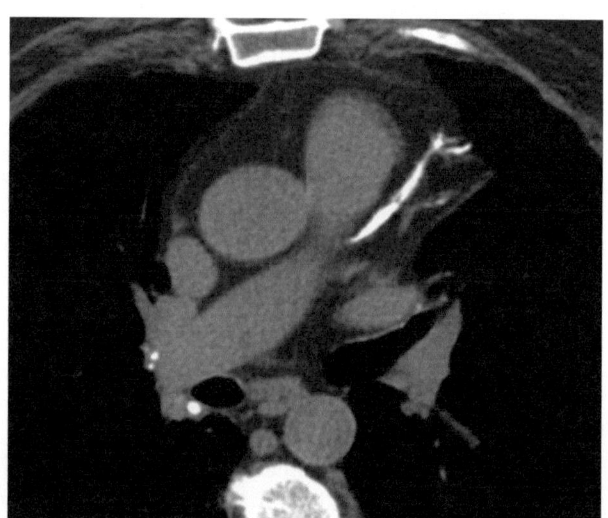

significant Ifs and the patients should receive a pulmonary consult. Fortunately, they usually respond favorably to smoking cessation.

Other forms of pulmonary fibrosis such as usual interstitial pneumonia (UIP) with reticulation, traction bronchiectasis, and honeycombing can be seen on LCS CT and are considered a significant IF. A recent report from an expert panel on ILD agreed that traction bronchiectasis and honeycombing warrant an S modifier in LCS and the patient should receive a pulmonary consult [32]. The group also recommended that even more mild forms of interstitial lung abnormality (ILA) with subpleural reticulation can progress and should be actively followed with yearly follow-up CT. In the setting of LCS, ILA can be re-evaluated on the next LCS CT.

Persons who smoke have an increased risk of coronary artery disease (CAD) which can be apparent on LCS-LDCT as CAC (Fig. 15.4). Multiple studies have shown CAC is a strong independent predictor of adverse future cardiac events

[33–37]. Morgan et al. reported CAC in 56% of patients undergoing LCS-LDCT [9]. Among National Lung Screening Trial (NLST) participants, 25% succumbed to cardiovascular disease [2]. Further analysis of CAC in the NLST confirmed the role LCS-LDCT can play in identifying CAC and indicated a visual scoring system (none, mild, moderate, and severe) is equivalent to the quantitative Agatston risk strata scoring [38]. The presence of moderate or severe CAC is considered significant and should be assigned an "S" modifier in Lung-RADS. Even patients with mild CAC, though not requiring an S-modifier, may benefit from ASCVD risk assessment as indicated in the Quick Guide.

The Quick Guide lists common IFs on LCS CT in the adrenal glands, kidneys, liver, pancreas, mediastinum, breast, and thyroid. As outlined in the Quick Guide, an abnormality in the imaged portions of these organs may or may not require further evaluation. Fortunately, the incidence of extrapulmonary malignancies in LCS is low, ranging from 0.4 to 1.6% [11, 39]. The most commonly diagnosed nonpulmonary malignancies found on LCS-LDCT are thyroid cancer, renal cancer, and lymphoma. Although LCS has the potential to identify unexpected malignancies or other disease, appropriate strategies should be used to avoid unnecessary testing. For example, while incidental thyroid nodules are commonly identified on chest CT, the overwhelming majority of thyroid nodules are benign. Management of thyroid nodules is primarily determined by the size of the nodule. In the LCS-eligible population, nodules <15 mm are typically benign with no need for follow-up. However, an ITN ≥ 15 mm (Fig. 15.5) is considered an actionable IF. An S modifier should be used and a thyroid ultrasound and clinical evaluation are recommended [14].

Another potentially significant IF on LCS-LDCT is low bone density. Individuals with a history of heavy cigarette smoking have an increased risk of osteoporosis [40]. CT attenuation values in vertebral bodies correlate with dual-energy X-ray absorptiometry (DEXA) values and are a useful tool to screen for osteoporosis [41].

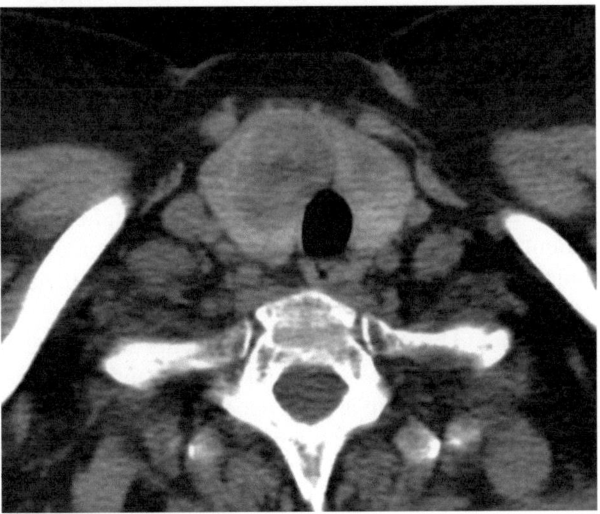

Fig. 15.5 60-year-old LCS patient with 3 cm right thyroid nodule

Bone density should be measured in the L1 vertebral body. Attenuation values <100 HU are consistent with osteoporosis and values 100–130 are concerning for osteopenia. Vertebral body fractures can be easily assessed on sagittal LDCT reconstructions [42, 43]. The LungRADS "S"-modifier should be used for these findings and further evaluation by the primary care provider is recommended.

Managing Incidental Findings in Centralized LCS Program

In some centralized screening Programs, the high likelihood of IF detection on LDCT is discussed with patients as part of the shared decision-making conversation. The dialogue should include the discovery of IFs but also potential additional testing/workup. Patients should be prepared and understand this risk before undergoing screening.

All prior imaging should be taken into consideration when assessing for stability or change in an IF. Any outside imaging should be obtained and uploaded to the patient's chart for a radiologist to review and make a formal comparison. After an IF has been reported, the LCS team performs a chart review to assess if the IF has been addressed by a PCP and/or specialist and if any diagnostic workup has been completed. For example, if a patient undergoes LDCT, and the radiologist reports an enlarged main pulmonary artery, the LCS team reviews the chart to determine if the patient recently completed an echocardiogram and whether pulmonary hypertension was noted. If severe coronary artery calcifications (CAC) are noted, the LCS team can look to see if the patient is on statin medication or is already followed by a cardiologist. If neither of these are present, LCS Programs can directly reach out to the PCP to discuss findings to ensure they will be addressed.

IFs should be reviewed in detail with the patient at an appropriate level for their health literacy. We encourage family members to be included in the discussion. It is important not to overwhelm them with information. After discussing each finding, we pause to confirm patient understanding. It is imperative to allow an opportunity for the patient and any family members to ask questions in a nonjudgmental space. When discussing findings, it is also crucial to describe clinical significance and whether any additional workup is needed. The information gathered from this chart review can help improve the patient's understanding and decrease their anxiety. The patient may feel more reassured knowing they are on a statin and followed by cardiology despite having severe CAC; therefore, their current care meets evidence-based guidelines [44].

IFs should be detailed in a results letter sent to the patient, PCP, and/or referring provider. We highlight or bold all findings and recommendations in the results letter, including IFs, making it stand out and more straightforward for providers to quickly identify results and recommendations.

In addition to the letters, our program sends additional communications via direct secure messaging and/or telephone calls to the PCP or referring provider for any actionable IFs. We discuss with the provider any additional imaging recommendations made by radiology before ordering subsequent testing. As part of the discussion, we determine whether the provider will be ordering the testing or if they would prefer the centralized program to place the order. Good communication and identification of the responsible provider are vital to ensure appropriate imaging and/or referrals are completed in a timely manner.

Multidisciplinary Team Approach

A multidisciplinary approach to IFs on LCS may not only improve outcomes but decrease unnecessary imaging. As a centralized LCS program, it is crucial to have an excellent collaborative and trusting relationship with primary care providers. Our program restructured our reporting process and letters based on feedback from their offices. We ensure any additional testing and referrals are made in partnership with the PCP.

To ensure we provide the best care to our patients, we collaborated with doctors and nurse practitioners from cardiology, pulmonary, vascular surgery, and thoracic surgery to create pathways for clinically significant IFs and better understand what constitutes a clinically significant finding as well as what requires further testing [45]. Working with each specialist allows us to efficiently identify individuals who require intervention.

In conjunction with various specialties, our LCS developed several pathways, including our cardiology-focused aortic aneurysm pathway, our thoracic surgery-based hernia/mediastinal pathway, our aortic aneurysm pathway in partnership with vascular surgery, and our pulmonary-driven interstitial lung disease and pulmonary hypertension pathway.

This multidisciplinary approach is not only reassuring to patients but also to their referring provider. Because it is not always clear which incidental findings are clinically significant or actionable, additional guidance from specialties can define IF management.

Additionally, these collaborative multispecialty pathways for incidental findings requiring a specialty referral make the referral process seamless. Curating relationships across specialties is crucial because when a clinically significant IF is identified, a referral is placed, and our pathway champions are contacted to ensure the patient is scheduled for further evaluation promptly. These multidisciplinary pathways take the onus off the patient and PCP and allow their appointments to focus on other health concerns while IFs are handled by the appropriate specialties. However, none of this is possible without having a strong foundation across specialties, a multidisciplinary team, and a willingness to work collaboratively. Without trust and confidence in your team, these referral processes will not work.

Conclusion

The main objective of lung cancer screening is to reduce lung cancer-related mortality through the early detection of lung cancer. It has a critical role in improving long-term outcomes and can decrease all-cause mortality. IFs detected on LDCT provide an opportunity to intervene and address abnormalities before disease progression. While there is a risk of additional, and at times unnecessary, imaging and workup based on findings, the benefits for some IFs outweigh the risks. It is part of the overall mission for centralized and decentralized LCS Programs, to appropriately manage IFs as part of comprehensive, high-quality screening care.

Collaboration with a multidisciplinary team to develop a structured and standardized approach to the handling of IFs helps ensure clinically significant findings are addressed. Furthermore, the standardization of IF reporting by radiologists is a crucial component of better management of IFs. It is imperative to remember that more than half of LDCT scans will likely identify a significant IF requiring intervention. This provides a valuable opportunity to impact outcomes and educate our patients on improving their overall health, which is the ultimate goal of preventative care.

References

1. American Cancer Society. American cancer society: cancer facts and figures 2021. Atlanta, GA: American Cancer Society; 2021.
2. The National Lung Screening Trial Research Team. Reduced lung-cancer mortality with low-dose computed tomographic screening. N Engl J Med. 2011;365(5):395–409.
3. Krist AH, US Preventive Services Task Force. Screening for lung cancer US preventive services task force recommendation statement. JAMA. 2021;325(10):962–70.
4. Mazzone PJ, Silvestri GA, Souter LH, Katki HA, Wiener RS, Detterbeck FC. Screening for lung cancer: CHEST guideline and expert panel report. Chest. 2013;160(5):E427–94.
5. Tsai EB, Chiles C, Carter BW, Godoy MCB, Shroff GS, Munden RF, et al. Incidental findings on lung cancer screening: significance and management. Semin Ultrasound CT MR. 2018;39(3):273–81; https://www.sciencedirect.com/science/article/pii/S0887217118300209.
6. O'Sullivan JW, Muntinga T, Grigg S, JPA I. Prevalence and outcomes of incidental imaging findings: umbrella review. BMJ. 2018;361:k2387; [cited 2021 Feb 23]. https://pubmed.ncbi.nlm.nih.gov/29914908/.
7. Powell DK. Patient explanation guidelines for incidentalomas: helping patients not to fear the delayed surveillance. AJR Am J Roentgenol. 2014;202:W602. https://doi.org/10.2214/AJR.13.12337.
8. American College of Radiology. ACR lung cancer screening CT incidental findings quick reference guide; 2021. https://www.acr.org/-/media/ACR/Files/Lung-Cancer-Screening-Resources/LCS-Incidental-Findings-Quick-Guide-Oct-2021.pdf.
9. Morgan L, Choi H, Reid M, Khawaja A, Mazzone PJ. Frequency of incidental findings and subsequent evaluation in low-dose computed tomographic scans for lung cancer screening. Ann Am Thorac Soc. 2017;14(9):1450–6.
10. U.S. Department of Health and Human Services. The health consequences of smoking—50 years of progress: a report of the surgeon general. Atlanta, GA: U.S. Department of Health and

Human Services, Centers for Disease Control and Prevention, National Center for Chronic Disease Prevention and Health Promotion, Office on Smoking and Health; 2014.
11. Nguyen XV, Davies L, Eastwood JD, Hoang JK. Extrapulmonary findings and malignancies in participants screened with chest CT in the national lung screening trial. J Am Coll Radiol. 2017;14(3):324–30.
12. Berland LL, Silverman SG, Gore RM, Mayo-Smith WW, Megibow AJ, Yee J, Brink JA, Baker ME, Federle MP, Foley WD, et al. Managing incidental findings on abdominal CT: white paper of the ACR incidental findings committee. J Am Coll Radiol. 2010;7:754–73.
13. Berland LL. Overview of white papers of the ACR incidental findings committee II on adnexal, vascular, splenic, nodal, gallbladder, and biliary findings. J Am Coll Radiol. 2013;10:672–4.
14. Hoang JK, Langer JE, Middleton WD, Wu CC, Hammers LW, Cronan JJ, Tessler FN, Grant EG, Berland LL. Managing incidental thyroid nodules detected on imaging: white paper of the ACR incidental thyroid findings committee. J Am Coll Radiol. 2015;12:143–50.
15. Megibow AJ, Baker ME, Morgan DE, et al. Management of the incidental pancreatic cysts: a white paper of the ACR incidental findings committee. J Am Coll Radiol. 2017;14:911–23.
16. Mayo-Smith WW, Song JH, Boland GL, et al. Management of incidental adrenal masses: a white paper of the ACR incidental findings committee. J Am Coll Radiol. 2017;14:1038–44.
17. Gore RM, Pickhardt PJ, Mortele KJ, et al. J management of incidental liver lesions on CT: a white paper of the ACR incidental findings committee. J Am Coll Radiol. 2017;13:1429–37.
18. Herts BR, Silverman SG, Hindman NM, et al. Management of the incidental renal mass on CT: a white paper of the ACR incidental findings committee. J Am Coll Radiol. 2018;15:264–73.
19. Munden RF, Carter BW, Chiles C, et al. Managing incidental findings on thoracic CT: mediastinal and cardiovascular findings. A white paper of the ACR incidental findings committee. J Am Coll Radiol. 2018;15:1087–96.
20. Munden RF, Black WC, Hartman TE, et al. Managing incidental findings on thoracic CT: lung findings. A white paper of the ACR incidental findings committee. J Am Coll Radiol. 2021;18(9):1267–79.
21. Blagev DP, Lloyd JF, Conner K, Dickerson J, Adams D, Stevens SM, et al. Follow-up of incidental pulmonary nodules and the radiology report. J Am Coll Radiol. 2016;13(2 Suppl):R18–24.
22. American College of Radiology. Lung CT screening reporting and data system. https://www. acr.org/Clinical-Resources/Reporting-and-Data-Systems/Lung-Rads.
23. McKee BJ. In: Muller NL, Finlay G, editors. Lung-RADS standardized reporting for low-dose computed tomography for lung cancer screening; 2022; https://www.uptodate.com/contents/lung-rads-standardized-reporting-for-low-dose-computed-tomography-for-lung-cancer-screening#H687802840.
24. Kinsinger LS, Anderson C, Kim J, et al. Implementation of lung cancer screening in the veterans health administration. JAMA Intern Med. 2017;177(3):399–406.
25. Janssen K, Schertz K, Rubin N, Begnaud A. Incidental findings in a decentralized lung cancer screening program. Ann Am Thorac Soc. 2019;16(9):1198–200.
26. Reiter MJ, Nemesure A, Madu E, et al. Frequency and distribution of incidental findings deemed appropriate for S modifier designation on low-dose CT in lung cnacer screening program. Lung Cancer. 2018;120:1–6.
27. Chung JH, Richards JC, Koelsch TL, et al. Screening for lung cancer: incidental pulmonary parenchymal findings. AJR. 2018;210:1–11.
28. Steiger D, Siddiqi MF, Yip R, et al. The importance of low-dose CT screening to identify emphysema in asymptomatic participants with and without a prior diagnosis of COPD. Clin Imaging. 2021;78:136–41.
29. Sverzellati N, Guerci L, Randi G, et al. Interstitial lung disease in a lung cancer screening trial. Eur Respir J. 2011;38:392–400.
30. Gy J, Lynch D, Chawla A, et al. Interstitial lung abnormalities in a CT lung cancer screening population: prevalence and progression rate. Radiology. 2013;268:563–71.
31. Salvatore M, Henschke CI, Yip R, et al. Evidence of interstitial lung disease on low-dose chest CT images: prevalence, patterns, and progression. AJR. 2016;206:487–94.

32. Hunninghake GM, Goldin JG, Kadoch MA, Kropski JA, Rosas IO, Wells AU, Yadav R, Lazarus HM, Abtin FG, Corte TJ, et al. Detection and early referral of patients with interstitial lung abnormalities an expert survey initiative. Chest. 2022;161(2):470–282.
33. Polonsky TS, McClelland RL, Jorgensen NW, et al. Coronary artery calcium score and risk classification for coronary heart disease prediction. JAMA. 2010;303:1610–6.
34. Shemesh J, Henschke CI, Shaham D, et al. Ordinal scoring of coronary artery calcifications on low-dose CT scans of the chest is predictive of death from cardiovascular disease. Radiology. 2010;257:541–8.
35. Malcolm KB, Dinwoodey DL, Cundiff MC, Regis SM, Borondy Kitts AK, Wald C, Lynch ML, Al-Husami W, McKee AB, McKee BJ. Qualitative coronary artery calcium assessment on CT lung screening exam helps predict first cardiac events. J Thorac Dis. 2018;10(5):2740–51. https://doi.org/10.21037/jtd.2018.04.76.
36. Mori H, Torii S, Kutyna M, et al. Coronary artery calcification and its progression: what does it really mean? J Am Coll Cardiol Img. 2018;11(1):127–42.
37. Schulman-Marcus J, Valenti V, et al. Prognostic utility of coronary artery calcium scoring in active smokers: a 15-year follow-up study. Int J Cardiol. 2014;177(2):581–3.
38. Chiles C, Duan F, Gladish GW, et al. Association of coronary artery calcification and mortality in the national lung screening trial: a comparison of three scoring methods. Radiology. 2015;276(1):82–90.
39. Rampinelli C, Preda L, Maniglio M, et al. Extrapulmonary malignancies detected at lung cancer screening. Radiology. 2011;261:293–9.
40. Bolland MJ, Grey AB, Gamble GD, Reid IR. Effect of osteoporosis treatment on mortality: a meta-analysis. J Clin Endocrinol Metab. 2010;95:1174–81.
41. Romme EAPM, Murchison JT, Phang KF, Jansen FH, Rutten EPA, Wouters EFM, et al. Bone attenuation on routine chest CT correlates with bone mineral density on DXA in patients with COPD. J Bone Miner Res. 2012;27:2338–43.
42. Woo EK, Mansoubi H, Alyas F. Incidental vertebral fractures on multidetector CT images of the chest: prevalence and recognition. Clin Radiol. 2008;63(2):160–4.
43. Chan PL, Reddy T, Milne D, Bolland MJ. Incidental vertebral fractures on computed tomography. N Z Med J. 2012;125:45–50.
44. Arnett DK, Blumenthal RS, Albert MA, et al. 2019 ACC/AHA guideline on the primary prevention of cardiovascular disease: a report of the American College of Cardiology/American Heart Association task force on clinical practice guidelines. Circulation. 2019;140:e596–646.
45. Majeed A, Ruane B, Shusted CS, Austin M, Mirzozoda K, Pimpinelli M, Vojnika J, Ward L, Sundaram B, Lakhani P, Kane G, Lev Y, Barta JA. Frequency of statin prescription among individuals with coronary artery calcifications detected through lung cancer screening. Am J Med Qual. 2022;37(5):388–95.

Chapter 16
Leveraging the Electronic Health Record for Continuous Quality

Bracken Babula

Background

Screening for lung cancer using low-dose computed tomography (LDCT) has been recommended by the United States Preventive Services Task Force (USPSTF) since 2014 [1]. Compared to other types of cancer, screening for lung cancer is particularly complex due to multipart inclusion criteria, associated risk and harms, regulatory requirements, and structured reporting needs [2]. Though small-scale screening programs may be able to address these complexities with basic tracking tools, most large institutions will need to leverage their electronic health record (EHR) to optimize the quality of care and reduce the morbidity and mortality associated with lung cancer. In this chapter, we detail the complexities involved in screening for lung cancer and how the EHR can be utilized to achieve continuous quality.

Screening Guidelines and Coverage

When identifying a cancer screening test, it is important to consider disease severity, the prevalence in the target population, the ability to diagnose and treat prior to the development of symptoms, and reduction of morbidity or mortality from the treatment [3]. These criteria have been used by organizations like the USPSTF to recommend screening tests for breast, cervical, colorectal, and lung cancers while finding insufficient evidence to support screening for ovarian, pancreatic, prostate, testicular, thyroid, bladder, oral, or skin cancers [4]. The evidence for breast, colon, and cervical cancer screening supports targeting a population-based primarily on

B. Babula (✉)
Department of Medicine, Thomas Jefferson University, Philadelphia, PA, USA
e-mail: Bracken.Babula@Jefferson.edu

G. C. Kane et al. (eds.), *Lung Cancer Screening*,
https://doi.org/10.1007/978-3-031-33596-9_16

age and/or gender. By contrast, the target population for lung cancer screening is significantly more complex with criteria that include age, smoking history, and other factors. Initial coverage determinations in 2015 from the Centers for Medicare and Medicaid Services (CMS) also added significant complexity to performing LDCT for the purposes of lung cancer screening [5].

The initial guidelines from the USPSTF found grade B evidence to support screening for lung cancer in current or former smokers aged 55 to 80 with a 30-pack-year smoking history [1], and a follow-up recommendation in 2021 amended the guidelines to include current or former smokers aged 50 to 80 with a 20-pack-year smoking history [6]. In both recommendations, the USPSTF recommends discontinuing screening when a person has not smoked for 15 years or has a health problem that substantially limits life expectancy. Similar recommendations have been released from other professional societies with slight variations, such as the American College of Chest Physicians [7] and the American Cancer Society [8].

In 2015, CMS released a coverage determination that approved LDCT for this patient population, but added additional requirements for insurance coverage. These requirements included specific elements necessary for the LDCT order, eligibility criteria for radiologists and radiology imaging facilities, and the use of a CMS-approved registry [5]. In 2022, CMS updated their coverage determination to match the 2021 USPSTF patient population and also to simplify the requirements for coverage of LDCT. The new coverage determination reduces the specific requirements for the LDCT order and reading radiologists and also removes the requirement that facilities participate in a CMS-approved registry [9]. Pursuant to the Patient Protection and Affordable Care Act passed in 2010, private health insurance must also cover screenings with a grade A or B recommendation from the USPSTF [10].

EHRs and Quality Metrics

There are a wide variety of options to address the complexities of lung cancer screening via the EHR. Some institutions will choose to implement large-scale programs with fully integrated EHR-based lung cancer screening programs. Alternatively, lung cancer screening can be supported by a third-party vendor or through standard computer database programs [11]. The larger the program, the more necessary it is to have an integrated EHR system that can track patients across the continuum of care, from identification to screening and onto follow-up. The National Lung Cancer Roundtable has identified a minimum list of features for an effective lung cancer screening software system (Table 16.1).

The features noted above serve two main functions in supporting a high-quality lung cancer screening program. The first is to ensure the collection of data required for reporting to CMS-approved registries such as the American College of Radiology's Lung Cancer Screening Registry (ACR-LCSR) (Table 16.2). The ACR-LCSR provides peer comparisons to participating institutions and physicians to help improve the quality of lung cancer screening programs [12]. The second function is

Table 16.1 Minimum recommended features and capability of a lung cancer screening software system [11]

Full integration and compatibility with existing EHR and patient portal
Patient registration and recall desk with full interface with EHR
Universal compatibility with all integrated digital imaging and communications in medicine software formats
Full capability of data extraction (lung-RADS category) from radiology reports
Lung nodule tracking and surveillance
Non-lung nodule (incidental findings) tracking
Automatic laboratory results interface and integration
Navigator dashboard
Complement of templated and customizable letters, integrated mail merge, and documentation of telephone communication with the EHR
Full automaticity in capturing all ACR-LCSR data elements
Full automaticity in routine batching and upload of ACR-LCSR data elements
Full capability to create data fields specific to individual screening program
Full capability to query and report data for lung cancer screening program quality and outcomes evaluation

Table 16.2 Required fields in the ACR-LCSR [13]

Patient data
Age
Sex
Height, weight
Smoking status
Pack years and years since quitting
Smoking cessation guidance?
Shared decision making?
Signs or symptoms of lung cancer
Exam data
Facility, radiologist, and ordering practitioner NPIs
CT scanner manufacturer and model
Radiation dose/modality
Screening date
Result data
Lung-RADS category
Other significant abnormalities (modifier S)
Prior history of cancer (modifier C)
Follow-up data (as applicable)
Follow-up date
Diagnostic test
Tissue diagnosis and histology
Location
Stage
Follow-up months

Table 16.3 Recommended quality metrics [14]

Access
Number referred
Number qualified
Number scanned
Number enrolled
Number discharged
Referral source
Smoking
Number current
Number former
Number quit
Number relapsed
Radiology
Lung-RADS category
"S" positive
Coronary calcifications
Emphysema
Cancer detection rate
Stage
Histology
Presumed by consensus
Noninvasive procedures
Pulmonary consults
PET/CT
Invasive procedures
Percutaneous biopsy
Bronchoscopy with biopsy
Surgery
Benign disease by modality

to allow for the collection of internal data that can be used by individual programs to ensure high-quality care. The American Thoracic Society has created a list of internal quality metrics that may be considered for use by individual institutions (Table 16.3).

Once an institution has identified the EHR, registry reporting requirements, and quality metrics that will be tracked internally, the next step is to identify the tools and workflows within the EHR to support high-quality care. In a lung cancer screening program, the EHR should be leveraged prior to screening, during the screening process, and for tracking and reporting purposes after screening.

Identification of Patients for Screening

The first step in leveraging the EHR for a successful lung cancer screening program is identifying appropriate patients for screening. The increased adoption of EHRs has contributed to a steady increase in cancer screening rates, with clear benefits related to using EHR tools for breast and colorectal cancer screening [15, 16]. Identifying patients for breast and colorectal cancer screening is accomplished by using two data points that exist in every EHR: age and gender. Additional EHR features also support custom recall frequencies based on recent results or allow providers to easily exclude patients for a variety of reasons. By contrast, identifying patients for lung cancer screening is significantly more complex.

In order to perform a LDCT for lung cancer screening, a minimum set of data must be identified and input into the EHR prior to placing the order. How that information is collected and who inputs the information into the EHR are important considerations for all lung cancer screening programs. It is also important to balance accuracy versus precision as programs consider how to collect the two most relevant discrete data points for lung cancer screening: current smoking status and pack-years smoked.

Smoking status is frequently documented in the EHR as part of smoking cessation quality improvement metrics from programs such as the Healthcare Effectiveness Data and Information Set (HEDIS), Consumer Assessment of Healthcare Providers and Systems (CAHPS), Medicare Access and CHIP Reauthorization (MACRA), and Meaningful Use [17]. There is some evidence to suggest that when present, smoking status and years since quitting are accurately recorded in the EHR [18]. But none of the quality programs listed above have ever emphasized the accuracy of smoking intensity. As a result, even if recorded at all, pack-year data in the EHR correlates less well with actual smoking history [18].

Lung cancer screening programs should attempt to balance the available resources in order to screen the most number of eligible patients. For example, a program with a large centralized staff may opt to identify all current and former smokers and collect accurate smoking data, while a smaller or decentralized program may opt to encourage staff and providers to update smoking information at the point of care. The latter approach may miss more than half of eligible patients due to inaccurate EHR data [19], but may be necessary if a centralized team is not available. To improve the accuracy and completeness of smoking data, consider using real-time alerts to staff or providers to update smoking data that is missing or out of date (Fig. 16.1).

Once data in the EHR has been updated as best as possible, there are two general approaches to the identification of patients for lung cancer screening. Using a "strict" identification criteria, the EHR can be used to identify patients in the correct

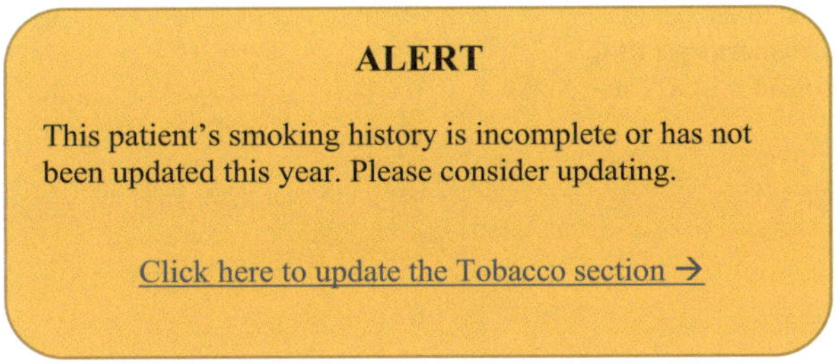

Fig. 16.1 Real-time EHR alert to encourage providers or staff to update tobacco information

age group, smoking status, pack years, and years since quitting if applicable. A more "broad" identification criteria might be used to identify all patients in a certain age group with a current or former smoking status, regardless of documented smoking intensity.

Shared Decision Making and Smoking Cessation Counseling

After patients have been identified for possible lung cancer screening, the next step is to perform shared decision making (SDM) and smoking cessation counseling, if applicable. Though SDM is commonly encouraged for other cancer screening studies, lung cancer screening is the first to have SDM required for insurance coverage [2, 5] and this requirement has been maintained in the updated CMS coverage determination [9]. A standardized approach to SDM within the EHR can help to ensure patient preferences are respected and providers properly document their conversations.

Various models exist to support SDM within EHRs, with one such model recommending the following four phases: (1) identifying the context for SDM and initiating the process, (2) exploring options for care, (3) deliberation between patient and provider on the risks and benefits of different approaches, and (4) monitoring of ongoing care to ensure treatments respect preferences [20]. Once patients are identified, real-time alerts should be used in the EHR to encourage providers to perform SDM or to refer to a centralized team to perform the SDM (Fig. 16.2). Consider whether or not to make these alerts a "pop-up" versus an asynchronous or silent alert based on the preferences of your institution and users.

Whether SDM is performed by the referring provider or a central team, the EHR should be configured to present the available options to the provider and patient and allow for documentation of the outcome in real time. At a minimum, approved options for SDM [14] should be hyperlinked from the EHR. If possible, the SDM tool should be configured to extract discrete data from the EHR to streamline the process.

In addition to SDM, patients who are currently smoking should receive smoking cessation guidance using similarly structured tools. EHRs should be used to send electronic referrals to smoking cessation programs and electronic prescriptions for

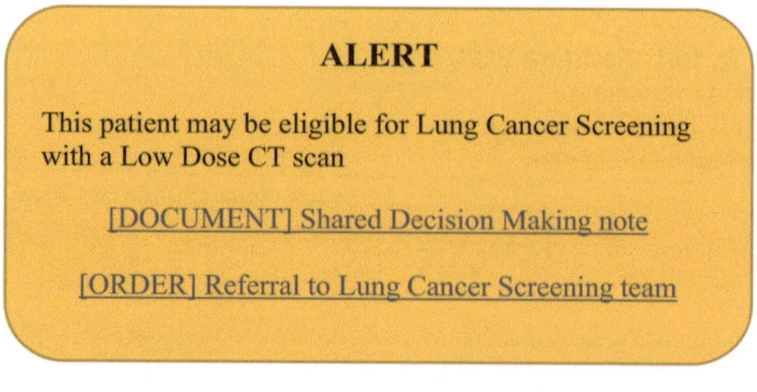

Fig. 16.2 Real-time EHR alert to encourage providers or staff to consider LDCT and SDM

smoking cessation medications. Some healthcare provider organizations have included a smoking cessation order set which might include various therapeutic options including doses as well as nicotine replacement therapy. By standardizing the identification, referral, and SDM process, lung cancer programs can ensure the proper collection of the standardized data required to order LDCT studies and properly follow patient outcomes.

Screening, Results, and Follow-up

As highlighted above, identifying and referring patients for lung cancer screening is one of the biggest barriers to a successful program. Once the order has been placed, most EHRs should be configured to manage the LDCT order similar to any other cancer screening or radiology request. Some of the most important considerations include ensuring an efficient and effective scheduling process, as well as maintaining tracking tools for screening completion and follow-up [2].

Scheduling for LDCT should be carefully protocolized to encourage proper tracking throughout the process. Work queues should be configured within the EHR to identify patients with an order that has not been scheduled, scheduled orders not yet completed, and scheduled orders that were subsequently canceled or no-showed. For programs seeing a large number of no-show appointments or last-minute cancellations, consider utilizing additional EHR functionality including patient education tools, dynamic scheduling, and/or more effective appointment reminders [21]. Distinguishing between initial LDCT, subsequent LDCT, or follow-up imaging is also an important aspect of the scheduling process that is often a challenge for lung cancer screening programs [22].

Once the LDCT is performed and read, it is important to properly route the results. Tracking tools in the EHR can be utilized to identify studies by their Lung-RADS category as well as any additional significant ("S") findings. EHRs have flexible routing tools to identify the proper recipient of results, which may include central team members, ordering providers, or primary care providers. Though guidelines often recommend routing incidental findings back to the patient's primary care physician [23], there may be insufficient data to support this as standard practice. In a recent analysis of primary care provider response to incidental findings, some "felt compelled but frustrated" to follow-up on these findings, while others report not acting on results that are unfamiliar or occur in an unusual clinical context [24]. This process can be aided by including standard guidelines from the American College of Radiology with regard to standard follow-up for typical incidental findings such as thyroid nodules, coronary artery calcification, unexpected pulmonary findings, and renal, pancreas, liver, or adrenal nodules or lesions [25].

In each step of the process, from identification, to referral, order, scheduling, and resulting, the EHR can be used to ensure high-quality care. It is important for lung cancer screening program leaders to maintain a close relationship with EHR analysts and architects to ensure the system is designed to achieve the desired outcomes.

Reporting and Maintaining Quality

EHRs contain a variety of tools for tracking and reporting outcomes from screening programs. Most large EHRs support robust population health tools, while smaller EHRs may support basic reports and analysis. Lung cancer screening programs should identify relevant quality metrics and create dashboards and reports to provide real-time feedback.

Dashboards for quality improvement have become ubiquitous in EHRs, but for a relatively new screening program such as lung cancer, EHR administrators may need to customize their own tools. Successful dashboards not only provide real-time quality metrics, but they should also provide benchmarks to compare to similar institutions or national averages [11]. The primary process measure should be the percentage of eligible patients that are screened, as a surrogate for the outcome measure of 20% reduction in lung-cancer mortality as measured by the National Lung Screening Trial [26]. Additional process measures on the dashboard should track how closely patients enrolled in the program adhere to the USPSTF and ACR guidelines.

Reporting tools should also be made available from the dashboards to allow program staff or individual providers to monitor their quality metrics. Providers can use reports to identify patients that may qualify but have not been screened, or patients that were screened but not appropriately followed-up. Robust data from the EHR can help to inform ways to approve each step of the process from identification, to screening, to follow-up.

The quality metrics associated with lung cancer screening programs should be used to highlight successes and identify weaknesses by taking advantage of data transparency within the EHR. Each institution may prioritize different aspects to define high-quality care, but the overall goal should be leveraging the EHR to maintain a highly effective screening program. Ideally, lung cancer screening programs would use HER quality data to create rapid cycle improvements and enhance important outcome measures such as follow-up rates and referrals. This will be particularly important since early cohort studies suggest that follow-up after initial scans may be less than 25%, representing an important opportunity for improvement guided by EHR data [27].

Conclusions

There is a balance to strike in lung cancer screening between collecting enough data to ensure high-quality care while not making data collection so burdensome that it prevents screening. The complexities of this screening compared to other cancer screenings have been cited as the greatest system-level barrier [2], and likely explain why only about one out of eight eligible patients have been recently screened for lung cancer [28]. Recent changes to CMS coverage determination simplify some of these complexities, but it remains to be seen if these changes are significant enough to improve screening rates. EHRs should be leveraged to increase screening rates and improve the quality of care, while also minimizing the associated complexities. While there is no universal solution for EHR configuration, there are several standards that can be implemented to support a high-quality lung cancer screening program.

References

1. Moyer V. Screening for lung cancer: US preventive services task force recommendation statement. Ann Intern Med. 2014;160:330–3.
2. Carter-Harris L, Gould M. Multilevel barriers to the successful implementation of lung cancer screening: why does it have to be so hard? Ann Am Thorac Soc. 2017;14(8):1261–5.
3. Herman C, Gill H, Eng J, Fajardo L. Screening for preclinical disease: test and disease characteristics. Am J Roentgenol. 2002;179(4):825–31.
4. United States preventive services taskforce. Uspreventiveservicestaskforceorg. 2022 [cited 26 February 2022]. https://www.uspreventiveservicestaskforce.org/uspstf/.
5. Final National Coverage Determination on Screening for Lung Cancer with Low Dose Computed Tomography (LDCT). Cms.gov. 2015 [cited 26 February 2022]. https://www.cms.gov/medicare-coverage-database/view/ncacal-decision-memo.aspx?proposed=N&NCAId=274.
6. Krist A, Davidson K, Mangione C, Barry M, Cabana M, Caughey A, et al. Screening for lung cancer: US preventive services task force recommendation statement. JAMA. 2021;325(10):962.
7. Mazzone P, Silvestri G, Souter L, Caverly T, Kanne J, Katki H, et al. Screening for lung cancer. Chest. 2021;160(5):e427–94.
8. American Cancer Society. Lung Cancer Screening Guidelines. Cancer.org. 2018 [cited 26 February 2022]. https://www.cancer.org/health-care-professionals/american-cancer-society-prevention-early-detection-guidelines/lung-cancer-screening-guidelines.html.
9. Final National Coverage Determination on Screening for Lung Cancer with Low Dose Computed Tomography (LDCT). Cms.gov. 2022 [cited 26 February 2022]. https://www.cms.gov/medicare-coverage-database/view/ncacal-decision-memo.aspx?proposed=N&ncaid=304.
10. Interim final rules for group health plans and health insurance issuers relating to coverage of preventive services under the patient protection and affordable care act. Office of the federal register, national archives and records administration. 2010.
11. Fathi J, White C, Greenberg G, Mazzone P, Smith R, Thomson C. The integral role of the electronic health record and tracking software in the implementation of lung cancer screening—a call to action to developers. Chest. 2020;157(6):1674–9.
12. Lung cancer screening registry. Acrorg 2022 [cited 26 February 2022]. https://www.acr.org/Practice-Management-Quality-Informatics/Registries/Lung-Cancer-Screening-Registry.
13. LCSR required data elements. ACR Support 2019 [cited 12 Feb 2022]. https://nrdrsupport.acr.org/support/solutions/articles/11000041252.
14. Thomson C, McKee A, Borondy-Kitts A, Kelley K, Cooke D, Lamb C et al. Lung cancer screening implementation guide. 2018 [cited 12 February 2022]. https://www.lungcancer-screeningguide.org/.
15. Shekelle P, Pane J, Agniel D, Shi Y, Rumball-Smith J, Haas A, et al. Assessment of variation in electronic health record capabilities and reported clinical quality performance in ambulatory care clinics, 2014-2017. JAMA Netw Open. 2021;4(4):e217476.

16. Kern L, Barrón Y, Dhopeshwarkar R, Edwards A, Kaushal R. Electronic health records and ambulatory quality of care. J Gen Intern Med. 2012;28(4):496–503.
17. American Lung Association. Tobacco cessation and quality measures: an overview. 2019. http://lung.org.
18. Patel N, Miller D, Snavely A, Bellinger C, Foley K, Case D, et al. A comparison of smoking history in the electronic health record with self-report. Am J Prev Med. 2020;58(4):591–5.
19. Modin H, Fathi J, Gilbert C, Wilshire C, Wilson A, Aye R, et al. Pack-year cigarette smoking history for determination of lung cancer screening eligibility. Comparison of the electronic medical record versus a shared decision-making conversation. Ann Am Thorac Soc. 2017;14(8):1320–5.
20. Lenert L, Dunlea R, Del Fiol G, Hall L. A model to support shared decision making in electronic health records systems. Med Decis Mak. 2014;34(8):987–95.
21. Marbouh D, Khaleel I, Al Shanqiti K, Al Tamimi M, Simsekler M, Ellahham S, et al. Evaluating the impact of patient no-shows on service quality. Risk Manag Healthc Policy. 2020;13:509–17.
22. Gould M, Sakoda L, Ritzwoller D, Simoff M, Neslund-Dudas C, Kushi L, et al. Monitoring lung cancer screening use and outcomes at four cancer research network sites. Ann Am Thorac Soc. 2017;14(12):1827–35.
23. American College of Radiology. ACR lung cancer screening CT incidental findings. 2021. http://acr.org/lungresources.
24. Zafar H, Bugos E, Langlotz C, Frasso R. "Chasing a ghost": factors that influence primary care physicians to follow up on incidental imaging findings. Radiology. 2016;281(2):567–73.
25. American College of Radiology. ACR lung cancer screening CT incidental findings quick reference guide. 2021. https://www.acr.org/-/media/ACR/Files/Lung-Cancer-Screening-Resources/LCS-Incidental-Findings-Quick-Guide-Oct-2021.pdf.
26. The National Lung Screening Trial Research Team. Reduced lung-cancer mortality with low-dose computed tomographic screening. N Engl J Med. 2011;365(5):395–409.
27. Silvestri GA, Goldman L, Burleson J, Gould M, Kazerooni A, Mazzone PJ, et al. Characteristics of persons screened for lung cancer in the United States. Ann Intern Med. 2022;175:1501–5. https://doi.org/10.7326/M22-1325.
28. Richards T, Soman A, Thomas C, VanFrank B, Henley S, Gallaway M, et al. Screening for lung cancer—10 states, 2017. MMWR Morb Mortal Wkly Rep. 2020;69(8):201–6.

Chapter 17
Minimizing Harms of Screening

Prarthna Chandar Kulandaisamy

Background

Nearly six decades have passed since the publication of the first Surgeon General's Report on Smoking and Health and the expansive tobacco control efforts that have followed, but lung cancer is still the leading cause of cancer-related deaths in the United States as well as worldwide [1, 2]. In 2020, an estimated 228,820 persons were diagnosed with lung cancer, and 135,720 persons died of the disease [3]. Lung cancer has generally a poor prognosis, with an overall 5-year survival rate of less than 20%. However, early stage lung cancer has a better prognosis than late-stage disease and is more amenable to treatment, with a 5-year survival rate of over 50%. Therefore, lung cancer screening has the potential to drastically reduce lung cancer mortality, but as with any widely applied preventive healthcare measure, lung cancer screening comes with potential risks.

Lung Cancer Screening

Lung cancer screening with low-dose computed tomography (LDCT) has been shown to improve the early detection of lung cancer and reduce mortality among screened individuals [4, 5]. The National Lung Screening Trial (NLST) resulted in a 20.0% reduction in lung cancer mortality for individuals at high risk of developing lung cancer when screened with LDCT compared to those screened with chest

P. C. Kulandaisamy (✉)
Division of Pulmonary, Critical Care, and Allergy, Department of Medicine, Jane and Leonard Korman Respiratory Institute, Thomas Jefferson University, Philadelphia, PA, USA
e-mail: Prarthna.Chandar@jefferson.edu

   169
G. C. Kane et al. (eds.), *Lung Cancer Screening*,
https://doi.org/10.1007/978-3-031-33596-9_17

radiography [6]. The United States Preventive Services Task Force (USPSTF) subsequently released a recommendation supporting LDCT, requiring private insurers to cover the cost of screening [7, 8]. In 2015, the US Centers for Medicare and Medicaid Services (CMS) also issued a coverage determination for annual lung cancer screening with low-dose CT [9]. In 2021, USPSTF updated its guidelines for screening, lowering the criteria for screening, and thereby significantly increasing the number of eligible persons [10].

Potential Harms of Lung Cancer Screening

In the years since the NLST, which showed a significant reduction in lung cancer mortality as well as an overall reduction in all-cause mortality in individuals screened with an LDCT, several additional trials have been conducted throughout the world. While many studies have been able to replicate the reduction in lung cancer deaths, none were able to establish a significant reduction in death from all causes, despite the NLST showing a 7% reduction in all-cause mortality [6]. This has led to debate around the world about the pros and cons of lung cancer screening, lung cancer screening programs, and costs associated with screening. The major risks associated with lung cancer screening are: (1) overdiagnosis, false positive results; (2) risks related to radiation exposure; and (3) patient economic and psychological impact.

Overdiagnosis

Overdiagnosis is an often underappreciated harm of screening. In the context of cancer screening, this term refers to the detection of cancers that appear histopathologically to be invasive malignant tumors but grow so slowly that they never would have become clinically evident during the usual lifetime of the patient or occur in a person who dies of another cause before the cancer symptoms appear [11, 12]. Factors contributing to overdiagnosis include the level of sensitivity of screening tests, biopsy rates, and thresholds for reporting abnormal-appearing cells in biopsy specimens as malignant.

The rate of overdiagnosis for lung cancer screening depends on the age and health status of the population (competing causes of mortality will increase overdiagnosis in older or sicker populations), the distribution of cancer types (bronchoalveolar cancers are more likely to be overdiagnosed due to its slow growth rate), and the screening protocol (more frequent screening or longer duration of screening will increase the overdiagnosis rate) [13]. Data from the NLST indicate approximately four cases of overdiagnosis (and three lung cancer deaths prevented) per 1000 people screened over 6.5 years [14].

Overdiagnosis has the potential to cause significant harm in these patients if they were to undergo more invasive or surgical interventions with no meaningful benefit added from these measures. Overdiagnosis is particularly problematic when patients experience complications from treatment. The concept of overdiagnosis has been discussed in depth by Dr. Peter Bach in his Thorax editorial [15]. He wrote, "overdiagnosis is potentially very harmful [to patients], given that surgery confers risks both short and long-term." But he went on to acknowledge that "current knowledge does not allow [physicians] to distinguish between those histological foci that pose a reduced threat repair with those that pose a very real and imminent threat" [15]. It is clear that at this juncture, detected cancers require prompt and effective treatment.

False Positive Results

Screening with LDCT identifies both cancerous and benign non-calcified nodules. The latter are often called "false positives". Although most LDCT screening studies have reported on nodules detected, the categorization and manner of reporting are inconsistent. Across various screening studies, the average nodule detection rate per round of screening was 20%, but varied from 3 to 30% in RCTs and 5 to 51% in cohort studies. Most studies reported that >90% of nodules were benign [5]. The false-positive rate in lung cancer screening is particularly problematic as these nodules have to be investigated, increasing expense and resource utilization, as well as frequently causing unnecessary morbidity, with reduced acceptance of screening among at-risk individuals. False-positive results can potentially lead to unnecessary tests (both invasive and non-invasive), incidental findings, and short-term increases in distress because of indeterminate results.

In the NLST 1.2% of patients who were not found to have lung cancer underwent an invasive procedure such as needle biopsy or bronchoscopy, while 0.7% of patients who were not found to have lung cancer had a thoracoscopy, mediastinoscopy, or thoracotomy [6]. Invasive nonsurgical procedures in patients with benign lesions were common (73% in NLST). These procedures have their own complications and adverse effects. The frequency of a major complication occurring during a diagnostic evaluation of a detected finding was 33 per 10,000 individuals screened by LDCT. In the NLST data, for patients who had nodules detected by LDCT that turned out to be benign, death occurred within 60 days among 0.06%, and major complications occurred among 0.36%. While these numbers are low, they give reason for pause because the deaths would not have occurred in the absence of screening and the detection of a false-positive result. The challenge for successful lung cancer screening programs is to minimize the number of false positives but also to achieve minimal rates of complication as result of various biopsy techniques.

Radiation Exposure

The effective dose of radiation in LDCT screening is estimated to be 1.5 mSv per examination, but there is substantial variation in actual clinical practice. However, diagnostic chest CT (~8 mSv)[47] or PET-CT (~14 mSv)[47–49] to further investigate detected lesions substantially increases exposure and accounts for most of the radiation exposure in screening studies. The lifetime attributable risk (LAR) varies based on the age of onset of screening and differs between men and women. Among COSMOS trial participants who received 10 years of CT screening procedures, the risk of a new lung cancer ranged between 5.5/10,000 participants (this would be equivalent to 1 in 1811) and 1.4/10000 participants (this would be equivalent to 1 in 6908), while the risk of major cancers among all organ systems could be up to twice is high [16]. Among other various cohort studies and RCTs, the incidence of lung cancer due to radiation exposure from screening varies between 0.05% and 1.8% [16, 17].

This is a challenging area of concern for multiple reasons, including that person's being screened are at higher risk by virtue of their inclusion in the screening cohort. In addition, some members of the scientific community have pointed out that for the most part, studies on the health effects of radiation have generally used data from higher dose exposures and extrapolated those results to lower dose circumstances such as would be the case here, in clinical use in lung cancer screening. Some have postulated that there may be a threshold or margin of safety associated with lower dose exposure as these have not been observed to consistently lead to cancer or other adverse health consequences [18]. There are studies that are now looking at using-ultra low dose CT for screening, which uses one-tenth of the radiation of an LDCT. In the future, this approach has the potential to decrease the radiation exposure-related risks from screening. For now, we must accept that there is uncertainty with regard to radiation exposure risks and rely on clinical trials in large populations guided by overall survival data in order to justify screening.

Economic and Psychological Impact

The economic and psychological impact of lung cancer screening is grossly underreported. The cost-benefit analysis is a subject of continued debate, especially due to decreasing smoking rates as one would expect the incidence of lung cancer to decline as well. False-positive and incidental findings, unnecessary surgical interventions, and over-screening in lower-risk individuals all have the potential for creating imbalance in the cost-benefit equation. Several researchers have analyzed the cost-effectiveness of LDCT screening based on the NLST. One study estimated that the cost of preventing one lung cancer death was US$240,000. A second study revealed that screening with LDCT would cost US$81,000 per quality-adjusted life year (QALY) gained [19].

The data on the psychological impact of screening is even more sparse. One study showed that 46% of the screened population reported psychological distress while awaiting results [20]. One can speculate about QOL benefits due to lower morbidity from advanced lung cancer, but there are also potential detriments due to anxiety, costs, and harms from the evaluation of both false positive scans and over-diagnosed cancers. Data on psychological distress scores the importance of sound shared decision making at the onset of lung cancer screening so that persons have a clear option to opt into screening, understand the risks and benefits, and the details of follow-up before engaging in the screening process.

Minimizing the Risks of Lung Cancer Screening

Minimizing the harms of screening requires a multifaceted approach as there are both direct and indirect risks as we have outlined above. This should be the focus of healthcare policymakers where in the era of rising healthcare costs, screening is being viewed as expensive and risky, thereby endangering the widespread implementation and acceptance of the screening program. Below are potential ways of overcoming the shortcomings of existing screening programs, some of which might remain just as wishful thinking.

Need for a Validated Risk Predictive Calculator

While most lung cancer screening guidelines (including USPSTF) take into account the major risk factors for cancer, these are not all inclusive resulting in the screening of a large number of persons with relatively low risk, which in turn leads to a high number of false positive results and overdiagnosis. To overcome, this a number of risk prediction models and calculators have been proposed [21, 22]. But none of these models have been validated and applied to a larger and more heterogeneous population. Development of one such calculator, which will catch the maximum number of early stage lung cancer while screening the lowest number of people, would be ideal. Future studies should be aimed at developing such a calculator and should be applicable to the population that it is applied to. This may require development of more than one calculator as the inherent risk of cancer varies widely among the population and depends on number of local variables of the population like their age, race, ethnicity, diversity, socio-economic status, and environmental exposures.

Shared Decision Making

Shared decision making (SDM) is an important component of any medical decision. In the United States, formal SDM, including use of a decision aid, is required by CMS to order a CT for lung cancer screening. SDM visits improve patients' understanding of the benefits and harms of lung cancer screening [23, 24]. However, some studies have shown that clinicians rarely use lung cancer screening decision aids, the quality of the shared decision-making discussions is poor and inconsistent, and they lack sufficient discussion on the harms of screening [25, 26]. A recent review of more than 100 randomized clinical trials concluded that decision aids increase patients' knowledge and result in decisions that are more likely to reflect their values. Patients can make informed choices about LDCT only if practitioners fully disclose all the potential harms of screening, including the risk of overdiagnosis. After an in-depth discussion, patients may decide against screening, if it is not something that is in line with their worldview and values. It will be important for researchers to continue to refine estimates of lung cancer overdiagnosis, allowing physicians to provide more accurate information to our patients. The fear associated with even a slight suspicion of lung cancer highlights the need for careful education of LDCT participants, and the need for carefully worded scan interpretations.

A Multidisciplinary Team Approach

Once a LDCT is completed, clinically concerning results from the screening CT should be presented and discussed before a multidisciplinary team. This is especially important when abnormal incidental findings are identified on LDCT. The multidisciplinary team will use both interdisciplinary review, standard algorithms, and detailed discussions with radiology, pulmonology, and thoracic surgery to arrive at a consensus for management. This approach allows for a collaborative effort that aims to find the balance between an overly aggressive workup, with high proportions of unnecessary procedures and the risk of overtreatment, and overly lax management with infrequent surveillance, resulting in delayed and late-stage diagnoses.

At our Philadelphia-based institution, all positive lung cancer screening results are discussed extensively in a weekly multidisciplinary conference with clinicians from pulmonology, interventional pulmonology, and thoracic surgery. As positive LDCT results (Lung-RADS 3, 4A, 4B, and 4X) have the potential to trigger additional imaging and/or invasive procedures, which is why we believe it is imperative to have a multidisciplinary discussion ahead of deciding on the next steps. Cases that result in a cancer diagnosis are then reviewed by a subsequent panel which includes providers from pulmonology, thoracic surgery, medical oncology, radiation oncology, radiology, and pathology to formulate an appropriate treatment plan. This heavily collaborative workflow has led to fewer patients undergoing invasive tests based on a positive screening result than would be expected by adhering to a strict protocol that doesn't allow for team discussion. Every patient is unique, hence management of each patient should be tailor-made for the patient; and a team-based approach allows for this flexibility by contextualizing each patient.

A multidisciplinary approach is not limited to clinical discussions surrounding interpreting results and developing treatment strategies. As the lung cancer screening process has been shown to create significant stress and anxiety, offering psychological guidance and support to patients is imperative. Lung cancer screening providers should seek input from colleagues in psychiatry, psychology, and social work, to help manage stressors related to the screening process and related barriers (e.g., parking costs, transportation, and child care) for patients undergoing screening. Additionally, working with mental health professionals to determine how to most effectively answer all questions and concerns from individuals considering LDCT may significantly psychological distress.

Another area for multidisciplinary collaboration in lung cancer screening is smoking cessation. Tobacco use is linked to approximately 90% of lung cancer cases; simply stated, smoking cessation is the most effective and inexpensive tool for reduction in lung cancer and lung cancer mortality. Smoking cessation counseling is required by CMS for lung cancer screening reimbursement, and programs should offer robust cessation programs run by certified tobacco cessation specialists with guidance from psychiatry, psychology, social work, primary care, and pulmonology.

Conclusion

Despite the potential risks of lung cancer screening, the benefits from screening far outweigh the known harms. It is the responsibility of the healthcare team and the policymakers to identify, manage, and mitigate these risks to improve outcomes and resource utilization. It will be essential for programs to monitor their outcomes and treatment-related complications in order to ensure that lung cancer screening programs have a positive impact on the community. A multidisciplinary team approach is an indispensable part of a successful screening program and goes a long way in minimizing the harms of screening.

References

1. Siegel RL, Miller KD, Jemal A. Cancer statistics, 2018. CA Cancer J Clin. 2018;68(1):7–30.
2. Boer R, Moolgavkar SH, Levy DT. Chapter 15: impact of tobacco control on lung cancer mortality in the United States over the period 1975–2000—summary and limitations. Risk Anal. 2012;32:S190–201.
3. Non-Small Cell Lung Cancer Treatment (PDQ®)–Health Professional Version. National Cancer Institute. Updated November 18, 2020. https://www.cancer.gov/types/lung/hp/non-small-cell-lung-treatment-pdq. Accessed 15 Jan 2021.
4. Henschke CI, Yankelevitz DF, Libby DM, Pasmantier MW, Smith JP, Miettinen OS. International early lung cancer action program Investigators1. International early lung cancer action program Investigators1. Survival of patients with stage I lung cancer detected on CT screening. N Engl J Med. 2006;355:1763–71.
5. Bach PB, Mirkin JN, Oliver TK, Azzoli CG, Berry DA, Brawley OW, Byers T, Colditz GA, Gould MK, Jett JR, Sabichi AL. Benefits and harms of CT screening for lung cancer: a systematic review. JAMA. 2012;307(22):2418–29.

6. Aberle D, Adams A, Berg C, Black W, Clapp J, Fagerstrom R, Gareen IF, Gatsonis C, Marcus PM, Sicks JD. Reduced lung-cancer mortality with low-dose computed tomographic screening. N Engl J Med. 2011;365(5):395–409. https://doi.org/10.1056/NEJMoa1102873.

7. Moyer VA, US Preventive Services Task Force. Screening for lung cancer: US preventive Services task force recommendation statement. Ann Intern Med. 2014;160(5):330–8.

8. Simard EP, Engels EA. Cancer as a cause of death among people with AIDS in the United States. Clin Infect Dis. 2010;51(8):957–62.

9. Services CfMM. Decision memo for screening for lung cancer with low dose computed tomography. 2015. https://www.cms.gov/medicare-coverage-database/details/nca-decision-memo.aspx?NCAId=274.

10. US Preventive Services Task Force. Screening for lung cancer: US preventive services task force recommendation statement. JAMA. 2021;325(10):962–70. https://doi.org/10.1001/jama.2021.1117.

11. Welch HG, Black WC. Overdiagnosis in cancer. J Natl Cancer Inst. 2010;102(9):605–13.

12. Marcus PM, Prorok PC, Miller AB, DeVoto EJ, Kramer BS. Conceptualizing overdiagnosis in cancer screening. J Natl Cancer Inst. 2015;107(4):djv014.

13. Ebell MH, Lin KW. Accounting for the harms of lung cancer screening. JAMA Intern Med. 2018;178(10):1422–3. https://doi.org/10.1001/jamainternmed.2018.3061.

14. Jonas DE, Reuland DS, Reddy SM, et al. Screening for lung cancer with low-dose computed tomography: an evidence review for the U.S. preventive services task force. Rockville, MD: Agency for Healthcare Research and Quality; 2021; (Evidence Synthesis, No. 198). https://www.ncbi.nlm.nih.gov/books/NBK568573/.

15. Bach PB. Overdiagnosis in lung cancer: different perspectives, definitions, implications. Thorax. 2008;63:298–300.

16. Rampinelli C, De Marco P, Origgi D, et al. Exposure to low dose computed tomography for lung cancer screening and risk of cancer: secondary analysis of trial data and risk-benefit analysis. BMJ. 2017;356:j347. https://doi.org/10.1136/bmj.j347; Published 2017 Feb 8.

17. Brenner DJ. Radiation risks potentially associated with low-dose CT screening of adult smokers for lung cancer. Radiology. 2004;231(2):440–5.

18. Uncertainty in risk assessment: position of the health physics society. Health physics society website 2013. http://hps.org/documents/riskassessment_ps008-2.pdf.

19. Goulart BH, Bensink ME, Mummy DG, Ramsey SD. Lung cancer screening with low-dose computed tomography: costs, national expenditures, and cost-effectiveness. J Natl Compr Cancer Netw. 2012;10(2):267–75.

20. van den Bergh KA, Essink-Bot ML, Bunge EM, Scholten ET, Prokop M, van Iersel CA, van Klaveren RJ, de Koning HJ. Impact of computed tomography screening for lung cancer on participants in a randomized controlled trial (NELSON trial). Cancer. 2008;113(2):396–404.

21. Tammemägi MC, ten Haaf K, Toumazis I, et al. Development and validation of a multivariable lung cancer risk prediction model that includes low-dose computed tomography screening results: a secondary analysis of data from the national lung screening trial. JAMA Netw Open. 2019;2(3):e190204. https://doi.org/10.1001/jamanetworkopen.2019.0204.

22. Chung K, Mets OM, Gerke PK, et al. Brock malignancy risk calculator for pulmonary nodules: validation outside a lung cancer screening population. Thorax. 2018;73:857–63.

23. Lillie SE, Fu SS, Fabbrini AE, Rice KL, Clothier B, Nelson DB, Doro EA, Moughrabieh MA, Partin MR. What factors do patients consider most important in making lung cancer screening decisions? Findings from a demonstration project conducted in the veterans health administration. Lung Cancer. 2017;104:38–44.

24. Mazzone PJ, Tenenbaum A, Seeley M, Petersen H, Lyon C, Han X, et al. Impact of a lung cancer screening counseling and shared decision-making visit. Chest. 2017;151:572–8.

25. Bellinger C, Pinsky P, Foley K, Case D, Dharod A, Miller D. Lung cancer screening benefits and harms stratified by patient risk: information to improve patient decision aids. Ann Am Thorac Soc. 2019;16(4):512–4.

26. Brenner AT, Malo TL, Margolis M, Elston Lafata J, James S, Vu MB, et al. Evaluating shared decision making for lung cancer screening. JAMA Intern Med. 2018;178:1311–6.

Chapter 18
A Multidisciplinary Approach

Tyler Grenda and Olugbenga Okusanya

Organizing a Multidisciplinary Team

As lung cancer screening recommendations have grown with expanded screening criteria, recommendations regarding comprehensive management of lung nodules with multidisciplinary expertise have been established [1, 2]. In order to realize the benefits of lung cancer screening, the findings of the low-dose chest CT must be managed appropriately [3]. As a result, success in lung cancer screening requires the engagement of a multidisciplinary lung cancer screening program that includes stakeholders, such as diagnostic radiology, pulmonology, and thoracic surgery [4]. When developing a lung cancer screening program, careful implementation is necessary in order to achieve a favorable balance of benefit and risk with respect to screening. As a result, prior literature has highlighted the importance of management of patients with pulmonary nodules should be performed in the context of a multidisciplinary team that includes radiologists, pulmonologists, thoracic surgeons, and cancer specialists [5].

In order to optimize the outcomes of a screening program, organizing a team around the key providers for lung nodule management across several phases of care (e.g. screening and surgery) is essential. For example, radiologists are key stakeholders across multiple aspects of lung cancer screening, including interpretation of radiographic studies and tissue biopsy [6]. In addition, surgeons play an important role in decisions related to planning and performing interventions for lung nodules. Nurse

T. Grenda (✉) . O. Okusanya
Division of Thoracic and Esophageal Surgery, Department of Surgery, Thomas Jefferson University, Philadelphia, PA, USA
e-mail: Tyler.Grenda@jefferson.edu; Olugbenga.Okusanya@jefferson.edu

  177
G. C. Kane et al. (eds.), *Lung Cancer Screening*,
https://doi.org/10.1007/978-3-031-33596-9_18

navigators are a crucial part of the multidisciplinary team, as they are essential in program development, tracking of outcomes, and providing patient care within screening programs [7]. As a result, lung cancer screening programs should utilize a multidisciplinary team, including chest radiology, pulmonology, and thoracic surgery [8, 9].

Prior literature has highlighted the importance of multidisciplinary team in areas such as lung cancer management, where significant benefits were observed with respect to guideline compliance and revisions to treatment plans [10]. When applied to lung cancer screening, there is no specific template that must be followed with respect to the composition of the "team." However, approaches to the multidisciplinary team for lung cancer screening have previously been described [11].

Strengths of a Multidisciplinary Team

The multidisciplinary team lends the expertise of individual specialties and the individual perspectives that each specialty provides to amplify the value of the lung cancer screening team. Previous literature has suggested that a multidisciplinary lung nodule clinic may promote guideline-concordant care for patients with incidentally detected lung nodules [12]. Furthermore, this study also highlighted the importance of the multidisciplinary team in guideline-discordant care in the setting of competing diagnoses that may affect typical patient management. As a result, the multidisciplinary team may be particularly important in navigating the management of patients with multiple comorbid conditions or complex medical issues.

In addition, the multidisciplinary team is best situated to navigate complex nodule management, such as the patient with multiple lung nodules or ground glass opacities, by leveraging the expertise of multiple specialties. For example, pulmonologists can contribute comprehensive differential diagnoses and evaluation strategies, particularly for nodules that have a high likelihood of being nonneoplastic, while thoracic surgeons can provide context regarding the extent of surgical resection that may be needed based on nodule location. Increased incidence of challenging clinical scenarios, such as the "multiple ground glass opacity patient" is anticipated with the expansion of lung cancer screening services, requiring expertise and a well-organized approach to ensure optimal management [13]. In addition, previous literature has demonstrated high rates of adherence to recommendations in the setting of a multidisciplinary approach for lung nodule management [11]. Ensuring adherence will be imperative to ensure recommendations are translated into clinical care management to ultimately result in patient mortality benefits.

Determining Optimal Management Strategy

While the benefits of lung cancer screening include improvement in mortality and quality of life, risks of screening include false positive results, overdiagnosis of incidental findings, and complications related to diagnostic evaluations [8]. A multidisciplinary team may promote efficient utilization of resources, such as selecting appropriate specialist consultations in the evaluation of lung nodules [14]. A focus on the utilization of services will be important as lung cancer screening services expand and the potential impact of the increased demand on limited services, such as surgical specialists [15]. Prior literature has suggested the multidisciplinary team may be able to recognize and mitigate procedures that are likely to have low diagnostic value, such as bronchoscopic biopsy of a pure ground-glass nodule that is growing in absolute size. As a result, a lung cancer screening program should review every biopsy decision in a multidisciplinary setting [3].

Similarly by including specialties that perform biopsy procedures, such as interventional radiologists, interventional pulmonologists, and thoracic surgeons, attention can be focused on the feasibility of biopsy and potential yield of biopsy in clinical management. More importantly, a multidisciplinary team that includes proceduralists can determine the best modality for biopsy. The importance of the multidisciplinary approach for tissue sampling in lung cancer has previously been highlighted [16]. Leveraging the expertise of the "team" may be particularly important for lung nodules that require special consideration for biopsy (e.g., located along the fissure or mediastinum). Furthermore, identification of lung nodules that would require diagnostic lobectomy for resection, due to anatomic considerations, can be stratified to the appropriate diagnostic modality based on a multidisciplinary discussion that includes key stakeholders.

In addition to diagnostic strategy, surgeon engagement is necessary to ensure low morbidity and mortality for patients undergoing surgical intervention for suspected or confirmed early-stage lung cancer [17]. Surgeons may provide a unique perspective on lung nodules, particularly in patients with previous lung surgery, differentiating postoperative changes from potential pathology. In addition, thoracic surgeons may offer value in minimizing potential risk and providing opinions on an efficient biopsy strategy, should intervention be required [18]. Finally, it is particularly important to ensure patients obtain the same survival benefits observed in screening trials, such as the NLST, that are predicated on low perioperative morality to ensure expected mortality benefits are realized [19].

Maximizing Efficiency

From a healthcare system perspective, utilization of services directed by the multidisciplinary team is important. The costs of services related to lung cancer screening need to be considered, particularly as events such as false-positive results may attribute additional costs and thus need to be efficiently navigated by the multidisciplinary team [8]. In addition, reducing delays in care of the patients with lung nodules detected during screening is essential as well. Previous literature has suggested that a coordinated multidisciplinary team may also provide benefits by reducing delays in care [20].

Quality Improvement

Optimizing quality is key to realizing the benefits of lung cancer screening. The multidisciplinary team may have unique opportunities for quality improvement initiatives in lung cancer screening programs. With a group that includes multiple engaged providers that span the spectrum of providers from screening to diagnosis/treatment, one can track metrics, such as nondiagnostic biopsy yield to inform quality improvement for the lung cancer screening program. In addition, the issues of false-negative screening results are an important consideration [21]. The review of a multidisciplinary team may also be beneficial in limiting potential false-negative results. As potential program-level metrics are developed for screening programs, the multidisciplinary team may be particularly important to ensure programs meet clinical performance benchmarks that are established to ensure quality [22]. The multidisciplinary team thus has a unique opportunity to improve quality over growing experience in order to optimize patient outcomes.

Conclusion

Lung cancer screening services should be provided in the setting of a multidisciplinary team that includes the expertise of a diverse group of providers engaged in the management of lung nodules, such as radiologists, pulmonologists, nursing, and surgeons. This approach may ensure adherence to established guidelines, improve the efficiency of care, navigate difficult clinical scenarios, and provide optimal decisions related to interventions. In addition, the multidisciplinary approach may assist in tracking of metrics and ensuring programs meet quality benchmarks.

References

1. Krist AH, Davidson KW, Mangione CM, Barry MJ, Cabana M, Caughey AB, et al. Screening for lung cancer: US preventive services task force recommendation statement. JAMA. 2021;325(10):962–70.
2. Mazzone PJ, Silvestri GA, Souter LH, Caverly TJ, Kanne JP, Katki HA, et al. Screening for lung cancer: CHEST guideline and expert panel report. Chest. 2021;160(5):e427–e94.
3. Mazzone PJ. Obstacles to and solutions for a successful lung cancer screening program. Semin Respir Crit Care Med. 2016;37(5):659–69.
4. Colson YL, Shepard JO, Lennes IT. New USPSTF guidelines for lung cancer screening: better but not enough. JAMA Surg. 2021;156(6):513–4.
5. Arenberg D, Kazerooni EA. Setting up a lung cancer screening program. J Natl Compr Cancer Netw. 2012;10(2):277–85.
6. Snoeckx A, Franck C, Silva M, Prokop M, Schaefer-Prokop C, Revel MP. The radiologist's role in lung cancer screening. Transl Lung Cancer Res. 2021;10(5):2356–67.

7. Hunnibell LS, Slatore CG, Ballard EA. Foundations for lung nodule management for nurse navigators. Clin J Oncol Nurs. 2013;17(5):525–31.
8. Wood DE, Kazerooni EA, Baum SL, Eapen GA, Ettinger DS, Hou L, et al. Lung cancer screening, version 3.2018, NCCN clinical practice guidelines in oncology. J Natl Compr Cancer Netw. 2018;16(4):412–41.
9. Field JK, Smith RA, Aberle DR, Oudkerk M, Baldwin DR, Yankelevitz D, et al. International association for the study of lung cancer computed tomography screening workshop 2011 report. J Thorac Oncol. 2012;7(1):10–9.
10. Gaudioso C, Sykes A, Whalen PE, Attwood KM, Masika MM, Demmy TL, et al. Impact of a thoracic multidisciplinary conference on lung cancer outcomes. Ann Thorac Surg. 2022;113(2):392–8.
11. Roberts TJ, Lennes IT, Hawari S, Sequist LV, Park ER, Willers H, et al. Integrated, multidisciplinary management of pulmonary nodules can streamline care and improve adherence to recommendations. Oncologist. 2020;25(5):431–7.
12. Verdial FC, Madtes DK, Cheng GS, Pipavath S, Kim R, Hubbard JJ, et al. Multidisciplinary team-based management of incidentally detected lung nodules. Chest. 2020;157(4):985–93.
13. Pedersen JH, Saghir Z, Wille MM, Thomsen LH, Skov BG, Ashraf H. Ground-glass opacity lung nodules in the era of lung cancer CT screening: radiology, pathology, and clinical management. Oncology (Williston Park). 2016;30(3):266–74.
14. Wrightson WR, Gauhar U, Hendler F, Joiner T, Pendleton J. Centralized lung nodule management at a veterans hospital using a multidisciplinary lung nodule evaluation team (LNET). Zhongguo Fei Ai Za Zhi. 2018;21(11):828–32.
15. van Meerbeeck JP, Franck C. Lung cancer screening in Europe: where are we in 2021? Transl Lung Cancer Res. 2021;10(5):2407–17.
16. Chang AC, Sundaram B, Arenberg DA. Lung cancer: multidisciplinary approach to tissue sampling. Radiol Clin N Am. 2012;50(5):951–60.
17. Stiles BM, Pua B, Altorki NK. Screening for lung cancer. Surg Oncol Clin N Am. 2016;25(3):469–79.
18. Randhawa S, Moore RF, DiSesa V, Kaiser L, Ma GX, Jaklitsch MT, et al. Role of thoracic surgeons in lung cancer screening: opportune time for involvement. J Thorac Oncol. 2018;13(3):298–300.
19. Aberle DR, Adams AM, Berg CD, Black WC, Clapp JD, Fagerstrom RM, et al. Reduced lung-cancer mortality with low-dose computed tomographic screening. N Engl J Med. 2011;365(5):395–409.
20. Albano D, Bilfinger T, Feraca M, Kuperberg S, Nemesure B. A multidisciplinary lung cancer program: does it reduce delay between diagnosis and treatment? Lung. 2020;198(6):967–72.
21. Bartlett EC, Silva M, Callister ME, Devaraj A. False-negative results in lung cancer screening-evidence and controversies. J Thorac Oncol. 2021;16(6):912–21.
22. Mazzone PJ, White CS, Kazerooni EA, Smith RA, Thomson CC. Proposed quality metrics for lung cancer screening programs: a national lung cancer roundtable project. Chest. 2021;160(1):368–78.

Chapter 19
Managing Lung Cancer Screening in a Major Healthcare System

James H. Finigan and Neha Agarwal

Background

In 2013, the US Preventative Services Task Force (USPSTF) released guidelines based on the National Lung Cancer Screening Trial (NLST) to screen patients aged 55–80 years who smoked 30-pack-years with a low-dose computed tomography (LDCT) [1, 2]. The Centers for Medicare and Medicaid Services (CMS) approved reimbursement for lung cancer screening in 2015, making millions of Americans eligible for this new service. Many community and academic healthcare settings across the nation quickly adopted lung cancer screening (LCS) programs with the hopes of replicating the 20% lung cancer mortality reduction seen in NLST trial participants. However, the establishment of an effective screening programs has been difficult and slow, especially in community-based healthcare settings [3]. Screening programs need to do more than simply order an imaging study on the right person, at the right time. They require dedicated financial resources, stakeholder engagement, compliance with guidelines, quality control, and of course, additional time to sufficiently counsel patients.

In 2015, Shepard et al. described the crucial elements that made a successful LCS program. Broadly, these include education, technological resources, and a robust team of physicians and program coordinators with access to software that enables tight communication with their patient population [4]. Coordinating all these resources across a large healthcare system, whether urban or rural, can be quite challenging.

J. H. Finigan (✉)
Pulmonary and Critical Care Medicine, National Jewish Health, Denver, CO, USA
e-mail: FiniganJ@NJHealth.org

N. Agarwal
Pulmonary and Critical Care Sciences, University of Colorado, Aurora, CO, USA
e-mail: Neha.2.agarwal@cuanschutz.edu

© The Author(s), under exclusive license to Springer Nature Switzerland AG 2023
G. C. Kane et al. (eds.), *Lung Cancer Screening*,
https://doi.org/10.1007/978-3-031-33596-9_19

Choosing the Appropriate Guideline

Although the USPSTF recommended guidelines were based on the results of the NLST, the proposed guidelines differ from CMS and the National Comprehensive Cancer Network (NCCN) recommendations [5] (Table 19.1). The upper age limit for screening eligibility according to the 2013 USPSTF guidelines is 80 years and for CMS is 77 years. Alternatively, the NCCN risk stratifies patients into two categories. The first group, NCCN1, is modeled after the NLST population (age 55–74), while the second group, NCCN2, has a lower age of eligibility ($\geq$50 years), reduced pack-year smoking history to $\geq$20 years, and requires one additional risk factor. Risk factors identified by the NCCN include exposures (to radon, silica, asbestos, cadmium, arsenic, beryllium, chromium, diesel, fume, or nickel), personal history of other cancer, family history of lung cancer, or personal history of lung disease (emphysema, chronic obstructive pulmonary disease, or pulmonary fibrosis).

Which set of guidelines accurately captures the at-risk population and should be implemented by a LCS program? In 2017, Nemesure et al. analyzed all biopsy-proven lung cancer cases seen at their institution over a 10-year period [5]. They found that only 49% of the studied patients met USPSTF screening criteria, 46% of patients met CMS screening criteria, and 70% of patients met NCCN screening criteria. Populations who were at risk of being missed included patients at the extremes of age (age < 55 and age > 77), patients who quit smoking over 15 years ago, or patients who never smoked. 15% of biopsy-proven cases were aged less than 55 and 15% of cases were over the age of 77. Additionally, 28% of patients quit smoking >15 years prior, thereby making them ineligible for screening based on USPSTF 2013, CMS, and NCCN1 guidelines. Furthermore, 13% of patients never smoked. These missed populations are consistent with a prior study performed in Olmstead County, Minnesota [6], suggesting the need to reevaluate the current guidelines especially amidst increasing life expectancy and decreasing smoking trends in the United States.

It is important to note that none of the aforementioned guidelines account for race or ethnicity. The NLST population had a very small percentage of minority patients, and in 2015 Fiscella et al. showed that CMS guidelines do not accurately assess lung cancer risk in the Black and Hispanic populations [7]. Black patients have a higher lung cancer incidence independent of pack-year history while Hispanic

Table 19.1 Lung cancer screening recommendations per society

	USPSTF 2021	USPSTF 2013	CMS	NCCN 1	NCCN 2
Age	50–80	55–80	55–70	55–74	$\geq$50
Pack-years	$\geq$20	$\geq$30	$\geq$30	$\geq$30	$\geq$20
Years quit	<15 years	<15 years	<15 years	<15 years	
Other					[a]1 additional risk factor

[a]Additional risk factors as defined by NCCN include history of lung disease, personal history of cancer, family history of lung cancer, exposure history (asbestos, silica, radon, cadmium, arsenic, beryllium, chromium, diesel fumes, nickel). (Adopted and modified [5])

patients have a lower incidence, possibly due to differences in environmental exposures and/or genetic susceptibilities [8–10]. Therefore, the application of USPSTF or CMS guidelines may increase racial disparities in lung cancer screening. Lung cancer risk prediction models that capture differences in race include that used in the Prostate, Lung, Colorectal, and Ovarian Cancer Screening Trial ($PLCO_{2012}$) and one developed by Etzel et al. [11, 12]. These risk models included factors such as COPD, history of hay fever, and exposure to asbestos and wood dust. Application of the $PCLO_{2012}$ model increased LCS eligibility amongst the Black population.

These studies clearly demonstrated the need for updated guidelines that capture high-risk patients at the extremes of age and patients from minority groups. In March 2021, the USPSTF updated lung cancer screening guidelines, lowering the age of eligibility from 55 years to 50 years, and the minimum pack-year smoking history from 30 years to 20 years [13]. The Cancer Intervention and Surveillance Modeling Network (CISNET) Lung Cancer Working Group estimated that these updated guidelines would increase the screening-eligible population by 87%, detect an additional 21% of lung cancers, and increase screening of underrepresented communities including women, non-Hispanic Black individuals, Hispanic individuals, Asian individuals, and lower-income individuals [14].

Ritzwoller et al. studied the impact of these updated screening guidelines on reaching these patients who are historically underserved [15]. Their cohort study analyzed patients engaged in any of five healthcare systems part of the Population-based Research to Optimize the Screening Process Lung Consortium (PROSPR); The Henry Ford Health System in Detroit Michigan, Kaiser Permanente Colorado in Aurora Colorado, Kaiser Permanente Hawaii in Oahu Hawaii, Marshfield Clinic Health System in Marshfield Wisconsin, and the University of Pennsylvania Health System in Philadelphia, Pennsylvania. Using electronic-health record derived clinical and demographic data, the group found that the updated guidelines increased overall lung cancer screening eligibility by 53.7%, increased identification of lung cancers by 30%, and increased the number of eligible women by 17.1%, Hispanic patients by 23.3%, Asian/Native Hawaiian/Pacific Islander patients by 21.8%, Black patients by 17.5%, and patients in the lowest socioeconomic status by 17.9%. Additional studies are needed to assess whether these updated eligibility criteria truly reduce barriers to LCS for high-risk populations.

It is important to consider that these updated LCS guidelines can potentially cause increased harm. Screening can generate false-positive results leading to unnecessary procedures and their complications, overdiagnosis, radiation exposure, and increased patient anxiety [13]. In the CISNET modeling studies, the 2021 expanded guidelines had a rate of 2.2 false-positive results per person over a lifetime of screening compared to 1.9 false-positive results in the 2013 guidelines [14]. This resulted in a mean 688 biopsies per 100,000 people compared to 518 biopsies using the prior eligibility criteria. Overdiagnosis ranged from 83 to 94 per 100,000 patients compared to 69 with the 2013 criteria.

Because Medicare and most insurers are required to reimburse USPSTF recommendations with a grade B or higher, most institutions follow the updated 2021 LCS guidelines. Nonetheless, ordering providers should recognize that these guidelines may not capture high-risk populations including patients over the age of 80 and ethnic minorities. Furthermore, there is also an increase in harms related to screening [14]. While the screening CT scan is covered by most insurers, the additional clinic visits, testing, and treatment may not be [16]. This further increases the complexity, cost, and burden for LCS [16].

Establishing Lung Cancer Screening Champions

Identifying the institution's champions for a lung cancer screening program is critical to overall success. Leaders help set the vision for a large program and encourage downstream innovations for continual quality improvement. Some studies have advocated for two project champions—an administrative leader who can help mobilize physical and financial resources, and a physician leader who can provide guidance on quality of care, implementation, and program monitoring [3, 17]. Because the number of patients eligible for screening is increasing, buy-in from healthcare administrators is crucial to secure the financial resources needed to access more equipment and space to accommodate the additional patient capacity. In rural and community healthcare settings, these project champions can also serve as ambassadors to foster relationships with higher-volume referral centers that have access to specialized diagnostic equipment, subspecialists, and additional procedural capabilities. Pulmonologists and radiologists are central to the lung cancer screening process and therefore are naturally suited to be institutional program champions.

Need for Radiology Equipment and Support

LCS requires certain radiologic capacity to perform screens as well as follow-up on results. LCS centers need the capacity to perform CT scans, PET scans, and magnetic resonance images (MRIs) of the brain. This requires enough CT technologists, CT technology aides, nurses to insert IVs for nuclear medicine studies, and MRI technologists. CT scanners must meet technical requirements as set forth by the American College of Radiology (ACR), such as a volumetric CT dose index $\leq$3 mGy for standard-sized patients with appropriate weight adjustments for other patients. By meeting these technical requirements, institutions are eligible for accreditation as a Designated Lung Cancer Screening Center [13].

In addition to scanning equipment, LCS centers need thoracic radiologists and radiologists who interpret nuclear medicine studies and MRIs. Previously, CMS dictated that radiologists at LCS centers needed continuing medical education credits and a minimum number of chest CT scans read per year. However, CMS removed these requirements when the 2021 USPSTF screening guidelines were published. Radiologists are still required to utilize a standardized lung nodule reporting identification and classification system such as Lung-RADS [13]. The electronic health record therefore should utilize software with access to reporting templates for radiologists.

Given the anticipated increase of screening CT examinations, image interpretation aids could be applied when possible. For example, computer-aided nodule detection has been shown to decrease interreader variability while automated volume measurement can assess nodule growth over time and thereby assist in evaluating malignant potential [18]. There is ongoing work to address the known limitations of these technological aides. Nonetheless, an LCS program should consider the use of these computer-based tools when able to improve standardization and nodule detection.

Creating the Multidisciplinary Pulmonary Nodule Review Board

Many low-risk lung nodules found on screening CT scans have clear, image-based, and management plans based on Lung-RADS recommendations. However, some findings are more concerning for malignancy and warrant prompt discussion among a multidisciplinary team (MDT) of physicians involved in all aspects of lung nodule care including initial detection, tissue sampling, staging, and cancer treatment. Increasingly, MDT teams are recommended for optimal management of numerous malignancies. Guidelines in breast [19], central nervous system [20], rectal [21], and laryngeal cancers [22] all recommend management through a MDT team due to improvements in time to treatment [23], patient satisfaction [23], cost-effectiveness [24], and patient survival [25]. Many lung cancer care guidelines also recommend management through a MDT [26–28], however, there is a paucity of randomized control trials studying the impact of a MDT in patients with lung cancer.

In 2008, Coory et al. performed a systematic review of MDTs in lung cancer care and found that there is currently limited evidence to demonstrate that multidisciplinary care has an impact on patient survival for lung cancer [29]. Sixteen studies were included in the review, but clinical heterogeneity precluded pooled statistics. One primary study reported an increase in survival from 3.2 to 6.6 months and an increase in chemotherapy use from 7% to 23% after the implementation of a MDT team [30]. However, the before and after design was weak evidence of a causal association. On the contrary, a single center, 3-year study performed in New South Wales, Australia, evaluated all patients with lung cancer. They found that patients presented through a MDT received more treatment, but there was no difference in survival [31]. However, patient survival is not the only outcome that must be considered. As elucidated by Patkar et al., the MDT establishes an environment that allows continuing medical education for all members [32], ensures adherence to guidelines, and improves coordination and efficient communication [30].

Therefore, successful LCS programs should have a multidisciplinary Pulmonary Nodule Review Group that ideally includes thoracic radiologists with Lung-RADS training, general pulmonologists, interventional pulmonologists, interventional radiologists, thoracic surgeons, pathologists, medical and radiation oncologists, palliative care, and lung cancer nurses [33]. In many tertiary centers, this group convenes weekly to formulate a diagnostic and management plan that can be discussed with a patient later that same day during their scheduled clinic visit. This structure allows the development of timely management plans with input from a variety of procedural subspecialists who can provide perspective on how to obtain a tissue diagnosis and staging while minimizing the number and risks of procedures. For patients ultimately diagnosed with metastatic non-small cell lung cancer, early referral to palliative care has demonstrated a 3-month survival benefit and significant improvements in quality of life and mood [34]. In one study, palliative care inclusion in MDT meetings increased the proportion of patients being managed by palliative care from 80% to close to 100% [35].

Effective MDT meetings result in accurate cancer staging with the fewest number of procedures, timely care [36], higher treatment rates, and better adherence to clinical guidelines [37]. In fact, Boxer et al. showed that patients newly diagnosed with lung cancer who were presented at a MDT review were better characterized in terms of malignancy stage and Eastern Cooperative Oncology Group (ECOG) performance status and were more likely to enroll in clinical trials [31]. This is consistent with another study which demonstrated that presentation at a MDT review resulted in better staging (79% vs. 93%), quicker treatment (29 days vs. 17 days), and adherence to evidence-based guidelines (81% vs. 97%) [38]. The percentage of patients undergoing surgical staging procedures was 72% with MDT presentation compared to 33% without a MDT. Lastly, patients with stage IIIA NSCLC were more likely to undergo surgery if presented in the MDT, suggesting that thoracic surgery might be underutilized in the absence of a MDT.

Plutyer et al. studied the application of a custom-made clinical decision support system (CDSS) to support multidisciplinary decisions [39]. The system paralleled clinical thinking and presented findings from radiology, biopsies, pathology, molecular diagnostics, patient medical history, functional status indicators, and patient preferences in a systematic fashion. All these data points could be visualized in one screen, enabling the identification of missing data and co-visualization of discordant findings (e.g., PET scan and histology results). Application of this CDSS provided clinicians with a more holistic perspective of each case, ensured relevant information was not overlooked, and stimulated critical thinking. As of now, this CDSS is in its infancy, and further studies are needed to evaluate its generalizability and adaptability to additional clinical settings.

The Nodule Review Board's Procedural Capabilities

Ideally, these subspecialists participating in weekly meetings are also the proceduralists ultimately performing the diagnostic procedure. With current advances in technology, there are several minimally invasive procedures this group can pursue.

Bronchoscopic interventions remain the preferred sampling modality due to their ability to diagnose and stage malignancies within one procedure. Interventional and often general pulmonologists are trained in bronchoscopy with endobronchial ultrasound-guided fine needle aspiration (EBUS-FNA) and more recently, robotic bronchoscopies. Since 2019, two robotic-assisted bronchoscopy (RAB) platforms are used to reach peripheral pulmonary nodules through bronchoscopic methods: the Ion (Intuitive Surgical) and the Monarch (Auris Health). The ongoing PRECIsE and completed BENEFIT trials demonstrated the feasibility and safety of the Ion and Monarch systems, respectively [40, 41]. In 2019, Fielding et al. studied the Ion platform in 17 patients with an average lesion size of 12.2 mm, and demonstrated an overall diagnostic yield of 79%, with a diagnostic yield for malignancy of 88% [42]. Similarly, the first feasibility study for the Monarch platform was conducted in 15 patients with an average lesion size of 26 mm (range 10–63 mm) [43]. Samples were collected in 93% of patients and no one suffered a pneumothorax or significant bleeding complication. Preliminary results from the BENEFIT trial with 56 patients demonstrated successful sampling in 96% cases, a diagnostic yield of 74%, and a pneumothorax rate of 3.6% [41]. Larger multicenter studies are needed to characterize the true diagnostic yield, complication rates compared to transcutaneous biopsies, and overall impact of the RAB platforms in being able to diagnose and stage lung cancers earlier. RAB platforms allow bronchoscopic sampling and staging of even T1a lesions, which have a better prognosis than larger stage T1 lesions [44]. Therefore, if a pathologist is available for rapid-one site evaluation (ROSE), the pulmonologist can sample the nodule of interest, obtain a real-time tissue diagnosis, and pursue lymph node biopsies for cancer staging if indicated. By the time, the patient has awoken from procedural anesthesia, the pulmonologist has a preliminary diagnosis and staging information.

Thoracic surgeons also play a central role in the management of lung nodules, especially since some nodules suggestive of malignancy warrant surgical resection without a biopsy. The Society of Thoracic Surgeons (STS) created a General Thoracic Surgery Task Force on CT Screening that published a clinical statement elucidating their role [45]. The Task Force suggests that all thoracic surgeons involved in a LCS program be trained in performing lobectomies, segmentectomies, wedge resections, and minimally invasive thoracic surgery including video-assist thoracoscopic surgery (VATS) and robotic approaches. With an increasing number of pulmonary nodules detected earlier, there is a concomitant increase in the number of malignancies amenable to surgical resection and cure. For example, the International Early Lung Cancer Action Program demonstrated an increase in the use of VATS from 10% to 34% [46]. In 2020, Nguyen et al. described trends in robotic-assisted lobectomy (RL), video-assisted thoracoscopic lobectomy (VL), and open lobectomy (OL) [47]. From the study period of 2008 to 2015, there was a decline in OL (71% to 43%) with a concomitant increase in RL (1% to 17%) and VL (28% to 41%). RL had lower rates of complications, conversions to an open procedure, and shorter length of stay compared to the other surgical modalities. In high-volume centers where more than 25 lobectomies were performed annually, the cost of RL was comparable to VL and OL. Therefore, there is a clear and growing need for access to thoracic surgeons in lung cancer screening programs [48].

Many smaller community and rural settings may not have access to interventional radiologists, interventional pulmonologists, or thoracic surgeons [33]. The National Lung Cancer Audit in the UK demonstrated that patients who are first presented in a MDT based in a thoracic surgery center are more likely to undergo surgical resection, and even more so when the thoracic surgeon regularly attends MDT meetings [49]. In 2012, Meyenfeldt et al. published a meta-analysis evaluating the association between surgeon specialty, surgeon volume, and hospital volume of lung resections as related to postoperative mortality and long-term survival [50]. The results of a pooled estimated effect size demonstrated improved postoperative mortality for thoracic surgeons over general surgeons (OR 0.78, CI 0.7–0.88), and for cardiothoracic surgeons over general surgeons (OR: 0.82, CI 0.69–0.96). Interestingly, there was no significant relationship between surgeon volume and postoperative mortality or survival. High-volume hospitals had better postoperative mortality and improved survival, though the survival outcome did not reach statistical significance. Interestingly, the analysis could not identify a cutoff value to distinguish high-volume hospitals from low-volume hospitals. The authors concluded that the improvements in postoperative mortality may be due to the surgical team's performance rather than the individual surgeon.

Should Screening Be Centralized?

Given the different postoperative mortality between surgeon specialties, some centers have suggested centralization of lung cancer care. LCS programs can be classified as centralized or decentralized programs. Centralized programs have a dedicated team of clinicians, patient navigators, and nurse coordinators who accept referrals for LCS, manage patient screening, nodule tracking, patient communication, and follow-up management. In decentralized programs, primary care providers refer patients directly to a clinician for LCS.

In 2007, the Dutch Cancer Society formed a "Quality of Cancer Care" taskforce that performed an extensive review on outcomes associated with pancreatectomies, bladder, lung, colorectal, and breast cancer resections [51]. Their study demonstrated that the quality of care varied by hospital and region as well as differences in infrastructure, procedural volume, and hospital specializations. Based on these findings, the Dutch Surgical Society established criteria for hospitals to be able to perform lung cancer surgery based on procedural volume, infrastructure, specialization, and outcome measures [52]. Centralizing these complex and high-risk surgical procedures may improve postoperative mortality, long term survival, and encourage further quality improvement.

Sakoda et al. studied adherence to lung cancer screening across 5 academic and community-based sites that had both centralized and decentralized programs [53]. Their study demonstrated 46% adherence in patients receiving care through a centralized system, compared to 35.3% adherence for patients in a decentralized system. Further analysis suggested that the independent factor strongly associated with adherence was the screening program type, with a 2.8-fold increased likelihood of adherence with centralized screening (adjusted odds ratio 2.78). Smith et al. found similar results in their retrospective study of the Medical University of South Carolina's hybrid LCS program [54]. Additionally, of all the patients screened, 90% of the ineligible patients were screened in the decentralized program, suggesting that centralized programs are better equipped to identify eligible patients.

Is there a role for decentralized programs? To date, no literature has yet elucidated a benefit to decentralized programs. However, the creation of a centralized program requires significant planning, leadership, and resources. In regions where available resources do not permit the creation of centralized programs, decentralized programs will continue to play an important role.

The Role of the Electronic Health Record and Nodule Tracking

For an LCS program to be truly successful, it must have systems in place to identify and screen eligible patients, manage detected nodules and incidental findings, follow patient adherence to annual screening, and encourage smoking cessation. The electronic health record (EHR) system can be a powerful tool that when utilized correctly and can decrease the complexities of LCS. Partnering with IT (Information technology) and clinical informatics specialists early on is crucial to developing a sustainable program within a large healthcare system [55].

The EHR can be used to identify patients eligible for LCS and can facilitate referrals to LCS programs, especially in decentralized healthcare settings, although inaccurate or incomplete smoking histories can limit utility. Dashboards with information on population health management and clinical decision support tools such as best practice advisories can be integrated into an EHR to ease identification of eligible patients. An EHR can also be designed with templated LCS referrals that require the ordering provider to verify key information such as smoking status, shared decision making, and smoking cessation counseling. Such templated referrals decrease inappropriate referrals and can also function as decision aide tools [55].

The EHR plays an important role in facilitating screening for eligible patients. Unfortunately, even the most sophisticated EHRs are unable to provide enough support to effectively manage detected nodules [55]. Larger screening programs with thousands of patients would benefit from purchasing a proprietary third-party software designed specifically for LCS and nodule tracking. Multiple tracking systems currently exist including Eon Health, LungView, PenLung, Medtronic's LungGPS, and Lung Health. These programs can create a file for each screened patient, capture and transfer digital imaging from testing facilities, automatically extract pertinent nodule characteristics from a radiologist's read, track the nodules' Lung-RADS score and any incidental findings, provide navigation and decision-making support, monitor diagnostic testing, and generate templated letters to facilitate patient communication [55]. When fully integrated with the EHR, these tracking programs have the capability of decreasing the total time spent per patient per year from an estimated 122 min to 11.5 min [56]. Furthermore, LCS software has analytic

Table 19.2 Minimum recommended features and capability of a lung cancer screening software system

Full integration and compatibility with existing EHR and patient portal
Patient registration and recall desk with full interface with EHR
Universal compatibility with all integrated digital imaging and Communications in Medicine software formats
Full capability of data extraction (lung-RADS category) from radiology reports
Lung nodule tracking and surveillance
Non-lung nodule (incidental findings) tracking
Automatic laboratory results interface and integration
Navigator dashboard
Complement of templated and customizable letters, integrated mail merge, and documentation of telephone communication with the EHR
Full automaticity in capturing all ACR-LCSR data elements
Full automaticity in routine batching and upload of ACR-LCSR data elements
Full capability to create data fields specific to individual screening program[a]
Full capability to query and report data for lung cancer screening program quality and outcomes evaluation

[a]Beyond the required elements of the ACR, high-quality programs collect quality metrics associated with clinical care and program evaluation that may be specific to local circumstances. (Adopted from Chest [55])

capabilities, thereby facilitating quality improvement and programmatic evaluation. Table 19.2 shows the minimum recommended features of a LCS software system [56].

Currently, many LCS tracking software programs cannot be fully integrated into the EHR [55]. There is increasing interest in building or revising existing EHRs so they can perform at the level of these software tracking programs. In the interim, it is crucial to partner with IT specialists who have intimate knowledge of the existing EHR and can analyze compatibility with the different LCS tracking software programs.

The cost of these organizational support systems varies depending on the LCS program size, program location, number of partnering radiology facilities, number of software updates, and maintenance needs [55]. Small LCS programs caring for fewer than a few hundred patients may instead use EHR-based tracking methods. Nonetheless, application of a LCS software allows a large program to track thousands of patients, monitor patient adherence, and ultimately provide better care.

Creating the Pulmonary Nodule Clinic and Team

Large LCS centers often have a designated pulmonary nodule clinic with pulmonary physicians, patient navigators, support staff, and schedulers. Each of these individuals serves a critical role in the care and management of screening eligible patients. The physician director of the clinic is often one of the LCS program champions. They work to establish a standardized workflow for the nodule clinic and provide oversight on guideline adherence and programmatic quality control. Clinical support staff are needed to obtain and upload imaging studies performed at other institutions, while front desk staff and schedulers promote timely follow-up [57]. Lastly, patient navigators are usually midlevel providers such as nurse practitioners or physician assistants who connect patients with the appropriate care team and ensure patients adhere to recommended follow-up. Their role in LCS programs has been well demonstrated in multiple studies.

The Kaiser Permanente Colorado Group (KPCO) analyzed their LCS implementation in 2019 and found that only 46% of patients undergoing a LDCT truly met CMS eligibility and reimbursement criteria [58]. To improve this low rate and ensure only eligible patients underwent screening, the group recruited nurse navigators. After receiving a LCS referral, nurse navigators confirmed a patient's smoking status, pack years, and time since quitting smoking. They then updated the electronic health records, and if the patient was eligible for screening, they ordered and scheduled a LDCT. Finally, the patient's information was added into an electronic tracking tool. Adoption of a nurse navigator in this program's LCS workflow increased their patient eligibility from 46% to 93%, and increased outreach to patients living in lower-income neighborhoods, those with lower levels of education, and patients with a higher comorbidity burden. This demographic difference may be because healthier patients were more likely to be engaged with the healthcare system and seek out LCS, as demonstrated previously in a California LCS center [59]. Nonetheless, the literature demonstrates ample evidence that patient navigators play a crucial role in improving patient adherence and ensuring the right patients are screened [60].

Patient Education and Resources

Shared decision making is at the forefront of LCS and requires providers to counsel patients on the aim of LCS, the possibility of false-positive results or incidental findings, and the risks of repeated radiation exposure. Although patients can be counseled by different types of providers including health educators or non-physician practitioners, thorough counseling takes significant time and can be anxiety provoking. Successful LCS programs should provide readily available resources such as waiting room pamphlets, online websites with answers to frequently asked questions, links to the literature, and contact information for their institution's lung nodule program navigator [57]. These tools can supplement shared decision making, encourage smoking cessation, and further prepare patients for incidentalomas or false-positive results. Among participants in NLST, 10.2% had baseline incidental clinical findings such as atherosclerosis, aneurysms, chronic obstructive pulmonary disease, and indeterminant breast, liver, kidney, and adrenal lesions [61]. Providing additional educational resources can help minimize patient anxiety and promote adherence in a LCS program.

LCS Outreach and Publicity

Batlle et al. describe the importance of a marketing campaign in growing a LCS program [62]. Educational seminars and presentations directed at referring physicians can foster PCP and subspecialist relationships, increase awareness of complex screening guidelines, and enhance exposure to the program. Similarly, there are numerous avenues to educate patients on the importance of screening. In addition to health fairs and community events [57], programs can also use online marketing to increase awareness. Opportunities include advertisements on social media, informational videos on the institution's website, and blogs of real patient stories. Batlle et al. observed that one-third of their patients were referred to their program through sources including newspaper/magazine advertisements (13%), internet/social media (9%), radio commercials (5%), and word of mouth (3%) [62]. It is important to note, however, that these methods may miss vulnerable populations including patients in low-income communities. Designated outreach to these vulnerable populations should be a component of all LCS programs.

Adhering to Societal Guidelines and Reimbursements

LCS centers must adhere to several requirements designed to promote large-scale improvements in screening and qualify for CMS reimbursement guidelines. As of 2021, CMS significantly reduced the requirements for coverage. To date, LCS programs are required to document pertinent patient eligibility information, a shared decision-making visit, and smoking cessation counseling [13]. Programs are no longer required to report their data to a national registry such as the ACR's Lung Cancer Screening Registry. These liberalized guidelines aim to increase LCS access to vulnerable populations and reduce administrative hurdles to accommodate the growing number of eligible patients.

References

1. Moyer VA, US Preventive Services Task Force. Screening for lung cancer: U.S. preventive services task force recommendation statement. Ann Intern Med. 2014;160:330–8.
2. National Lung Screening Trial Research Team, Aberle DR, Adams AM, et al. Reduced lung-cancer mortality with low-dose computed tomographic screening. N Engl J Med. 2011;365:395–409.
3. Allen CG, Cotter MM, Smith RA, Watson L. Successes and challenges of implementing a lung cancer screening program in federally qualified health centers: a qualitative analysis using the consolidated framework for implementation research. Transl Behav Med. 2021;11(5):1088–98.
4. Baile JC, Maroules CD, Latif MA, Cury RC. A five-step strategy for building an LDCT lung cancer screening program. Appl Radiol. 2018;47(1):12–8.

5. Nemesure B, Plank A, Reagan L, Albano D, Reiter M, Bilfinger TV. Evaluating efficacy of current lung cancer screening guidelines. J Med Screen. 2017;24(4):208–13.
6. Wang Y, Midthun DE, Wampfler JA, et al. Trends in the proportion of patients with lung cancer meeting screening criteria. JAMA. 2015;313:853–5.
7. Fiscella K, Winters P, Farah S, et al. Do lung cancer eligibility criteria align with risk among blacks and hispanics? PLoS One. 2015;10:e0143789.
8. Benowitz NL, Dains KM, Dempsey D, Wilson M, Jacob P. Racial differences in the relationship between number of cigarettes smoked and nicotine and carcinogen exposure. Nicotine Tob Res. 2011;13:772–83.
9. St Helen G, Dempsey D, Wilson M, Jacob P, Benowitz NL. Racial differences in the relationship between tobacco dependence and nicotine and carcinogen exposure. Addiction. 2012;108:607–17. https://doi.org/10.1111/j.1360-0443.2012.04077.x. PMID: 22971134 26.
10. Berg JZ, Mason J, Boettcher AJ, Hatsukami DK, Murphy SE. Nicotine metabolism in African Americans and European Americans: variation in glucuronidation by ethnicity and UGT2B10 haplotype. J Pharmacol Exp Ther. 2010;332:202–9. https://doi.org/10.1124/jpet.109.159855. PMID: 19786624.
11. Etzel CJ, Kachroo S, Liu M, et al. Development and validation of a lung cancer risk prediction model for African-Americans. Cancer Prev Res. 2008;1:255–65.
12. Zhu CS, Pinsky PF, Kramer BS, et al. The prostate, lung, colorectal, and ovarian cancer screening trial and its associated research resource. J Natl Cancer Inst. 2013;105(22):1684–93.
13. US Preventive Services Task Force, Krist AH, Davidson KW, et al. Screening for lung cancer: us preventive services task force recommendation statement. JAMA. 2021;325(10):962.
14. Meza R, Jeon J, Toumazis I, et al. Evaluation of the benefits and harms of lung cancer screening with low-dose computed tomography: modeling study for the US preventive services task force. JAMA. 2021;325(10):988–97. https://doi.org/10.1001/jama.2021.1077.
15. Ritzwoller DP, Meza R, Carroll NM, et al. Evaluation of population-level changes associated with the 2021 us preventive services task force lung cancer screening recommendations in community-based health care systems. JAMA Netw Open. 2021;4(10):e2128176.
16. Melzer AC, Wilt TJ. Expanded access to lung cancer screening—implementing wisely to optimize health. JAMA Netw Open. 2021;4(3):e210275.
17. Miech EJ, Rattray NA, Flanagan ME, Damschroder L, Schmid AA, Damush TM. Inside help: an integrative review of champions in healthcare-related implementation. SAGE Open Med. 2018;6:2050312118773261.
18. Jeon KN, Goo JM, Lee CH, et al. Computer-aided nodule detection and volumetry to reduce variability between radiologists in the interpretation of lung nodules at low-dose screening computed tomography. Investig Radiol. 2012;47(8):457–61.
19. National Breast and Ovarian Cancer Centre. Multidisciplinary meetings for cancer care: a guide for health service providers. National Breast and Ovarian Cancer Centre, 2005. http://www.nbocc.org.au/view-document-details/mdm-multidisciplinarymeetings-for-cancer-care. Accessed 8 Mar 2022.
20. National Institute on Clinical Excellence Guidance on cancer services: improving outcomes for people with brain and other CNS tumours. National institute on clinical excellence, 2006. http://guidance.nice.org.uk/CSGBraincns/Guidance/pdf/English. Accessed 8 Mar 2022.
21. Burton S, Brown G, Daniels IR, et al. MRI directed multidisciplinary team preoperative treatment strategy: the way to eliminate positive circumferential margins? Br J Cancer. 2006;94:351–7.
22. Pfister DG, Laurie SA, Weinstein GS, et al. American society of clinical oncology clinical practice guideline for the use of larynx-preservation strategies in the treatment of laryngeal cancer. J Clin Oncol. 2006;24:3693–704.
23. Gabel M, Hilton NE, Nathanson SD. Multidisciplinary breast cancer clinics. Do they work? Cancer. 1997;79:2380–4.

24. Westin T, Stalfors J. Tumour boards/multidisciplinary head and neck cancer meetings: are they of value to patients, treating staff or a political drain on healthcare resources? Curr Opin Otolaryngol Head Neck Surg. 2008;16:103–7.
25. Birchall M, Bailey D, King P, South west cancer intelligence service head and neck tumour panel. Effect of process standards on survival of patients with head and neck cancer in the south and west of England. Br J Cancer. 2004;91:1477–81.
26. American College of Chest Physicians, Health and Science Policy Committee. Diagnosis and management of lung cancer: ACCP evidence-based guidelines. American College of Chest Physicians. Chest. 2003;123(suppl 1):1S–337S.
27. Cancer Council Australia Clinical Practice Guidelines for the Prevention, Diagnosis and Management of Lung Cancer. Cancer Council Australia, 2004. http://www.nhmrc.gov.au/publications/subjects/cancer.htm. Accessed 8 Mar 2022.
28. The lung Cancer Working Party of the British Thoracic Society Standards of Care Committee. BTS recommendations to respiratory physicians for organising the care of patients with lung cancer. The lung cancer working party of the british thoracic society standards of care committee. Thorax. 1998;53(suppl 1):S1–8.
29. Coory M, Gkolia P, Yang IA, et al. Systematic review of multidisciplinary teams in the management of lung cancer. Lung Cancer. 2008;60:14–21.
30. Bydder S, Nowak A, Marion K, Phillips M, Atun R. The impact of case discussion at a multidisciplinary team meeting on the treatment and survival of patients with inoperable non-small cell lung cancer. Intern Med J. 2009;39:838–41.
31. Boxer MM, Vinod SK, Shafiq J, Duggan KJ. Do multidisciplinary team meetings make a difference in the management of lung cancer? Cancer. 2011;117(22):5112–20.
32. Patkar V, Acosta D, Davidson T, Jones A, Fox J, Keshtgar M. Cancer multidisciplinary team meetings: evidence, challenges, and the role of clinical decision support technology. Int J Breast Cancer. 2011;2011:831605, 1.
33. Prabhakar CN, Fong KM, Peake MD, Lam DC, Barnes DJ. The effectiveness of lung cancer MDT and the role of respiratory physicians. Respirology. 2015;20(6):884–8.
34. Rich AL, Tata LJ, Free CM, Stanley RA, Peake MD, Baldwin DR, Hubbard RB. Inequalities in outcomes for non-small cell lung cancer: the influence of clinical characteristics and features of the local lung cancer service. Thorax. 2011;66:1078–84.
35. Horvath LE, Yordan E, Malhotra D, Leyva I, Bortel K, Schalk D, Mellinger P, Huml M, Kesslering C, Huml J. Multidisciplinary care in the oncology setting: historical perspective and data from lung and gynecology multidisciplinary clinics. J Oncol Pract. 2010;6:21–6.
36. Stone CJL, Robinson A, Brown E, et al. Improving timeliness of oncology assessment and cancer treatment through implementation of a multidisciplinary lung cancer clinic. J Oncol Pract. 2019;15(2):e169–77.
37. Pillay B, Wootten AC, Crowe H, et al. The impact of multidisciplinary team meetings on patient assessment, management and outcomes in oncology settings: a systematic review of the literature. Cancer Treat Rev. 2016;42:56–72.
38. Freeman RK, Van Woerkom JM, Vyverberg A, Ascioti AJ. The effect of a multidisciplinary thoracic malignancy conference on the treatment of patients with lung cancer. Eur J Cardiothorac Surg. 2010;38:1–5.
39. Pluyter JR, Jacobs I, Langereis S, et al. Looking through the eyes of the multidisciplinary team: the design and clinical evaluation of a decision support system for lung cancer care. Transl Lung Cancer Res. 2020;9(4):1422–32.
40. https://clinicaltrials.gov/ct2/show/NCT03893539.
41. Chen A, Silvestri GA, Gildea TR, et al. Robotic bronchoscopy for peripheral pulmonary lesions: a multicenter pilot and feasibility study (BENEFIT). Chest. 2021;159(2):845–52.
42. Fielding DIK, Bashirzadeh F, Son JH, et al. First human use of a new robotic-assisted fiber optic sensing navigation system for small peripheral pulmonary nodules. Respiration. 2019;98:142–50.
43. Rojas-Solano JR, Ugalde-Gamboa L, Machuzak M. Robotic bronchoscopy for diagnosis of suspected lung cancer: a feasibility study. J Bronchology Interv Pulmonol. 2018;25:168–75.

44. Goldstraw P, Chansky K, Crowley J, et al. The iaslc lung cancer staging project: proposals for revision of the tnm stage groupings in the forthcoming (eighth) edition of the tnm classification for lung cancer. J Thorac Oncol. 2016;11(1):39–51.
45. Rocco G, Allen MS, Altorki NK, et al. Clinical statement on the role of the surgeon and surgical issues relating to computed tomography screening programs for lung cancer. Ann Thorac Surg. 2013;96(1):357–60.
46. Flores R, Bauer T, Aye R, et al. Balancing curability and unnecessary surgery in the context of computed tomography screening for lung cancer. J Thorac Cardiovasc Surg. 2014;147:1619–26; Kumar R, Kavuru MS. Lung cancer.
47. Nguyen DM, Sarkaria IS, Song C, et al. Clinical and economic comparative effectiveness of robotic-assisted, video-assisted thoracoscopic, and open lobectomy. J Thorac Dis. 2020;12(3):296–306.
48. Randhawa S, Moore RF, DiSesa V, et al. Role of thoracic surgeons in lung cancer screening: opportune time for involvement. J Thorac Oncol. 2018;13(3):298–300.
49. Lau KK, Rathinam S, Waller DA, Peake MD. The effects of increased provision of thoracic surgical specialists on the variation in lung cancer resection rate in England. J Thorac Oncol. 2013;8:68–72.
50. von Meyenfeldt EM, Gooiker GA, van Gijn W, et al. The relationship between volume or surgeon specialty and outcome in the surgical treatment of lung cancer: a systematic review and meta-analysis. J Thorac Oncol. 2012;7(7):1170–8.
51. Wouters MWJM, Jansen-Landheer MLEA, van de Velde CJH. The quality of cancer care initiative in The Netherlands. Eur J Surg Oncol. 2010;36(Suppl 1):S3–S13.
52. Dutch Surgical Society. Minimal criteria for surgical treatment (Dutch). (Dutch Surgical Society (NVvH) web site), 2011. http://www.heelkunde.nl/uploads/5O/5H/5O5H5htx15bBtD FNcBEmkw/nvvh-normen-januari-2011.pdf. Accessed 21 Mar 2022.
53. Sakoda LC, Rivera MP, Zhang J, et al. Patterns and factors associated with adherence to lung cancer screening in diverse practice settings. JAMA Netw Open. 2021;4(4):e218559.
54. Smith HB, Ward R, Frazier C, Angotti J, Tanner NT. Guideline-recommended lung cancer screening adherence is superior with a centralized approach. Chest. 2021;161:818; Published online September 15, S0012–3692(21)03856–3.
55. Fathi JT, White CS, Greenberg GM, Mazzone PJ, Smith RA, Thomson CC. The integral role of the electronic health record and tracking software in the implementation of lung cancer screening-a call to action to developers: a white paper from the national lung cancer roundtable. Chest. 2020;157(6):1674–9.
56. Eon—lung cancer screening software solution. Eon. https://eonhealth.com/lung-cancer-screening-software. Accessed 7 Mar 2022.
57. Fintelmann FJ, Bernheim A, Digumarthy SR, et al. The 10 pillars of lung cancer screening: rationale and logistics of a lung cancer screening program. Radiographics. 2015;35(7):1893–908.
58. Carroll NM, Burnett-Hartman AN, Joyce CA, et al. Real-world clinical implementation of lung cancer screening-evaluating processes to improve screening guidelines-concordance. J Gen Intern Med. 2020;35(4):1143–52.
59. Li J, Chung S, Wei EK, Luft HS. New recommendation and coverage of low-dose computed tomography for lung cancer screening: uptake has increased but is still low. BMC Health Serv Res. 2018;18(1):525. https://doi.org/10.1186/s12913-018-3338-9.
60. Spalluto LB, Lewis JA, LaBaze S, et al. Association of a lung screening program coordinator with adherence to annual CT lung screening at a large academic institution. J Am Coll Radiol. 2020;17(2):208–15. https://doi.org/10.1016/j.jacr.2019.08.010.
61. McKee BJ, McKee AB, Flacke S, Lamb CR, Hesketh PJ, Wald C. Initial experience with a free, high-volume, low-dose CT lung cancer screening program. J Am Coll Radiol. 2013;10(8):586–92.
62. Batlle JC, Maroules CD, Latif MA, Cury RC. A five-step strategy for building an LDCT lung cancer screening program. Appl Radiol. 2018;47(1):12–8.

Chapter 20
Cost Considerations

Gregory C. Kane

Cost is broadly defined as the amount of money paid or charged for something of value. Cost considerations in lung cancer screening (LCS), however, have implications that go well beyond the simple charge or fee to obtain an initial scan. In this chapter, we will discuss the relative value or charges for some of the basic medical services involved in LCS and also discuss the downstream value of medical services and revenue that may ultimately flow to hospitals, clinics, and healthcare systems. The goal is to shed light on the economic factors, primarily from the healthcare organization or health system perspective that are part of the landscape of lung cancer screening. Understanding this impact will be necessary as health systems plan for the growth of LCS in the balance of this decade. This chapter will not discuss costs related to other aspects of screening such as radiation exposure, economic costs associated with over-diagnosis, unnecessary medical procedures, or anxiety created by false-positive scans. Furthermore, patient financial and emotional costs experienced by patients who undergo screening are not addressed. These other costs are important but are beyond the scope of this chapter. Here, we will be focusing principally on the economic costs and revenue of medical testing and interventions for lung cancer and suspected lung cancer from an institutional perspective.

Prior to discussing fees or payments, which patients or consumers must pay for medical services, unless covered by insurance, it is necessary to understand the process of how Medicare pays for physician services. For each medical service, whether it be a physician visit, radiological study or medical procedure; a *workRVU* (a *relative value unit* of work) is designated which represents the relative value of a particular service among the multitude of evaluations, medical tests, and medical procedures a patient might potentially undergo for any medical reason [1]. The payment formula is further divided into three RVUs, one for *physician work*, one for

G. C. Kane (✉)
Department of Medicine, Thomas Jefferson University, Philadelphia, PA, USA
e-mail: gregory.kane@jefferson.edu

practice expense (PE), and one for *malpractice expense* (ME). While beyond the scope of this discussion, all workRVUs are geographically adjusted to reflect unique costs in different locales across the country. The workRVU for any medical service reimbursed by Medicare is then multiplied by a Medicare conversion factor, usually expressed in dollars, to obtain a final price. Historically, Medicare's physician workRVU, the relative value of one physician's service compared to another's for any particular physician visit, radiological study, or medical procedure are determined by a committee of the American Medical Association. This body, composed largely of specialty physicians, wields substantial influence over the relative value of different services in American Medicine [2]. The actual cost of a medical service independent of any insurance coverage is determined by the workRVU and the Medicare multiplier with which the workRVU is multiplied to get the actual dollar cost of a service. While this multiplier is specific to Medicare, many private insurers follow Medicare's lead in pricing their own coverage for medical services. With a budget neutrality adjustment to account for changes in RVUs, the current 2022 multiplier is $33.59, down $1.30 from 2021 [3].

Another foundational element of cost relates to "profit" or "margin contribution" and these terms can be defined in multiple ways. One reason for the challenge of this discussion is that hospitals and health systems typically have a very high overhead for infrastructure costs when compared to stand-alone radiology facilities and community-based surgical centers where there is lower overhead principally related to focused facility design and staffing models. For purposes of the discussion in this chapter, we will assume that the evaluation of a positive low-dose CT scan with further diagnostic radiology, staging procedures, biopsies, and any necessary surgeries will be performed in a hospital or within a health system. The reader should understand that some assumptions would contribute to lower contribution margins as compared to outpatient radiology facilities or outpatient surgical centers, such as facilities that are prevalent for orthopedic procedures or gastrointestinal endoscopies.

Recognizing the variable background of our readership, a glossary of economics may be helpful and is provided in Table 20.1.

The first level of costs associated with lung cancer screening relates to intake and performance of the initial screening study. There are two aspects of this initial step in LCS. They are a review of the risks, benefits, and alternatives as part of shared decision making with the patient. The second aspect is the actual performance of the low-dose CT scan. This initial scan is often referred to as the "T0" scan or baseline scan. The reasons for this designation relate to the fact that the significance of this scan may not be fully appreciated until the follow-up or "T1" scan is completed. The comparison allows clinicians to assess the presence or absence of nodule growth—a key finding that suggests a high likelihood of lung cancer. These designations are most applicable to research studies or other published analyses. For patients with either Medicaid or Medicare coverage (including dual eligible persons) or persons with private insurance, a low-dose CT (LDCT, CPT code 7121 effective January 2021) is a covered service. While there is a cost as demonstrated in Table 20.2, the cost is not a barrier because federal law considers cancer screening tests for eligible enrolled persons as covered services. The cut-off age for lung

Table 20.1 Glossary of basic economic terms (adapted from the National Library of Medicine's Glossary of Frequently Encountered Terms in Health Economics [4])

Term	Meaning	Significance or example
workRVU	The assigned relative value of a particular service compared to other healthcare services	Product of the workRVU and a multiplier leads to a monetary value established by CMS. The actual price for medicare beneficiaries is established
Charge	Monetary value for service requested by the seller/hospital	This can vary widely and may be more than CMS might designate for the service
Cost	The actual amount of resource is that it would take to perform service	This can very based on utilization. For example, when a PET scanner is used twice is much each month, cost of the PET scan would go down
Fee	A charge for a service rendered	Such as fee for a physician visit
Fixed cost	This cost relates to the investment in equipment or necessary staffing in a healthcare setting	For example, cost of the PET-CT machine
Variable cost	This cost relates to factors tied to the individual frequency of use of the service	For example, cost of the nuclear pharmaceutical for the PET scan which will be administered to each individual patient
Health insurance	A method of providing coverage to pay for specific types of healthcare expenses incurred by an insured person. Policies typically designate what services will be covered, what amount will be paid, can be referred to as a "third party payer"	Private insurance such a blue cross and blue shield or government provided insurance such as medicare or medicaid are examples
Medicaid	A federal health insurance program managed by the states which provide medical and healthcare coverage for poor	States determine who is eligible for this program
Medicare	A federal health insurance program begun in the 1960s which provides medical and healthcare coverage for the elderly and disabled. Persons with end-stage renal disease who require dialysis are also eligible	Typically for persons 65 and older in the United States
Overhead	Refers to fixed costs that apply to the overall organization	Examples of overhead would include the cost of maintaining parking facilities, security, HVAC systems, and routine maintenance
Physician practice pattern	An approach to diagnosing a specific illness that may be unique to a particular physician (or surgeon) or group of physicians	For example, some surgeons recommend a brain MRI be performed prior to resection for an early stage lung cancer, while other do not

(continued)

Table 20.1 (continued)

Term	Meaning	Significance or example
Profit	A financial gain is determined by the amount of revenue minus the cost of producing that service	Profit (or loss) can be assigned to specific service lines or specific business units. It can also apply to the global organization
Quality-adjusted life year (QALY)	The life years gained as a result of any particular health interventions with consideration of the quality of these life years gained	For example, the years gained because a cancer was found at an early stage and successfully resected for cure instead of allowing this cancer to progress and metastasize
Contribution margin	Revenue minus expense for a particular type of service such as a surgery including assignment of appropriate overhead	The contribution margin may be calculated for a lung cancer surgery or treatment with radiation for primary lung cancer such as SBRT

Table 20.2 CPT codes and professional workRVU for typical services performed at the initial stage of lung cancer screening

Service (CPT code)	Professional component workRVU[a]	Fee schedule	Total workRVU professional and facility	Fee schedule
Shared decision making (G0296)	1.51	$52.69		
LDCT (71271)	1.52	$53.04	4.32	150.74
Diagnostic CT thorax (71260)	1.63	$56.89	5.29	184.58

[a]The designation includes workRVU plus practice expense (PE) workRVU and malpractice workRVU combined

cancer screening was initially 55 years meaning that certain individuals may qualify for screening eligibility and yet lack healthcare insurance through their employer or because they are out of work. These individuals are most commonly 55 years through 64 years. This creates particular challenges for these individuals, not only to cover the cost associated with the initial scan but also with regard to follow-up. Newer United States Preventive Services Task Force (USPSTF) guidelines created additional eligibility for persons as young as 50 years of age, thus leading to a larger proportion of patients below Medicare age (65 years) who might be without insurance and unable to afford a low-dose CT [5, 6]. For this group, the cost of self-pay would represent a significant barrier for access to screening [7]. If we are to realize the promise of lung cancer screening, it is essential that we remain cognizant of this potential insurance gap for persons at risk for lung cancer between ages 50 and 64. For those who do have coverage, Table 20.2 outlines initial services often encountered at the early referral phase of lung cancer screening.

One conclusion based upon the above workRVU data is that a low-dose CT is reimbursed comparably, but slightly below, a traditional diagnostic CT scan which may include the administration of contrast media. Not included in the presented calculations are costs associated with follow-up including the follow-up of incidental nodules or suspicious findings. Persons undergoing low-dose CT screening should be expected to have substantial smoking history and therefore are anticipated to have multiple important findings which require appropriate follow-up, which at least requires a T1 scan at a 12-month interval. One barrier for health systems is assuring that the cost for those necessary follow-ups is addressed to minimize malpractice risks and assures optimal outcomes for screened persons. For persons lacking insurance, the total cost for the shared decision making visit and the low-dose CT combined ($202.73) would be unreasonably high, especially when one considers that a follow-up scan most certainly will be required in order to assure that any detected lesion is followed appropriately for at least 1 year.

The impact of lung cancer screening would be negligible if cancers were not detected. The methodology of cancer diagnosis typically involves additional imaging with contrast-enhanced CT chest, FDG PET-CT, or chest X-ray. Based upon results of these studies and comparison to the T0 scan, bronchoscopy (with or without biopsy) and/or needle aspiration biopsy might be performed. Definitive studies are often surgical and may include mediastinoscopy for staging followed by VATS or robotic surgery with lung tissue resection.

The frequency of these studies in any cohort of screened individuals could be estimated in two ways. First, data from the NLST can be extrapolated. Second, data from actual screening programs (published or unpublished) might also form the basis of such analyses [8]. It is necessary, however, for healthcare executives to understand how these estimates might be calculated so that they might understand the impact of launching or expanding a lung cancer screening program, based upon the frequency of subsequent radiological, biopsy, and surgical interventions. In the NLST, 649 cancers were detected among 26,722 enrolled subjects over the T0, T1, and T2 scans or 3 years of follow-up. On average, this scenario would amount to approximately 216 patients diagnosed with lung cancer each year of the NLST among the 26,722 enrolled subjects. It is important to note that this is an average, as the number of cases in the NLST varied considerably each year [9].

The author team for the NLST cataloged the diagnostic studies performed among persons with positive low-dose CT scans, though they did not enumerate the CPT codes for the procedures. Moreover, in clinical practice, one would expect certain local practice variations, all of which would still be within the standard of care. For example, an FDG PET scan might be ordered with CT (designated as FDG PET-CT, CPT code 78492) or a biopsy may be more likely to be performed via bronchoscopy than needle aspiration depending on local resources. When considering these variations, this author will make certain assumptions. For example, we will assume that all follow-up CT scans will be conducted with contrast even though this might not necessarily be the case and all FDG PET scans will be carried out with CT for lesion localization. The authors of the NLST did not quantitate brain imaging with MRI or essential blood work prior to biopsy or surgery, but all subjects undergoing such interventions would typically have blood studies. This is not meant as criticism, but just to point out that this presentation will not comment on routine blood work as part of the cost of LCS. The cost of follow-up studies, then, can be estimated from the frequency of such follow-up studies in the NLST or other series [8, 9].

The methods of this analysis are based upon the following sequence of estimates. We have chosen to make the measure as *"per 1000 persons screened"* as this approach should prove facile for public health planners and health systems administrators. As mentioned above, among the active screened group over 3 years, the NLST identified 649 cancers in the low-dose CT arm of the trial in 26,722 persons compared to 279 cancers in the control group. Annualized this experience would represent 216 cancers per year in the 26,722 screened subjects or approximately 8 cancers per 1000 subjects screened annually [8]. We acknowledge that this estimate is the average number of cancers. For comparison, Shusted and colleagues reported on 1276 subjects followed over 33 months with 32 cancers detected resulting in a slightly higher frequency of approximately 12 cancers/year per 1000 subjects, representing real-life data from a diverse population in an inner-city academic screening program [9]. I also point out that additional cases of malignancy occurred in 367 subjects including in some subjects who were never screened, and a significant number who were diagnosed during the post screening period. With these cases added in, one could anticipate up to 13 cancers/year per 1000 subjects. The comparison should be considered illuminating, as the range of 8–13 cancers might be expected among every 1000 patients screened annually in a typical risk population at least early in a screening program's existence. In the midst of all this discussion about economic costs, wRVU, and contribution margin, this author would like to highlight the fact that these 8–13 cases of lung cancer represent patients with a high likelihood of surgical cure. They would have otherwise gone on to develop more advanced stages of lung cancer were it not for the advent of CT imaging-based LCS. The costs of life years lost are substantial and medical costs of more advanced-stage symptomatic tumors would most likely exceed those costs associated with the evaluation of positive scans during the screening process. It would also be important for the reader to understand that other investigators, including Claudia Heschke and colleagues, identified 27 cancers in 1000 subjects with an initial scan and subsequent imaging based on the findings and follow-up that continued for up to two years. This reminds us that the yield of continuing to follow patients over time, including following abnormalities seen on the initial CT scan, at an appropriate interval, yields additional cancer diagnoses from the original cohort. Based on this study some might suggest that 27 cancers would be anticipated upon screening 1000 patients annually, though this yield requires additional follow-up studies that extend beyond the first year. Thus, the reader should realize the number of cancers at an early phase of lung cancer screening may increase once patients with suspicious nodules complete the requisite follow-up [10].

The economic value of LCS to health systems is influenced by "downstream revenue," which is the volume of additional clinical procedures including radiography, biopsy, and surgeries and the associated revenues genrated. In some cases, when advanced tumors are diagnosed, this would include radiation treatments and/ or chemotherapy, molecular therapy, or immunotherapy administration. While the realization of revenue is straightforward, it is important to emphasize that the margin on surgeries and complex biopsy procedures often creates a favorable financial bottom-line view of screening for health systems. Therapy from radiation treatments and chemotherapy, however, is also important. The frequency of non-lung

Table 20.3 Estimated numbers of key medical services (per 1000 screening examinations) and WorkRVUs (per individual study or service) for typical downstream services associated with suspicious findings on lung cancer screen

Service by CPT code[a]	Service	Number per 1000 enrolled annually	Work RVUs [2]	Non-facility PE RVUs[b]	Facility PERVUs[b]	Mal-practice RVUs[b]	Total non-facility RVUs[b]	Total facility RVUs[b]
71,046	Chest X-ray	32	0.22	0.08	0.08	0.01	0.31	0.31
71,260	Chest CT with contrast	109	1.16	0.42	0.42	0.05	1.63	1.63
78,492	FDG PET or FDG PET CT[c]	18	1.80	0.61	0.61	0.07	2.48	2.48
A9597	FDG PET tracer code[d]	18	N/A	N/A	N/A	N/A	N/A	N/A
99,204	Level 4 new visit with pulmonologist	13[e]	2.6	2.09	1.12	0.24	4.93	3.96
32,408	Percutaneous transthoracic needle aspiration	3	3.18	24.82	0.98	0.28	28.28	4.44
38,505	Percutaneous extrathoracic needle biopsy (i.e., lymph node)	1	1.14	2.40	0.77	0.11	3.65	2.02
31,645	Bronchoscopy without biopsy	4	2.88	5.05	1.14	0.27	8.20	4.29
31,628	Bronchoscopy with biopsy	5	3.55	7.63	1.31	0.29	11.47	5.15
99,205	Level 5 new visit with surgeon	10[f]	3.5	2.69	1.56	0.32	6.51	5.38
39,401	Mediastinoscopy	1	3.5	NA	2.28	1.30	NA	9.02
32,607	Thoracoscopy	3	5.5	NA	2.21	1.34	NA	9.05
32,100	Thoracotomy	6	13.75	NA	6.71	3.33	NA	23.79

A "facility" place-of-services thought of as a hospital, ambulatory surgery center, or skilled nursing facility.

A "non facility" is typically associated with the physician's office as the place of service

[a] CPT codes and descriptors only are copyright 2020 American Medical Association. All Rights Reserved. Applicable FARS/DFARS apply

[b] If values are reflected for a code with a status indicator other than "A," "R," or "T," the RVUs generally reflect recommendations submitted to CMS processed through the PFS methodology without modification

[c] Author of this chapter made in assumption that FDG PET scan will be performed with CT scan for tumor localization based on typical but not universal physician practice patterns

[d] The nuclear pharmaceutical is essential to this test and is billed separately as a pharmacy drug could charge (prices may vary based on the market)

[e] The number of new visits with pulmonologist is not described in the NLST, however, it would be anticipated that associated with every percutaneous biopsy or bronchoscopy, a visit with pulmonologist would occur

[f] The number of new visits with a surgeon is not described in the NLST, however, it would be anticipated that associated with every percutaneous biopsy or bronchoscopy, a visit with pulmonologist would occur

cancer malignancies is also important in the lung cancer screening program, but the numbers are smaller relative to the total number of cancers detected and are not addressed in this presentation.

In Table 20.3, we used NLST data to estimate the annual incidence of specific follow-up tests or procedures per 1000 persons screened. We have also included workRVU for professional fees and total workRVU to include the facility or non-facility component. Table 20.3 utilizes the frequency of these studies reported among the screened cohort in the NLST. For example, among 1000 screened subjects there would be, on average, approximately 109 CT scans (beyond the screening studies) of the thorax and 18 PET-CT scans with 13 biopsy procedures and up to 10 surgeries expected each year. These numbers should be considered as estimates, as actual experience is expected to vary. The value of this analysis may be greatest for planners in health systems that are building out their programs and are looking to estimate the volume of associated procedures. A weakness of this analysis is that the NLST did not comment on comprehensive therapies beyond those described above.

In an unpublished series, this author asked an institutional economic analysis team at Jefferson Health to assess revenue, both inpatient DRG revenue as well as professional fees, from select interventions across our actual insurance mix from the calendar year 2019. The number of downstream evaluations at our center city urban location included 34 PET scans yielding $1167 revenue per case or $39,678. Seven patients underwent biopsy with average net revenue that included any necessarily associated studies of $3515 per case for a net revenue of $ 24,605. Twelve patients underwent surgery with an average net revenue of $23,967/case or $287,604. In addition, one patient had severe coronary artery calcifications detected and required lifesaving CABG due to critical left main disease yielding $51,994 in net revenue (personal communication). More recently, the editors expanded their analysis of the contribution margin for LCS among 593 patients screened. The sum of inpatient and outpatient Current Procedural Terminology (CPT) codes for each patient was accounted, and the net revenue was calculated. These revenues were balanced against costs across all 593 patients, leading to a contribution margin of approximately $1,160,000 for the cohort (personal communication).

Why are financial considerations so important to health systems? The oft-quoted mantra of "no margin no mission," first coined by a religious leader, Sister Irene Krause, in a faith-based health system, provided a very simple and straightforward view of how health systems set priorities. This view underscores the reality that unless they can stay financially solvent, there is no way to fund essential interventions or new programs (such as lung cancer screening) [11]. The finances of lung cancer screening are actually quite appealing. For a small investment in a centralized program with a nurse navigator and an infrastructure to track and follow results, health systems can benefit from the "downstream" revenue of thoracic surgeries and cancer care. These services typically already provide revenue that drives health systems—it just occurs at a more accelerated rate through lung cancer screening programs while treating patients at an earlier stage as a result of a successful case identification that will support better outcomes and long-term survival. Thus, lung cancer screening is a true "win-win" and an example where doing well for patients and communities translates into increased revenue for health systems, while improving lung cancer mortality and saving lives.

In the early years after the publication of the NLST, even before most medical societies came on board to support lung cancer screening, the cost-effectiveness was suggested and supported by a number of investigations [12]. One analysis estimated that the cost would be approximately $19,000/life year saved. This compares favorably to recently published estimate for breast cancer, at $26,880.00 per life-year saved [13]. Other assessments of the quality-adjusted life-year saved (QALY) ranged higher ($81,000 per QALY gained) as analyzed by the NLST Research Team, but they also found widely variable results based upon modest adjustments in the screening group (such as specific age cohorts) or based on variable surgical mortality associated with the lung resection from 1.2% to 8% [14].

In summary, cancer care is a major part of the business of medicine, and LCS will generate activity (and contribution margins) for those health systems that add this service and promote its growth. Such added activity will lead to predictable healthcare services for diagnostic studies, biopsies, and surgeries for individual with suspicious lesions. While having reviewed the financial activity that can be expected to follow from these medical services, this author concludes by focusing attention on the lives saved. Indeed, saving 8–12 lives per 1000 screened each year should be judged as worth the cost. While prior actuarial analyses of the total number of saved lives have been published, the true reduction in lung cancer mortality is challenged by the need to expand lung cancer screening to all eligible persons [14]. An important question that is raised by the findings reported here is, "What are the societal costs of not rapidly expanding lung cancer screening to serve the majority of at risk Americans?."

References

1. Reinhardt U. How medicare pays physicians. New York, NY: The New York Times; 2010. Accessed 6 Feb 2022.
2. Anna Wilde Matthews and Thomas McGinty 2010 "Physician panel prescribes the fees set by medicare. Accessed 6 Feb 2022.
3. www.cms.gov/newsroom/fact-sheets/calendar-year-cy-2022-medicare-physician-fee-schedule-final-rule. Accessed 1 Mar 2022.
4. https://www.nlm.nih.gov/nichsr/edu/healthecon/glossary.html. Accessed 3 Mar 2022.
5. Meza R, Jeon J, Toumazis I, et al. Evaluation of the benefits and harms of lung cancer screening with low-dose computed tomography: modeling study for the US preventive services task force. JAMA. 2021;325(10):988–97.
6. Rivera MP, Katki HA, Tanner NT, et al. Addressing disparities in lung cancer screening eligibility and healthcare access. An official American thoracic society statement. Am J Respir Crit Care Med. 2020;202(7):e95–e112.
7. Wang GX, Baggett TP, Pandharipande PV, Park ER, Percac-Lima S, Shepard J-AO, et al. Barriers to lung cancer screening engagement from the patient and provider perspective. Radiology. 2019;290(2):278–87.

8. National Lung Screening Trial Research Team, Aberle DR, Adams AM, Berg CD, Black WC, Clapp JD, Fagerstrom RM, Gareen IF, Gatsonis C, Marcus PM, Sicks JD. Reduced lung-cancer mortality with low-dose computed tomographic screening. N Engl J Med. 2011;365(5):395–409. https://doi.org/10.1148/radiol.2018180212.

9. Shusted CS, Evans NR, Juon H, Kane GC, Barta JA. Association of race with lung cancer risk among adults undergoing lung cancer screening. JAMA Netw Open. 2021;4(4):e214509. https://doi.org/10.1001/jamanetworkopen.2021.4509.

10. Henschke CI, McCauley DI, Yankelevitz DF, Naidich DP, McGuinness G, Miettinen OS, et al. Early Lung Cancer Action Project: overall design and findings from baseline screening. The Lancet. 1999;354(9173): 99–105.

11. Pellegrini Vincent D Jr, Guzick DS, Wilson DE, Evarts CMC. Governance of academic health centers and systems: a conceptual framework for analysis. Acad Med. 2019;94(1):12–6. https://doi.org/10.1097/ACM.0000000000002407.

12. Pyenson BS, Henschke CI, Yankelevitz DF, Yip R, Dec E. Offering lung cancer screening to high-risk medicare beneficiaries saves lives and is cost-effective: an actuarial analysis. Am Health Drug Benefits. 2014;7(5):272–82. PMID: 25237423; PMCID: PMC4163779.

13. Pashayan N, Morris S, Gilbert FJ, Pharoah PDP. Cost-effectiveness and benefit-to-harm ratio of risk-stratified screening for breast cancer: a life-table model. JAMA Oncol. 2018;4(11):1504–10. https://doi.org/10.1001/jamaoncol.2018.1901.

14. Black WC, Gareen IF, Soneji SS, National Lung Screening Trial Research Team, et al. Cost-effectiveness of CT screening in the national lung screening trial. N Engl J Med. 2014;371(19):1793–802.

Part IV
Taking Care of the Patient

Chapter 21
Using Health Literacy Principles to Engage Patients from Diverse Backgrounds in Lung Cancer Screening

Rickie Brawer and Kristine Pham

Background

Health disparities are exacerbated by underlying social determinants of health, resulting in poorer overall health and outcomes from diseases such as cancer. Findings from many studies confirm that lower health literacy is one of the social determinants of health associated with cancer-related disparities, and that expanding partnerships with community-based organizations and consumers addresses unmet needs associated with cancer disparities [1–5]. Nearly 9 out of 10 adults may struggle with health literacy, but even those with proficient health literacy may experience difficulty with understanding and acting on health information, such as when they are stressed, sick, or were just told they have cancer. Examples of populations that may experience higher rates of lower health literacy include individuals with less education, older adults, individuals on Medicaid, and people with limited English proficiency (LEP) such as those for whom English is a second language [6–8]. According to studies, nearly half of all cancer patients may have difficulty understanding information related to their disease or treatment, potentially resulting in poorer health and treatment outcomes [6, 9, 10]. Recent studies have shown poorer cancer outcomes are associated with decreased adherence to treatment plans [11] and higher rates of missed appointments [10, 12]. In addition, as noted by the 2020–2021 President's Cancer Panel, screening barriers specific to lung cancer

R. Brawer (✉) · K. Pham
Department of Medical Oncology, Thomas Jefferson University, Philadelphia, PA, USA
e-mail: Rickie.Brawer@Jefferson.edu; kristine.pham@jefferson.edu

    211
G. C. Kane et al. (eds.), *Lung Cancer Screening*,
https://doi.org/10.1007/978-3-031-33596-9_21

include patient lack of awareness, fear of cancer diagnosis, stigma, and challenges related to accessing health care [13]. Provider unfamiliarity with lung cancer screening guidelines and difficulty identifying eligible patients were also cited. The President's Cancer Panel developed four strategic goals and recommendations to enhance lung screening access and utilization for all populations [13]. Three of these goals directly address communication with patients and are described in the following text.

- Goal 1: *Improve and align cancer screening communication* to increase general community awareness about this relatively new screening, and enhance understanding about lung cancer and screening (knowledge, attitudes, beliefs) and utilization of lung cancer screening.
- Goal 2: *Facilitate equitable access to cancer screening* through community outreach and use of trusted messengers such as trained community health workers and others with lived experience.
- Goal 3: *Strengthen workforce collaborations to support cancer screening and risk assessment.* This goal calls for training all team members so they have the knowledge and skills needed to support cancer screening.

While training in health literacy is not specifically mentioned, being able to communicate in ways that patients understand, that consider cultural beliefs, and that patients can easily act on is key to increasing lung cancer screening.

Health Literacy Overview

The initial definition of health literacy, developed for the National Library of Medicine and used by the Institute of Medicine and Healthy People 2010 and 2020, is "the degree to which individuals have the capacity to obtain, process, and understand basic health information and services needed to make appropriate health decisions" [7, 14]. A key focus of the Healthy People 2030 plan (HP 2030) is to "*eliminate health disparities, achieve health equity, and attain health literacy to improve the health and well-being of all.*" Given this major focus, the U.S. Department of Health has expanded the definition of health literacy for HP 2030 to include both personal health literacy and organizational health literacy. As defined in the HP 2030 initiative, personal health literacy is "the degree to which individuals have the ability to find, understand, and use information and services to inform health-related decisions and actions for themselves and others." Personal health literacy includes understanding the doctor's instructions and being able to navigate the complex health system including the use of digital health technology. Organizational health literacy is defined as "the degree to which organizations equitably enable individuals to find, understand, and use information and services to inform health-related decisions and actions for themselves and others." Organizational health literacy includes the ease of navigating the health system such as scheduling appointments, increasing the use of evidence-based practices like Teach-back and motivational interviewing to enhance patient understanding and commitment, and organizational commitment to providing health communication materials that utilize best practices. Patients, community members, and providers should be continuously engaged in all aspects of the material development, implementation, and dissemination process [15–17].

The expansion of the health literacy definition promotes health equity and decision making by emphasizing peoples' ability to not only understand information, but to be able to use that information to make informed decisions [16]. The revised definition also stresses the role and responsibilities of organizations in addressing health literacy and aligns with efforts of other national plans and guidelines [3] such as the National Academy of Medicine's Ten Attributes of a Health Literate Organization [18], the Guide to Community Preventive Services [19], recommendations for the U.S. Preventive Services Task Force [20], the National Standards for Culturally and Linguistically Appropriate services in Health and Health Care (CLAS Standards) [11], and the Health and Human Services National Action Plan to Improve Health Literacy [15].

In 2019, the National Cancer Policy Forum and the Roundtable on Health Literacy brought together patients, advocates, clinicians, and representatives from health care organizations, academic medical centers, insurers, and federal agencies to explore opportunities to improve cancer communication across the continuum of care [10]. Suggestions for improving patient-provider communication include implementing effective training programs for providers that enhance listening skills, and build clinician skills to simplify complex information when communicating with patients about cancer prevention, risk reduction, screening, and treatment.

Training should also include evidence-based practices, such as motivational interviewing and shared decision-making, which promote patient-centered open dialogue that is culturally and linguistically sensitive.

Community-based outreach was noted as critical to building trust and improving the health of individuals and communities. Recommendations for improving cancer communication for the general public encourage engagement and collaboration with diverse members of the population, including patients, family members, and representatives from community organizations, in all stages of the development and dissemination of strategies and tools for communicating cancer information that is in plain language, actionable, and tailored to people in the community for whom the information is intended. To promote health literacy at the organizational level, training of all employees in communication that focuses on health literacy and implementing policies that regularly assess patient education and practices was advised. Patient navigation programs to address access barriers to care, including health literacy and other social determinants of health, were also proposed [10].

As part of the effort to achieve health equity and eliminate preventable health disparities, the CDC created *Health Equity Guiding Principles for Inclusive Communication* to support the development of communication materials and strategies that are culturally and linguistically appropriate. Examples of these principles include [21]:

- Use a health equity lens that considers racism, and other forms of discrimination. Recognize that individuals do not view their lives or health through a single identity lens and may belong to one or more racial, ethnic, or demographic groups with varying health and social inequities and assets. Acknowledge that diversity exists within and across populations and communities.
- Acknowledge that access to information is necessary but not sufficient if people cannot understand or use it, or it is not culturally and linguistically appropriate. Avoid language that implies blame based on an individual's or population's increased risk of poorer health outcomes. Consider how to improve access to information based on preferences of the population of interest.
- Tailor communication strategies to the population one is trying to reach. Community engagement and leadership is fundamental to the development of outreach materials and strategies that are culturally relevant, unbiased, and resonate with the intended audience. Pretest and revise materials with the intended audience before disseminating. Review the materials for language that the audience may find offensive, marginalizing, or stigmatizing. Sources for key principle and preferred terminology resource include: Key Principles|Gateway to Health Communication|CDC; Preferred Terms for Select Population Groups & Communities|Gateway to Health Communication|CDC; NCI dictionary of cancer terms https://www.cancer.gov/publications/dictionaries/cancer-terms/expand/N. International Association for the Study of Lung Cancer: Language Guide (https://www.iaslc.org/IASLCLanguageGuide).
- Recognize that health literacy within a population of interest can vary depending on factors such as disability status, a primary language other than English, and access to technology and/or the ability to use it.

Integrating Health Literacy into Health Care Systems

The 10 attributes of health literate health care organizations highlight what health care organizations can do to make it easier for people to navigate, understand, and use information and services to take care of their health [22, 23]. These attributes can serve as a measure of progress in advancing health literacy in an organization.

The Health Literate Care Model integrates health literacy into the evidence-based Care Model (previously called the Chronic Care Model). The Care Model is a systems approach to achieving productive communication between clinical care and patients. This approach necessitates cooperative engagement of health system leadership, clinical practice, the community and patients, including their families and caregivers, to attain the information and resources needed to improve patient and community health outcomes [22, 23]. The Agency for Healthcare Research and Quality (AHRQ) Health Literacy Precautions Toolkit provides information and tools for integrating health literacy into the various components of the Care Model [24].

Health literacy universal precautions assume that all patients may have difficulty at some point in understanding health information and navigating the complex health system. Given this assumption, practice-wide changes and simplifying oral and written communication are needed for patients of all health literacy levels. Universal precautions promote [24, 25]:

- Improving patient-provider communication by simplifying oral, written, and web-based information and confirming patient understanding through tools such as Teach-Back.
- Enhancing clinical practice and health system environments so they are easier to navigate.
- Creating environments that are patient-centered and engage and support patients' efforts to improve their health.

Personal Health Literacy: Communication Strategies

Productive patient-provider communication enables patients to be actively engaged in their health care. To achieve productive communication, health care providers need to convey information to patients orally and in writing that it is easily understood, actionable, and empowers the patient in making decisions related to their health. The NIH Clear Communication strategy outlines five basic steps for developing health information for all populations, with particular emphasis on reaching those with lower health literacy [26]: define the intended audience (population of interest); conduct the research; develop a concept for the product; develop content and visual design of materials; pretest and revise material. Chapter 25 in this toolkit describes how this strategy was used to develop materials and public awareness strategies by the Lung Cancer Learning Community (LC2) initiative developed by Thomas Jefferson University.

Advisory groups give credibility to the research conducted and increase the likelihood that the materials, programs, and services developed will engage and meet the needs of patients and families. An advisory group that involves patients from the intended audience(s) and representatives from community organizations who serve these populations is key to informing and conducting community-based participatory research designed to understand what patients from the intended audiences may already know and believe about lung cancer including myths and misinformation, cultural preferences and sensitivities, motivators for lung cancer screening uptake, and social determinants of health and barriers that may impact lung cancer screening. The advisory group is essential not only to inform the research process, but also the development, pretesting, and dissemination of communication materials and strategies based on the research findings. They also play a key role in helping health systems identify community resources and services that address screening barriers such as those related to social determinants of health.

Raising patient and public awareness about lung cancer screening requires a multi-pronged approach including strategies such as tailoring oral and written communication to meet the needs of patients and the community; creating web-based material that is easy to find, use, and understand; and health literacy training for health system personnel.

Health Literacy Strategies in Interpersonal Communication

It is difficult to determine which patients may have lower health literacy. Studies show that patients immediately forget 40–80% of the medical information they are given and about 50% of information is not remembered correctly [27, 28]. Patients with limited health literacy may even have completed high school or college, be well spoken, be employed in professions such as health care, and may indicate they understand written materials provided [29]. While methods to assess health literacy exist, they are not accurate in all situations, and the process can be stigmatizing for patients, for example, having health literacy status documented in the patient health record. Using universal precautions means that health care providers communicate with all patients and families assuming that they will have difficulty understanding some health information. Ultimately, this approach recognizes that everyone benefits from communication that is clear, easy to understand, and actionable [24].

Principles for effective oral communication with patients include [30, 31]:

- *Create a shame-free environment* that encourages questions, shares concerns and problems, protects patients from embarrassment in front of others, is respectful, and builds trust.
- *Ask the patient how she prefers to receive information* (reading, hearing, or viewing).
- *Speak in plain language*—speak slowly with patients in a conversational manner that uses simple easy to understand language and avoids medical jargon. Include examples whenever possible and use visual models such as diagrams, pictures, and videos to illustrate the information. Table 21.1 provides common terminology used when discussing lung cancer and lung cancer screening and suggestions for plain language substitutions.
- Common terminology to describe lung cancer test results can also be confusing to patients. For example, in everyday life "positive" usually indicates something that is good or desired and "negative" is not good or desired. Yet for cancer test results the opposite is true. A positive test result means that one may have cancer and that further testing may be indicated. False-positive is also a misunderstood term and given the frequency of lung cancer test results that are false-positives, this term needs to be better explained for most people.

Table 21.1 Common lung cancer terminology

Cancer terminology	Simplified
Pulmonology	Having to do with the lungs
Carcinogen	Cancer causing
Low-dose computed tomography scan (also known as low-dose CT scan or LDCT)	A procedure that uses a computer linked to an X-ray machine that uses a low dose of radiation to take detailed pictures of tissues and organs in the body
Metastasis	The spread of cancer cells from the place in the body where they first formed to another part of the body
Nodule	A growth or lump that may be malignant (cancer) or benign (not cancer)
Malignant	Cancerous. Malignant cells can invade nearby tissue and spread to other parts of the body
Benign	Not cancerous
Pack-year	A way to measure how much a person has smoked over a long period of time. To determine the pack year multiply the number of packs of cigarettes smoked per day times the number of years the person has smoked. For example: 1 pack per day for 20 years is 20 pack-years. ½ pack per day for 40 years is 20 pack-years

(Source [39]: NCI Dictionary of Cancer Terms—National Cancer Institute)

- *Focus on what the patient needs to know and needs to do.* Limit, organize, and repeat the 3–5 most important key points. Teach 1 step at a time. Break down complex instructions.
- *Communicate in ways that encourage patient engagement* such as using pictures, videos, interactive computer programs, and personal risk assessments. Prepare patients for their health care visit by encouraging them to write down their questions or providing a list of suggested questions to ask their health care providers. Motivational interviewing, cited as an evidence-based practice by the Robert Wood Johnson Foundation, National Committee for Quality Assurance, and the Joint Commission [32], facilitates patient-centered discussion and fosters collaboration by asking patients open-ended questions about their goals, concerns, and other constraints in making a health care decision or behavioral change such as getting screened for lung cancer or giving up smoking. The role of the provider is to listen, affirm, and reflect what the patient says; elicit, clarify, and resolve ambivalence; summarize the discussion and help the patient create a personal plan for next steps. Providers should emphasize patient action, motivation, and self-empowerment rather than detailed facts [32]. Motivational interviewing and shared decision making communication strategies can be used sequentially to support the decision making process. Shared decision-making, a required component of lung cancer screening, also uses reflective listening to explore treatment options and help patients make informed decisions based on their preferences [33]. Chapters 4 and 11 in this

toolkit provide in-depth information regarding shared decision making and lung cancer screening.

- *Confirm patient understanding and encourage questions* using methods such as Teach-back. The Teach-back method assesses understanding by asking the patient to explain in his or her own words the information the staff provided, or by asking the patient to demonstrate a skill that was taught. Refrain from simply asking the patient "Do you understand?" Regardless of one's ability to understand the information, many people who do not understand may still answer "Yes." Teach-back is not about testing the patient's knowledge. It is about how well the provider explained the information [29]. Consider asking questions such as:

  - *We discussed a lot today and want to make sure I explained things clearly. When you go home today, what will you tell your wife about our conversation concerning lung cancer screening?*
  - *We have gone over a lot of information; and I want to make sure I explained it correctly. Can you tell me about the plan we discussed for getting screened for lung cancer?*

Language Assistance

Providing language assistance for those with limited English Proficiency (LEP) and other communication needs, including translating health materials into commonly spoken languages, providing sign language and braille, and providing interpreter services for in-person encounters, is required by Section 504 of the Rehabilitation Act of 1973 and Title VI of the Civil Rights Act of 1964 [34]. In 2013, the Office of Minority Health released the enhanced National CLAS Standards, a comprehensive set of 15 guidelines that inform, guide, and facilitate practices related to culturally and linguistically appropriate health services. Four of these standards (standards 5–8) directly relate to *Communication and Language Assistance* and apply to both oral and written communication [11]. These standards endorse providing language assistance to all LEP individuals at no cost; informing individuals about the availability of language assistance services in writing, verbally, and in preferred languages; ensuring that competently trained and tested bilingual interpreters are used and that American Sign Language (ASL) standards are met by individuals providing sign language; and providing easy-to-understand print and multimedia materials and signage in the most commonly spoken languages.

Using a Health Literacy Lens to Develop and Improve Written Health Materials

The Plain Writing Act of 2010 requires the federal government, including all health agencies, to apply health literacy plain writing principles to all documents in print and online [35]. As a result, the government and many other organizations, such as Medline Plus, have increased access to a variety of health materials written at or below a sixth grade level, that are accurate, easy to understand, and actionable. Whether one is using existing health education materials, revising materials, or developing new materials, assessing materials for readability, accuracy and relevance, and design is necessary.

Your document is written in plain language when your intended audience understands it. Engaging patients and members of the intended audience in the process is essential to ensuring documents are suitable, understandable, and actionable. Readability level alone is not an indicator that the document meets the health literacy guidelines for plain language. Patient education materials are *understandable and actionable* when consumers of diverse backgrounds and varying levels of health literacy can process and explain key messages, and identify what they can do based on the information presented. The following information provides a brief overview for developing written materials; extensive toolkits such as the AHRQ Health Literacy Universal Precautions Toolkit [24], the Center for Healthcare Strategies [35], and the CMS Toolkit for Making Written Material Clear and Effective [36] are available.

Assessing suitability of existing lung cancer screening materials:

- Utilize preexisting tools to provide guidance on health literacy assessment of written materials and videos, such as the Suitability Assessment of Materials (SAM). SAM addresses content, literacy demand, graphics, layout and type, learning simulation, and motivation and cultural appropriateness [37]. The Patient Education Materials Assessment Tool (PEMAT) is a systematic method to evaluate and compare *understandability* and *actionability* of patient education materials and assesses content, word choice and style, use of numbers, organization, layout and design, and use of visual aids [38]. Conducting a readability assessment for print materials in conjunction with the PEMAT is recommended.
- Conduct readability assessments using readability formulas such as SMOG, Fry, and Flesch-Kincaid. These assessments provide an estimate of the reading difficulty and are generally based on the number of multi-syllable words and sentence length. Assessing by hand is recommended; however, free online tools do exist (http://www.readabilityformulas.com/free-readability-formula-tests.php) and Flesch-Kincaid is available as part of MS Word. Readability scores should be interpreted as a range of difficulty rather than a specific grade level [35].

- Finally engage the intended audience in the review process and rely on their expertise and feedback to determine whether the material is clear and effective.

Processes for developing written materials to promote lung cancer screening: [26, 35].

- *Identify the intended population and conduct research* to understand their knowledge, attitudes, beliefs, and perceived barriers to lung cancer screening. Engage the intended audience through the formation of an advisory group and other methods such as focus groups, surveys, and key informant interviews.
- *Develop key concepts, messages, and strategies based on research findings.* Develop materials and pretest with the intended audience. Conduct readability assessments. Revise according to readability assessment and pretesting feedback from the intended audience.
- *Disseminate and evaluate materials based on input from the advisory group and intended audiences.* Evaluate satisfaction and understanding, and the impact on the intended audience using focus groups, surveys, and related tools.

Principles for developing written materials to promote lung cancer screening [24, 26, 35]:

- *Create text that is action and goal oriented.* Explain the purpose and limit content: create personal relevance by describing the purpose and benefits of screening from the patient viewpoint. Consider the following: What is it that the patient wants and needs to know? Is the information sensitive to the patient's gender, sexual orientation, and cultural or ethnic background? Emphasize desired patient actions, behaviors, and review key points. What is the least amount of information needed to provide the reader with the knowledge and motivation to get screened?
- *Utilize plain language principles for easy-to-read materials.* Write in a friendly, conversational style using active voice to motivate patients to action. Use short sentences (10–15 words) and limit paragraphs to three to five sentences. Use medical jargon sparingly and instead focus on plain language that defines and explains medical terms simply and clearly as shown in Table 21.1 [39]. To address numeracy, limit the use of statistics and use general words like most, many, half. Mathematical concepts, such as risk, normal, and range, may not be easily understood by the intended audience. If possible, use words such as "chance" or "possibility" instead. Repeat and summarize important messages.
- *Utilize design principles that make it easier for patients to read and navigate print materials.* Written materials that appear dense and difficult may overwhelm patients and discourage their use. Materials should provide content that is logically structured, using bulleted lists with subheadings that organize information. Materials should be designed so that the ratio of white space to words and images is maximized by using strategies such as 1-in. margins, 1½ to double spaced text, and a font size that is 12 point or larger. Other design strategies that help poorer readers and older adults navigate written materials include: strong contrast between background and text colors; left justified margins; using fonts that are

easy to read; and avoiding *italics*, all CAPITAL LETTERS, and *underlining which can make text appear blurry.* For more guidance regarding strategies to develop written materials refer to the AHRQ Health Literacy Universal Precautions Toolkit [24], NIH Clear Communication—Clear and Simple [26], and the Center for Health Care Strategies Health Literacy Fact Sheets [35].

- *Provide visual cues, illustrations, and interaction to help the reader focus on what is important.* Incorporating visual images and patient interaction into written materials increases the likelihood that the information will be remembered and focuses attention on what is important. To build trust in the information, visual images should establish a familiar context showing people and settings that are familiar to the intended audience. Visual cues use color, boxes, arrows, and other features to draw attention to important information and highlight the positive actions that individuals should do, rather than what they should not do. The inclusion of a question and answer section, opportunities to consider how the patient will resolve a problem, and writing action plans help patients determine their personal risk, and address their barriers to seeking care. Using visuals with testimonials from people with lived experience and photonovels (a comic book style publication based on the experiences of the intended audience about a health concern, such as lung cancer or smoking) provides realism and helps build patient self-efficacy.
- *Translate materials into common languages spoken.* In addition to information discussed in the oral communication section in the preceding text regarding meaningful access for those with limited English proficiency, written materials should be translated into desired languages by qualified individuals, back-translated into English by a different translator to identify any discrepancies, and then pre-tested with individuals from the intended audience to ensure they are accurate, understandable, and culturally relevant and appropriate.
- *Design websites for lower literacy users.* Increasing access to quality online information is a priority. Websites should conduct usability testing with intended audiences to ensure the information is understandable and the site is easy to navigate. Lower literacy website users face the same obstacles as poorer readers and principles for developing plain language written materials apply. In addition, many people experience decreased reading speed by as much as 25% on computers. Scrolling, drop-down menus, pop-ups, and text or visuals that move can impact visual concentration and website navigation and should be avoided or limited. Simplifying navigation is key to digital literacy and usability. The following usability guidelines provide specific steps/details to enhance accessibility for all patients, including those with disabilities, and should be employed to develop and evaluate existing and new websites: Research-Based Web Design & Usability Guidelines developed by the U.S. General Services Administration [40]; the Customer Usability Toolkit at digital.gov [41]; and the Web Accessibility Evaluation Tools List [42].
- *Pretest and revise.* Conduct a review of materials using appropriate tools (SAM, PEMAT, readability tests). Pretest the draft and the final materials for comprehension, attractiveness, and acceptability with patients from the intended audi-

ences. Revise and disseminate. Potential topics for pretesting include patient understanding of key messages; identifying anything that may be offensive or inappropriate; relatability of visual images; opportunities to improve the materials, and other information that should be included. The Centers for Disease Control and Prevention (CDC) have several resources and toolkits to support educational material pretesting [43].

Organizational Health Literacy and Lung Cancer Screening

Healthy People 2030 and the National Action Plan to Improve Health Literacy emphasize the responsibility of organizations to equitably address health literacy. The intent of the enhanced National CLAS standards is to improve health equity and quality and reduce health disparities through the development of a blueprint that provides a structure for health care organizations to "provide effective, equitable, understandable, and respectful quality care and services that are responsive to diverse cultural health beliefs and practices, preferred languages, health literacy, and other communication needs." The National CLAS standards for *Governance, Leadership, and Workforce* are to: advance and sustain governance and leadership that promotes CLAS and health equity (standard 2); recruit, promote, and support a diverse governance, leadership, and workforce (standard 3); and educate and train governance, leadership, and workforce in CLAS (standard 4). In addition, standards 9–15 provide guidance on establishing and assessing organizational engagement, continuous improvement efforts, and accountability [44].

Health organizations will have different goals and expectations for implementing CLAS standards based on the size, type, and mission of the organization as well as the strategies that are already in place. A shared vision and necessary resources to successfully implement planned strategies should be determined prior to implementation. For example, how will responsibilities for plan implementation be distributed throughout the organization and what resources are needed to effectively support and sustain this effort? Specific implementation strategies that organizations can undertake to establish or enhance culturally and linguistically appropriate services can be found in the CLAS Blueprint. Examples of strategies to promote CLAS at the organizational level that also support lung cancer screening efforts include [44]:

- *Leadership support:* Identify informed and committed champions of cultural competency throughout the organization to focus and sustain efforts around providing culturally competent care. Develop and commit to system-wide policies, practices, procedures, and programs that support CLAS. For example, policies that support review of patient education materials and ensure usability of health information systems.
- *Training:* Increase organizational awareness about lung cancer screening and smoking cessation services. Increase organizational capacity to provide CLAS

services through training focused on culture and health literacy, such as implicit bias, health literacy basics, motivational interviewing, and shared decision-making.

- *Patient navigation support:* Provide patient navigation programs to address access barriers to care, including health literacy and other social determinants of health, such as transportation, insurance access, and scheduling future appointments.
- *Language assistance:* Assess the language and communication proficiency of staff to determine fluency and appropriateness for serving as interpreters.
- *Community outreach and engagement:* Identify and partner with trusted community organizations and messengers, such as community health workers, to serve as a bridge between the community and health and social services, and facilitate access to and enrollment in services such as lung cancer screening.
- *Evaluation:* Work with information technology to support and track efforts such as lung cancer screening referrals and screening rates and integration of the pack year calculator into electronic medical records. Implement ongoing organizational assessment of CLAS-related activities such as training and patient satisfaction with provider communication (patient focus groups; CAPHS survey questions related to patient satisfaction with communication).

Conclusion

The Healthy People 2030 objective for lung cancer screening is to increase the proportion of adults who receive a lung cancer screening based on the most recent guidelines to 7.5%. While lung cancer screening can help prevent lung cancer deaths in high risk individuals, estimated lung cancer screening rates across the United States for 2019 are low at about 6.6%, or 1 out of 15 eligible individuals [45]. Low cancer screening rates have been linked to patient lack of awareness, fear of cancer diagnosis, stigma, and challenges related to accessing health care [13]. Increasing knowledge about screening recommendations among health care providers, people at risk for lung cancer, and the general public can help lower the lung cancer mortality rate. As reviewed throughout this chapter, integrating health literacy principles and training into care models and health systems can play a significant role in increasing awareness about and uptake of lung cancer screening and reducing health disparities. This approach also supports the National Action Plan to Improve Health Literacy, the enhanced National CLAS standards, and goals of the President's Cancer Panel to improve and align cancer screening communication, facilitate equitable access to screening, and strengthen the knowledge and skills of the workforce to support cancer screening and risk assessment. Most importantly, patient and community engagement is essential to developing and implementing effective health communication materials and strategies that are respectful of and responsive to the needs of diverse populations and ultimately can reduce lung cancer disparities.

References

1. Arnold CL, Rademaker A, Bailey SC, et al. Literacy barriers to colorectal cancer screening in community clinics. J Health Commun. 2012;17(3):252–64. https://doi.org/10.1080/1081073 0.2012.713441.
2. Hart TL, Blacker S, Panjwani A, Torbit L, Evans M. Development of multimedia informational tools for breast cancer patients with low levels of health literacy. Patient Educ Couns. 2015;98(3):370–7. https://doi.org/10.1016/j.pec.2014.11.015.
3. Simmons RA, Cosgrove SC, Romney MC, Plumb JD, Brawer RO, Gonzalez ET, Fleisher LG, Moore BS. Health literacy: cancer prevention strategies for early adults. Am J Prev Med. 2017;53(3S1):S73–7; 2017 American Journal of Preventive Medicine. Published by Elsevier Inc. This is an open access article under the CC BY-NC-ND license (http://creativecommons.org/licenses/by-nc-nd/4.0/).
4. Mazor KM, Rubin DL, Roblin DW, et al. Health literacy-listening skill and patient questions following cancer prevention and screening discussions. Health Expect. 2015;19(4):920–34. https://doi.org/10.1111/hex.12387.
5. Ownby RL, Acevao A, Waldrop-Valverde D, Jacobs RJ, Caballero J. Abilities, skills and knowledge in measures of health literacy. Patient Educ Couns. 2014;95(2):211–7. https://doi.org/10.1016/j.pec.2014.02.002.
6. Kutner M, Greenburg E, Jin Y, Paulsen C. The health literacy of America's adults: results from the 2003 national assessment of adult literacy. (NCES 2006-483). Washington, DC: U.S. Department of Education; 2006.
7. Nielsen-Bohlman L, Institute of Medicine. Health literacy: a prescription to end confusion. Washington, DC: National Academies Press; 2004.
8. Rudd RE, Anderson JE, Oppenheimer S, Nath C. Health literacy: an update of public health and medical literature. In: Comings JP, Garner B, Smith C, editors. Review of adult learning and literacy, vol. 7. Mahwah, NJ: Lawrence Erlbaum Associates; 2007. p. 175–204.
9. Heckinger EA, Bennett CL, Davis T, Wolf MS. Health literacy and cancer care: do patients really understand. J Clin Oncol. 2004;22(14 Suppl):6045.
10. National Academies of Sciences, Engineering, and Medicine. Health Literacy and communication strategies in oncology: proceedings of a workshop. Washington, DC: The National Academies Press; 2020. https://doi.org/10.17226/25664.
11. Rust CF, Davis C, Moore MR. Medication adherence skills training for African-American breast cancer survivors: the effects on health literacy, medication adherence, and self-efficacy. Soc Work Health Care. 2015;54(1):33–46.
12. Knolhoff JB, Djenic B, Hsu CH, Bouton ME, Komenaka IK. Missed appointments in a breast clinic: patient-related factors. Am J Med Sci. 2016;352(4):337–42.
13. Closing Gaps in Cancer Screening: Connecting People, Communities, and Systems to Improve Equity and Access. Lung cancer companion brief. 2022. Lung cancer companion brief. https://PresCancerPanel.cancer.gov/report/cancerscreening.
14. Ratzan SC, Parker RM. Introduction. In: Selden CR, Zorn M, Ratzan SC, Parker RM, editors. National library of medicine current bibliographies in medicine: health literacy. Bethesda, MD: National Institutes of Health, U.S. Department of Health and Human Services; 2000. NLM pub. No. CBM 2000–1.
15. U.S. Department of Health and Human Services, Office of Disease Prevention and Health Promotion. National Action Plan to Improve Health Literacy. Washington, DC, 2010. National Action Plan to Improve Health Literacy|health.gov.
16. Healthy People. 2030. https://health.gov/our-work/national-health-initiatives/healthy-people/healthy-people-2030/health-literacy-healthy-people-2030.
17. National Library of Medicine, An Introduction to Health Literacy. An Introduction to Health Literacy|NNLM

18. Brach C, Keller D, Hernandez LM, et al. Ten attributes of health literate organizations, institute of medicine roundtable. 2012; www.ahealthyunderstanding.org/Portals/0/Documents1/IOM_Ten_Attributes_HL_Paper.pdf. Accessed 17 Feb 2017.
19. CDC. The Guide to Community Preventive Services (The Community Guide). www.thecommunityguide.org/about/conclusionreport.html. Accessed 17 Feb 2017.
20. U.S. Preventive Services Task Force. www.uspreventiveservicestaskforce.org/Page/Name/uspstf-a-and-b-recommendations/. Accessed 17 Feb 2017.
21. Centers for Disease Control and Prevention. Health equity guiding principles for inclusive communication health equity guiding principles for inclusive communication|gateway to health communication|CDC. https://www.cdc.gov/healthcommunication/Health_Equity.html.
22. Attributes of a Health Literate Organization. https://www.cdc.gov/healthliteracy/planact/steps/index.html. Accessed 9 Mar 2022.
23. Brach C, Keller D, Hernandez LM, Baur C, Parker R, Dreyer B, Schyve P, Lemerise AJ, Schillinger D. Ten attributes of health literate health care organizations. NAM perspectives. Washington, DC: Discussion Paper, National Academy of Medicine; 2012. https://doi.org/10.31478/201206a.
24. AHRQ Health Literacy Universal Precautions Toolkit, 2nd ed. Health Literacy Universal Precautions Toolkit, 2nd Edition|Agency for Healthcare Research and Quality (ahrq.gov).
25. Koh HK, Brach C, Harris LM, Parchman ML. A proposed 'health literate care model' would constitute a systems approach to improving patients' engagement in care. Health Aff (Millwood). 2013;32(2):357–67. https://doi.org/10.1377/hlthaff.2012.1205; PMID: 23381529; PMCID: PMC5102011. https://www.ncbi.nlm.nih.gov/pmc/articles/PMC5102011/.
26. NIH Clear Communication. Clear & Simple|National Institutes of Health (NIH).
27. Anderson JL, Dodman S, Kopelman M, Fleming A. Patient information recall in a rheumatology clinic. Rheumatology. 1979;18(1):18–22.
28. Kessels RP. Patients' memory for medical information. J R Soc Med. 2003;96(5):219–22.
29. DeWalt DA, Callahan LF, Hawk VH, Broucksou KA, Hink A, Rudd R, Brach C. Health literacy universal precautions toolkit. Rockville, MD: Agency for Healthcare Research and Quality; 2010. p. 10–37; (Prepared by North Carolina Network Consortium, The Cecil G. Sheps Center for Health Services Research, The University of North Carolina at Chapel Hill, under Contract No. HHSA290200710014.) AHRQ Publication No. 10-0046-EF).
30. The Joint Commission. Advancing effective communication, cultural competence, and patient- and family-centered care: a roadmap for hospitals. Oakbrook Terrace, IL: The Joint Commission; 2010.
31. Weiss BD. Health literacy and patient safety: help patients understand. Manual for clinicians. 2nd ed. Chicago, IL: AMA Foundation; 2007. p. 30–4. http://www.partnershiphp.org/Providers/HealthServices/Documents/Health%20Education/CandLToolKit/2%20Manual%20for%20Clinicians.pdf
32. Motivational interviewing: an emerging trend in medical management, professional patient advocate institute dorland health, page 10. https://cupdf.com/document/motivational-interviewing-an-emerging-trend-in-medical-management.html.
33. Elwyn G, Dehlendorf C, Epstein RM, Marrin K, White J, Frosch DL. Shared decision making and motivational interviewing: achieving patient-centered care across the spectrum of health care problems. Ann Fam Med. 2014;12(3):270–5. https://doi.org/10.1370/afm.1615.
34. How does low health literacy, non-literacy, non-written languages, blindness and deafness among LEP populations affect the responsibilities of federal fund recipients? https://www.hhs.gov/civil-rights/for-individuals/faqs/how-do-literacy-vision-or-hearing-impairment-among-lep-populations-affect-the-responsibilities-of-federal-fund-recipients/711/index.html.
35. Center for Health Care Strategies, Health Literacy Fact Sheets, 2013. https://www.chcs.org/media/CHCS_Health_Literacy_Fact_Sheets_2013.pdf.
36. CMS toolkit for making written material clear and effective. https://www.cms.gov/outreach-and-education/outreach/writtenmaterialstoolkit?redirect=/writtenmaterialstoolkit.

37. Doak, Doak & Root's Teaching Patients with Low Literacy Skills, Second Edition, J.B. Lippincott Company, 1996, chapter 4. http://www.hsph.harvard.edu/healthliteracy/resources/teaching-patients-with-low-literacy-skills.
38. Shoemaker SJ, Wolf MS, Brach C. The patient education materials assessment tool (PEMAT) and user's guide. (Prepared by Abt Associates, Inc. under Contract No. HHSA290200900012I, TO 4). Rockville, MD: Agency for Healthcare Research and Quality; 2013. AHRQ Publication No. 14–0002-EF. https://www.ahrq.gov/sites/default/files/publications2/files/pemat_guide_0.pdf
39. NCI Dictionary of Cancer Terms. NCI Dictionary of Cancer Terms—National Cancer Institute; Lung Cancer Screening (PDQ®)–Patient Version—National Cancer Institute.
40. Research-Based Web Design & Usability Guidelines, U.S. General Services Administration (GSA). ISBN 0–16–076270-7. https://www.usability.gov/sites/default/files/documents/guidelines_book.pdf.
41. Customer usability toolkit. https://digital.gov/resources/customer-experience-toolkit/?dg.
42. Web accessibility initiative—web accessibility evaluation tools list. http://www.w3.org/WAI/RC/tools/complete.
43. CDC Health Literacy Testing. https://www.cdc.gov/healthliteracy/developmaterials/testing-messages-materials.html.
44. National Standards for Culturally and Linguistically Appropriate Services in Health and Health Care: A Blueprint for Advancing and Sustaining CLAS Policy and Practice. Think Cultural Health, U.S. Department of Health and Human Services. https://thinkculturalhealth.hhs.gov/.
45. Fedewa SA, Bandi P, Jemal A, Smith RA, Silvestri GA. Lung cancer screening rates during the COVID-19 pandemic. Chest. 161(2):586. https://doi.org/10.1016/j.chest.2021.07.030; Copyright:2021 American College of Chest Physicians. Published by Elsevier Inc. all rights reserved. https://journal.chestnet.org/action/showPdf?pii=S0012-3692%2821%2901364-7.

Chapter 22
Local Therapy for Early-Stage Lung Cancer

Nathaniel R. Evans III and Maria Werner-Wasik

Surgical Therapy to Early-Stage Lung Cancer

Surgical resection for lung cancer was first performed in the 1930s catalyzed by the availability of sulfa-based antibiotics which greatly enhanced the surgical outcomes [1]. In the near century since that innovation, surgical resection has evolved significantly. Both the procedures performed and the approach by which they accomplished has radically changed. Additionally, improvements in radiological detection, pre-operative care, anesthetic techniques, and post-operative care have drastically improved the morbidity and mortality of lung cancer operations. This combined with advanced in-targeted therapy, adjuvant and "neo-adjuvant" systemic therapies for high-risk early-stage patients has markedly improved the outlook and prognosis for lung cancer surgery patients.

The Evolution of Surgical Procedures for Lung Cancer

Evarts Graham performed the first surgical removal of a lung for lung cancer (which he called Pneumectomy) in 1932 [1]. This procedure, now known as pneumonectomy, was the standard of surgical care for lung cancer resection until the 1950s. By that time several groups including Churchill at Massachusetts General Hospital showed that resection of the lobe a cancer arose from (lobectomy) was adequate if

N. R. Evans III
Department of Surgery, Thomas Jefferson University, Philadelphia, PA, USA
e-mail: nathaniel.evans@jefferson.edu

M. Werner-Wasik (✉)
Department of Radiation Oncology, Thomas Jefferson University, Philadelphia, PA, USA
e-mail: Maria.Werner-Wasik@jefferson.edu

© The Author(s), under exclusive license to Springer Nature Switzerland AG 2023 227
G. C. Kane et al. (eds.), *Lung Cancer Screening*,
https://doi.org/10.1007/978-3-031-33596-9_22

the entire cancer could be removed that way, and that the stage of the cancer was a much better predictor of survival than the type of operation performed [2]. Thus, from the 1950s on, lobectomy became the standard for surgical resection of lung cancer.

With the advent of computed tomography, many more small lung cancers were identified. With that, the ability to remove less than a lobe of the lung, still removing the entire cancer and saving more functioning lung gained popularity [3]. Many practitioners argued that a lobectomy for very small lung cancer was more aggressive than necessary. To address this concern, The Lung Cancer Study Group comparted lobectomy to "sublobar resection" in patients with small cancers and no lymph node involvement. This study found that although survival was similar, lobectomy patients were less likely to have recurrence of their cancers in the lung [4]. Thus, lobectomy remains the standard of care for resection of early-stage lung cancer.

Recently there is renewed interest in "sublobar" resections especially segmentectomy (removal of one of the anatomic segments of a lobe rather than the entire lobe). Continued improvements in imaging and the adoption of lung cancer screening has helped identify more small early stage lung cancers. Additionally, as treatment for lung cancers improves, there is a growing population of patients with second and third primary lung cancers [5]. Given all of this, a recently completed international trial that compared lobectomy to sublobar resection in stage IA lung cancer with modern staging, imaging, and surgical techniques promises to inform the approach to early stage lung cancer. Initial reports from this study suggest that in appropriately selected patients, sublobar resection may be as effective as lobectomy in controlling local disease and improving survival [6].

Screen Detected Lung Cancers

It is imperative to keep in mind that screen detected lung cancers represent a subset of lung cancers that are generally earlier stage and thus have a markedly improved prognosis. This is one of the factors that makes lung cancer screening so powerful. Screening is most effective when there is a distinct set of risk factors that can be used to identify those at risk and there is a clear advantage to finding and treating that screen detected disease earlier. In the case of lung cancer screening, both are emphatically true [7].

Surgical Approach to Lung Cancer Surgery

Not only has the operation performed for lung cancer evolved over time. The approach used to perform that operation has also been the subject of constant change, innovation, and controversy. Until the 1990s, all thoracic surgery including lung cancer resection was performed via an incision on the chest that divided the muscles of the chest and spread the space between the ribs to allow access to the chest. The advent of video thoracoscopes allowed for many thoracic procedures to be performed in a minimally invasive fashion. Although direct comparisons between VATS and thoracotomy lobectomy have been plagued with selection bias and poor accrual, many studies have shown equal mortality, improved morbidity, and faster recovery with VATS lobectomy [8]. More recently, the introduction of surgical robotic technology has introduced another minimally invasive option for lung cancer surgery. According to the National Cancer Centers Network (NCCN), minimally invasive surgery is the treatment of choice for early stage lung cancer [9].

Outcomes After Lung Cancer Surgery

Surgical resection remains the standard of care for those patients who are fit for an operation because it provides excellent local control of tumor and improvement in overall survival. The expected perioperative mortality for surgical resection for lung cancer is currently 2.2%. The most common post-operative complication is atrial arrhythmia which occurs in nearly 11% of patients [10]. Most importantly, the 10-year survival for resected stage I lung cancer has been estimated at at least 88% [7]. At higher stages, there is the expected decrease in median survival, however advances in adjuvant therapy, including immunotherapy, and targeted therapy have improved survival in this subset of patients as well [11–13].

Challenges in Lung Cancer Surgery

Despite excellent overall results after resection for lung cancer, there remains a subset of patients who recur both locally and with distant disease [5]. Although multiple small studies have shown histologic and molecular markers that predict recurrence, there is not a widely established or accepted way to predict recurrence after surgical resection (or radiation or ablation) that is more accurate than pathologic staging. Although each version of the staging system becomes more specific, it remains a crude tool to predict recurrence [14]. The ability to predict recurrence and detect it earlier is one of the most pressing needs in research in early-stage lung cancer.

Surgical Candidacy and Alternatives to Surgery

Given the excellent expected outcomes from surgical resection for early stage disease, it is of paramount importance to objectively determine who is a candidate for surgical resection in terms of cardiopulmonary reserve and medical comorbidities. Guidelines for pre-operative assessment are well established. While most patients can be stratified using only a history and physical exam and pulmonary function tests, for those in whom the determination is less clear, a stepwise escalation of testing modalities is often employed, considering examinations such as 6-min walk tests and quantitative perfusion [15]. For those patients who are deemed not to be candidates for resection, stereotactic body radiation is the mainstay of therapy. Other treatment modalities such as cryoablation and radio frequency ablation continue to be investigated as alternatives to surgery and radiation [16–18].

Stereotactic Body Radiation Therapy (SBRT) for Treatment of Early-Stage Lung Cancer

Over the last two decades, Stereotactic Body Radiation Therapy (SBRT) has become an everyday tool for curative radiation in patients with small (usually defined as not exceeding 5 cm) node-negative non-small cell lung cancer (NSCLC) tumors. SBRT is used in medically inoperable patients (or those who refuse surgery), while lobectomy with mediastinal lymph node dissection remains the gold standard otherwise. Overall, the popularity of SBRT represents a great success story for radiation oncology due to its "high tech" noninvasive nature, requiring a minimum of visits and being associated with a high expectation of tumor control, as well as low toxicity [9, 19–21].

Current NCCN guidelines v.2–2022, recommend "definitive radiation therapy (RT), preferably stereotactic ablative radiotherapy (SABR, which is another term for SBRT) for medically inoperable patients with Stage IA and Stage IB node-negative NSCLC" [19]. In comparison to standard fractionated thoracic RT, which prescribes a total radiation dose of 60 Gy in 30 daily doses, or fractions, SBRT uses few fractions, commonly 54 Gy in three fractions of 18 Gy each, or 60 Gy in five fractions of 10–12 Gy each in peripheral tumor locations, with other dosing/fractionation schemes also acceptable [19]. Radiation dose distribution around the treated tumor is very tight, sparing therefore the normal surrounding lung parenchyma to minimize toxicity and exposure to surrounding normal lung. However, tumors in central locations, close to the large airways, large vessels, the esophagus, require special care in order to avoid potentially severe late toxicity, such as tracheomalacia, airway narrowing, or hemorrhage. A radiation dose escalation prospective trial of SBRT (RTOG 0813) studied a five-fraction regimen for central tumors with fraction sizes up to 12 Gy and was deemed safe [20].

Successful delivery of SBRT is not vendor-specific, allowing for use of a linear accelerator, CyberKnife, a proton unit, tomotherapy unit, etc. However, it is a sophisticated therapy, requiring a team expertise of radiation oncologists, medical dosimetrists, medical physicists, and radiation therapists, mostly to assure precise tumor targeting and honoring the tolerances of normal thoracic organs, in view of large fraction sizes.

A wide introduction of SBRT in the Dutch population resulted in survival improvement (from 16 to 21 months) among patients with Stage I NSCLC, who otherwise would have not be treated at all, presumably due to the inability to undergo surgery [21]. The effectiveness of SBRT vs standard RT was compared in two randomized trials [22, 23]. The SPACE trial demonstrated equivalent progression-free survival (PFS), which was the study's primary endpoint, as well as overall survival (OS), when standard RT to 70 Gy was compared to SBRT (66 Gy in three fractions) [22]. In a similar CHISEL trial, SBRT was superior to standard RT with regard to freedom from local failure, as well as OS [23].

The first American prospective Phase II study of SBRT was the RTOG 0236, which has enrolled 59 medically inoperable patients with multiple comorbidities, mostly pulmonary and cardiac (e.g., 40% of patients had severely reduced diffusion capacity and 43% had severe cerebral, cardiac, or peripheral vascular disease) [24]. An impressive local tumor control of 98% at 3 years was accomplished, without severe adverse events, and with median survival time of 4 years. Therefore, a new effective treatment modality was established for those patients, who had few viable options previously. SBRT has not been demonstrated to cause a decline in pulmonary function studies, such as the FEV1 and diffusion capacity [25]. Similarly, poor lung function should not prevent patients from being offered SBRT if the perceived risk of pneumothorax is too high to allow a biopsy, since the outcomes of biopsied vs non-biopsied patients were similar in large retrospective series [26]. However, a reasonable attempt at biopsy should be always performed, unless it is considered medically dangerous. In patients with evidence of an enlarging lung nodule, as well as an increasing hypermetabolic uptake on PET scan, a biopsy can be probably omitted, if contraindicated. Specific radiologic characteristics, such as tumor spiculations on a CT scan, are highly suspicious for a primary lung malignancy. Advanced age is not a contraindication for lung SBRT, since octo- and nonagenarians seem to derive the same benefit from SBRT as younger patients [27].

Distant tumor spread remains a dominant failure pattern (20% at 5 years in the Dutch experience), and medically inoperable patients may not always be candidates for chemotherapy following SBRT due to their comorbidities [28]. With the recent success of immunotherapy (IO) in Stage III lung cancer, prospective randomized studies were initiated of IO as adjuvant therapy after SBRT [29–31]. The SWOG 1914 trial is planning to enroll 480 high-risk patients with Stage I NSCLC, defined as having tumor size of at least 2 cm, or with a maximum Standardized Uptake Value (SUV) on a PET scan of at least 6.2, or a moderately or poorly differentiated histology. This should result in a higher chance of demonstrating benefit of the IO than allowing enrollment of unselected patients with lower likelihood of tumor recurrence. The primary study endpoint is overall survival.

The question whether SBRT would provide similar loco-regional control and survival as surgery for operable patients with early stage lung cancer remains unresolved. Several large Phase III randomized trials comparing surgery to SBRT (ROSEL; ACOSOG Z4009/RTOG 1021) were closed due to poor accrual [32]. SBRT has been delivered for early stage peripheral lesions in medically operable patients in the setting of a single-arm Phase II clinical trial, RTOG 0618, with 26 patients evaluated and achieving relatively high local tumor control (96%), low rates of surgical salvage and adverse events while preserving pulmonary function [33, 34].

In a pooled analysis of the STARS and ROSEL trials, which looked at operable Stage I NSCLC patients, SBRT was found to have a higher overall survival of 95% at 3 years compared to patients who had received lobectomy and mediastinal lymph node dissection at 75%, with similar recurrence-free survival [35]. Patients who had received surgery had more Grade 3 or higher events than the SBRT arms (44% vs 10%). This analysis supports the idea that further studies are necessary. In fact, the ongoing US VALOR trial (SBRT vs lobectomy) is accruing patients well and is expected to complete enrollment by 2026 [36]. Patients eligible for VALOR need to have adequate lung function, that is, FEV1 > 40% and DLCO>40%. In any case, the availability of exciting surgical and non-surgical treatment options for screen-detected and other early stage lung cancers promise to improve survival while maximizing lung function and minimizing side effects.

References

1. Graham EA, Singer JJ. Successful removal of an entire lung for carcinoma of the bronchus. J Am Med Assoc. 1933;101(18):1371–4.
2. Churchill ED, Sweet RH, Soutter L, Scannell JG. The surgical management of carcinoma of the lung; a study of the cases treated at the Massachusetts general hospital from 1930 to 1950. J Thorac Surg. 1950;20(3):349–65.
3. Carr SR, Schuchert MJ, Pennathur A, Wilson DO, Siegfried JM, Luketich JD, et al. Impact of tumor size on outcomes after anatomic lung resection for stage 1A non-small cell lung cancer based on the current staging system. J Thorac Cardiovasc Surg. 2012;143(2):390–7.
4. Ginsberg RJ, Rubinstein LV. Randomized trial of lobectomy versus limited resection for T1 N0 non-small cell lung cancer. Lung cancer study group. Ann Thorac Surg. 1995;60(3):615–22; discussion 22–3.
5. Lou F, Huang J, Sima CS, Dycoco J, Rusch V, Bach PB. Patterns of recurrence and second primary lung cancer in early-stage lung cancer survivors followed with routine computed tomography surveillance. J Thorac Cardiovasc Surg. 2013;145(1):75–81; discussion −2.
6. Van den Heuvel M, Altorki N. Sub-lobar resection as new standard-of-care for cT1aN0 NSCLC? In: 2022 World conference on lung cancer. Vienna: IASLC; 2022.
7. Henschke CI, Yankelevitz DF, Libby DM, Pasmantier MW, Smith JP, Miettinen OS. Survival of patients with stage I lung cancer detected on CT screening. N Engl J Med. 2006;355(17):1763–71.
8. Villamizar NR, Darrabie MD, Burfeind WR, Petersen RP, Onaitis MW, Toloza E, et al. Thoracoscopic lobectomy is associated with lower morbidity compared with thoracotomy. J Thorac Cardiovasc Surg. 2009;138(2):419–25.
9. National comprehensive cancer network. Non-small cell lung cancer. 2022.
10. Kozower BD, Sheng S, O'Brien SM, Liptay MJ, Lau CL, Jones DR, et al. STS database risk models: predictors of mortality and major morbidity for lung cancer resection. Ann Thorac Surg. 2010;90(3):875–81; discussion 81–3.
11. Pignon J-P, Tribodet H, Scagliotti GV, Douillard J-Y, Shepherd FA, Stephens RJ, et al. Lung adjuvant cisplatin evaluation: a pooled analysis by the LACE collaborative group. J Clin Oncol. 2008;26(21):3552–9.

12. Felip E, Altorki N, Zhou C, Csőszi T, Vynnychenko I, Goloborodko O, et al. Adjuvant atezolizumab after adjuvant chemotherapy in resected stage IB-IIIA non-small-cell lung cancer (IMpower010): a randomised, multicentre, open-label, phase 3 trial. Lancet. 2021;398(10308):1344–57.
13. Wu Y-L, Tsuboi M, He J, John T, Grohe C, Majem M, et al. Osimertinib in resected EGFR-mutated non–small-cell lung cancer. N Engl J Med. 2020;383(18):1711–23.
14. Amin MBES, Greene F, Byrd DR, Brookland RK, Washington MK, Gershenwald JE, Compton CC, Hess KR, et al. AJCC cancer staging manual(8th edition). 8th ed. Cham: Springer International Publishing; 2017.
15. Bolliger CT, Perruchoud AP. Functional evaluation of the lung resection candidate. Eur Respir J. 1998;11(1):198–212.
16. Murphy MC, Wrobel MM, Fisher DA, Cahalane AM, Fintelmann FJ. Update on image-guided thermal lung ablation: society guidelines, therapeutic alternatives, and postablation imaging findings. AJR Am J Roentgenol. 2022;219(3):471–85.
17. Rakovich G, Carignan S, Caty V, Bujold A. Thoracoscopic ultrasound-guided radiofrequency ablation for lung cancer. Can J Respir Crit Care Sleep Med. 2018;2(2):84–6.
18. Baisi A, De Simone M, Raveglia F, Cioffi U. Thermal ablation in the treatment of lung cancer: present and future. Eur J Cardiothorac Surg. 2013;43(4):683–6.
19. Guckenberger M, Andratschke N, Alheit H, Holy R, Moustakis C, Nestle U, et al. Definition of stereotactic body radiotherapy: principles and practice for the treatment of stage I non-small cell lung cancer. Strahlenther Onkol. 2014;190(1):26–33.
20. Grills IS, Hope AJ, Guckenberger M, Kestin LL, Werner-Wasik M, Yan D, et al. A collaborative analysis of stereotactic lung radiotherapy outcomes for early-stage non-small-cell lung cancer using daily online cone-beam computed tomography image-guided radiotherapy. J Thorac Oncol. 2012;7(9):1382–93.
21. Bezjak A, Paulus R, Gaspar LE, Timmerman RD, Straube WL, Ryan WF, et al. Safety and efficacy of a five-fraction stereotactic body radiotherapy schedule for centrally located non–small-cell lung cancer: NRG oncology/RTOG 0813 trial. J Clin Oncol. 2019;37(15):1316–25.
22. Haasbeek CJA, Palma D, Visser O, Lagerwaard FJ, Slotman B, Senan S. Early-stage lung cancer in elderly patients: a population-based study of changes in treatment patterns and survival in The Netherlands. Ann Oncol. 2012;23(10):2743–7.
23. Nyman J, Hallqvist A, Lund J, Brustugun OT, Bergman B, Bergström P, et al. SPACE—a randomized study of SBRT vs conventional fractionated radiotherapy in medically inoperable stage I NSCLC. Radiother Oncol. 2016;121(1):1–8.
24. Ball D, Mai GT, Vinod S, Babington S, Ruben J, Kron T, et al. Stereotactic ablative radiotherapy versus standard radiotherapy in stage 1 non-small-cell lung cancer (TROG 09.02 CHISEL): a phase 3, open-label, randomised controlled trial. Lancet Oncol. 2019;20(4):494–503.
25. Timmerman RD, Hu C, Michalski JM, Bradley JC, Galvin J, Johnstone DW, et al. Long-term results of stereotactic body radiation therapy in medically inoperable stage I non-small cell lung cancer. JAMA Oncol. 2018;4(9):1287–8.
26. Guckenberger M, Kestin LL, Hope AJ, Belderbos J, Werner-Wasik M, Yan D, et al. Is there a lower limit of pretreatment pulmonary function for safe and effective stereotactic body radiotherapy for early-stage non-small cell lung cancer? J Thorac Oncol. 2012;7(3):542–51.
27. Louie AV, Senan S, Patel P, Ferket BS, Lagerwaard FJ, Rodrigues GB, et al. When is a biopsy-proven diagnosis necessary before stereotactic ablative radiotherapy for lung cancer?: a decision analysis. Chest. 2014;146(4):1021–8.
28. Giuliani M, Hope A, Guckenberger M, Mantel F, Peulen H, Sonke JJ, et al. Stereotactic body radiation therapy in octo- and nonagenarians for the treatment of early-stage lung cancer. Int J Radiat Oncol Biol Phys. 2017;98(4):893–9.
29. Senthi S, Lagerwaard FJ, Haasbeek CJ, Slotman BJ, Senan S. Patterns of disease recurrence after stereotactic ablative radiotherapy for early stage non-small-cell lung cancer: a retrospective analysis. Lancet Oncol. 2012;13(8):802–9.

30. Antonia SJ, Villegas A, Daniel D, Vicente D, Murakami S, Hui R, et al. Durvalumab after chemo-radiotherapy in stage III non-small-cell lung cancer. N Engl J Med. 2017;377(20):1919–29.
31. Clifford Robinson M, editor. Durvalumab vs placebo with stereotactic body radiation therapy in early stage unresected non-small cell lung cancer patients (PACIFIC-4). In: Principal investigator. RTOG Foundation Study. p. 3515.
32. A randomized phase III trial of induction/consolidation atezolizumab (NSC #783608) + SBRT versus SBRT alone in high risk, early stage NSCLC.
33. Fernando HC, Timmerman R. American College of Surgeons oncology group Z4099/radiation therapy oncology group 1021: a randomized study of sublobar resection compared with stereotactic body radiotherapy for high-risk stage I non-small cell lung cancer. J Thorac Cardiovasc Surg. 2012;144(3):S35–8.
34. Timmerman RD, Paulus R, Pass HI, Gore EM, Edelman MJ, Galvin J, et al. Stereotactic body radiation therapy for operable early-stage lung cancer: findings from the NRG oncology RTOG 0618 trial. JAMA Oncol. 2018;4(9):1263–6.
35. Chang JY, Senan S, Paul MA, Mehran RJ, Louie AV, Balter P, et al. Stereotactic ablative radiotherapy versus lobectomy for operable stage I non-small-cell lung cancer: a pooled analysis of two randomised trials. Lancet Oncol. 2015;16(6):630–7.
36. Veterans Affairs Lung Cancer Surgery or Stereotactic Radiotherapy (VALOR).

Chapter 23
The Revolution of Lung Cancer Therapeutics

Zachary French, Jennifer Johnson, and Rita Axelrod

Background

Lung cancer remains one of the most common cancers and tops the list for causes of cancer-related deaths worldwide. Though decreased rates of smoking in the United States may help reduce the number of cases, and increased rates of lung cancer screening may help us diagnose lung cancers at an earlier stage, we continue to diagnose and treat many patients with advanced stage disease. The development of targeted and immune therapies has changed the landscape for how we treat these patients and have helped improve outcomes. Choosing the right treatment (or combination of treatments), for the right patient, at the right time, has become increasingly complex. Here we will review the advances in lung cancer therapeutics and the outlook for future research.

Non-small Cell Lung Cancer

The central modalities of treatment for early-stage non-small cell lung cancer (NSCLC) have been surgical resection and radiation therapy. These approaches offer an opportunity for cure for early localized disease. With increased rates of screening, we hope to diagnose more patients in this stage. The use of drug therapy begins with identifying patients who have resectable disease but may benefit from neoadjuvant or adjuvant chemotherapy. Chemotherapy has failed to show a benefit

Z. French · J. Johnson · R. Axelrod (✉)
Department of Medical Oncology, Sidney Kimmel Cancer Center, Thomas Jefferson University, Philadelphia, PA, USA
e-mail: zachary.french@jefferson.edu; ennifer.m.johnson@jefferson.edu; rita.axelrod@jefferson.edu

G. C. Kane et al. (eds.), *Lung Cancer Screening*,
https://doi.org/10.1007/978-3-031-33596-9_23

in very early-stage disease (stage IA and stage IB <4 cm). The role of targeted agents or immunotherapy in is under investigation and not yet established.

The standard of care for patients with stages IB to IIIA disease and reasonable performance status is actively evolving. Surgical resection followed by adjuvant chemotherapy has been the most common approach [1]. Histology helps to guide the choice of chemotherapy, but platinum doublets have proven to be most effective while minimizing toxicity. Cisplatin or carboplatin provides the backbone of the doublet. The second agent is often pemetrexed for non-squamous histology, namely, adenocarcinomas [2]. For squamous histology, there are several acceptable second agents, including gemcitabine [3], docetaxel [4], and vinorelbine [5]. The standard estimate for adjuvant chemotherapy in these patients is that there is a 50% chance of relapse after surgery, and the addition of adjuvant therapy may decrease the chance of relapse by an additional 5–15% [6–10]. While not a marked improvement, this strategy is recommended for all patients who may tolerate it regardless of age [11]. Adjuvant immunotherapy and targeted therapy with the EGFR-directed agent osimertinib are now approved in selected populations. The immunotherapy atezolizumab is given for 1 year following adjuvant chemotherapy for patients that are PD-L1 positive and do not have molecular targets for treatment [12]. In this trial, the median disease-free survival was not met for the atezolizumab arm, and 35.5 months in the best supportive care arm. Osimertinib, a third generation anti-EGFR tyrosine kinase inhibitor (TKI), is approved for adjuvant therapy for stages II-IIIA disease [13]. Median disease-free survival was not reached and 90% of patients were alive at 2 years in the osimertinib arm, compared to median disease-free survival 19.6 months and 44% of patients alive at 2 years in the placebo arm.

Neoadjuvant (or induction) chemotherapy has been studied and proven effective as well but is not currently standard of care and only used in select patient populations. In one study, the use of neoadjuvant chemotherapy prior to surgery compared to surgery alone had a marked impact on survival [14]. In patients with potentially resectable disease (N2 nodal stage), neoadjuvant chemotherapy may increase the likelihood of successful surgical resection [15, 16]. Neoadjuvant chemotherapy is also the preferred strategy in patients with superior sulcus (Pancoast) tumors [17]. Neoadjuvant concurrent chemoradiation has also been studied and can be used in select cases, but has not been shown to be more effective than neoadjuvant chemotherapy alone for patients with stage IIIA(N2) disease [18], and this strategy actually led to increased morbidity and mortality when used prior to pneumonectomy [16]. For patients undergoing pneumonectomy, neoadjuvant chemotherapy without radiation is the preferred treatment modality [19, 20].

Some small studies have also investigated the role of neoadjuvant immunotherapy without chemotherapy, though this is also not standard practice [21, 22]. Very recently, the FDA approved the combination of nivolumab with platinum doublet chemotherapy in the neoadjuvant setting. This strategy has the potential to become a new standard of care given the significant increase in median event-free survival by almost 11 months. As for neoadjuvant targeted therapy, there have been a few trials exploring the use of anti-EGFR TKIs erlotinib or gefitinib in this setting. Data from this small sample suggest neoadjuvant targeted therapy was feasible with acceptable toxicity, and may lead to improved downstaging and complete resection rates, though more robust studies are needed [23, 24]. The incorporation of immunotherapy and targeted drug therapy in early-stage disease will require broader and earlier adoption of molecular characterization of tumors for individualized patient care.

Stage IIIA(N2) and IIIB NSCLC are most often considered unresectable due to size or location of the primary tumor, the extent of lymph node station involved, or poor lung function. The recommended strategy for these patients is definitive concurrent chemoradiation, which was shown to be better than radiotherapy alone, and better than sequential therapy [25]. Similar to the chemotherapy selection for adjuvant disease, concurrent regimens are most often a platinum doublet, with cisplatin or carboplatin for the platinum agent, and pemetrexed or paclitaxel as the second agent [26, 27]. Newer evidence also supports the use of maintenance durvalumab following the completion of concurrent chemoradiation for a duration of 1 year [28]. The addition of durvalumab significantly extended median progression-free survival (PFS) from 5.6 to 16.8 months.

Metastatic stage IV NSCLC management requires a personalized approach for each case incorporating personal preferences of care, patient comorbidities, distribution of disease, and predictive biomarkers. Balancing efficacy and toxicity is particularly important as this treatment is given with palliative and not curative intent. Systemic therapies with palliative intent are the mainstay of treatment for metastatic NSCLC.

A portion of metastatic disease may be considered "oligometastatic," meaning there are only 1–5 sites of metastatic disease. In this setting, consolidative surgery or radiation may be added to systemic therapy, and this has been shown to significantly improve PFS [29]. Similarly, some patients experience "oligoprogression," where most sites of disease stabilize or improve, but a limited number of sites progress [30]. This is most common in patients treated with targeted therapies and can also be seen with immunotherapy [31, 32]. Oligoprogression can be successfully treated with local radiation while continuing the original systemic therapy.

Regardless of whether patients have limited or diffuse metastatic disease, biomarker testing can help to choose the systemic therapy regimen with the most favorable risk/benefit ratio. Molecularly targeted therapy has allowed us to treat patients with medications that are specific to alterations in their cancer [33]. Identifying patients that have these targets is essential, as this will drastically alter management and outcomes. Ideally, comprehensive testing of all targetable mutations would be performed on all pathology samples at the time of diagnosis. If this has not been completed, obtaining this information should be pursued. Additionally, retesting for these targets at the time of relapse or progression should be considered as new targets can develop. As a generalization, these targets are more commonly found in adenocarcinomas than squamous cell carcinomas, and non-smokers more than smokers, but this is not absolute. The most common targets include *EGFR, ALK, ROS1, MET, RET, BRAF V600E, KRAS G12C, NTRK,* and *HER2* [34–36]. Figure 23.1 demonstrates the relative frequency of these targets in the USA, though it is important to note that the distribution of these mutations does vary with

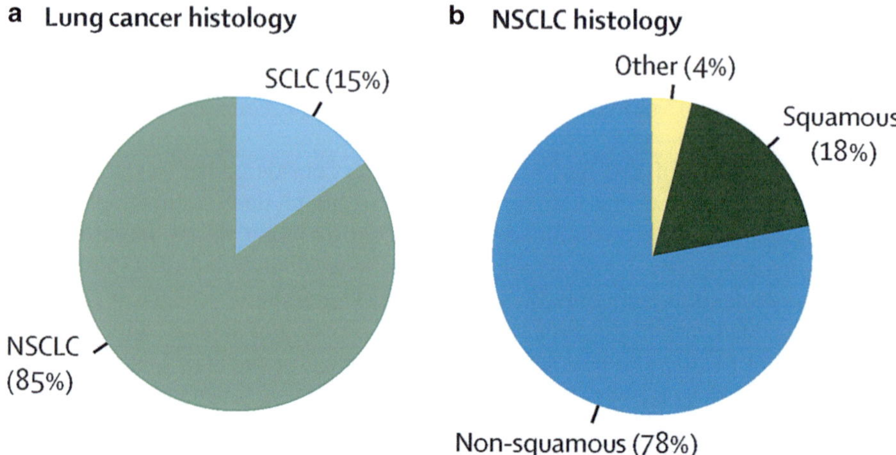

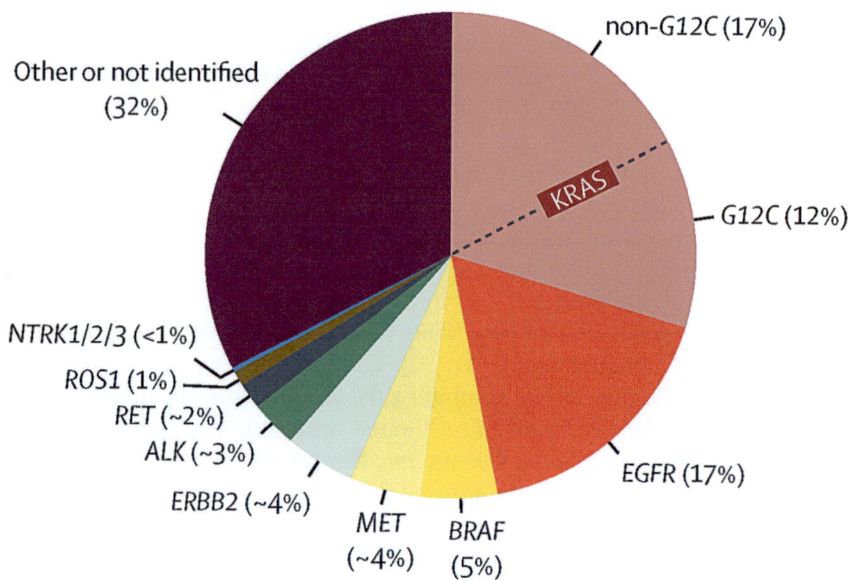

Fig. 23.1 Lung cancer histology (**a**), NSCLC histology (**b**), and oncogenic mutations in NSCLC (**c**) in the USA. (Used with permission from Thai et al. [84])

geography. Most often these targets are mutually exclusive and do not occur together. Not all alterations within these genes predict response to specific agents. For example, different agents are used to treat the two most common *EGFR* pathogenic variants, exon 19 deletion and L858R mutation, than are used to treat exon 20 insertions [37]. Similarly, therapies directed at *BRAF* V600E are often ineffective against other non-V600E *BRAF* mutations [38]. *KRAS* G12C is currently the only pathogenic variant responsive to an oral TKI (sotorasib) with other drugs in development for G12A, G12D, and G12V.

Most of the agents used for these targets are oral, well tolerated, and produce a longer duration of response than chemotherapy. Drawbacks of these agents can include cardiac toxicity, pulmonary toxicity, rash, diarrhea, fatigue, and the eventual development of resistance mutations requiring an alternate strategy. Progression on targeted therapy is often slow and oligometastatic, and these sites of progression can be treated with local approaches like radiation or surgery while continuing the targeted therapy agent. When tumors ultimately stop responding to targeted therapy, there are sometimes identifiable mechanisms of resistance, for which some have alternative targeted therapies available. For example, the first-generation tyrosine kinase inhibitors (TKIs) against *EGFR* including gefitinib and erlotinib were effective, but approximately 60% of tumors developed a second mutation in the *EGFR* gene, T790M, conferring resistance. Osimertinib is a third-generation anti-*EGFR* TKI that specifically targeted this mutation and was initially approved in the second line setting [39]. Subsequently, osimertinib was studied as a first-line agent and was proven to be more effective with improved overall survival (OS), and has now become the standard of care first-line agent for *EGFR* mutated NSCLC [40, 41]. Other secondary EGFR mutations and alterations in other genes involved in *EGFR* signaling are under investigation for the development of new agents [42]. In most cases, first-line treatment for metastatic NSCLC with an identified target will be an agent directed at that target. This often reserves chemotherapy for the time of disease progression. Unfortunately, patients with these mutations often do not respond to immunotherapy as well as those without them.

The other revolutionary change in NSCLC was the introduction of immunotherapy in 2015. In addition to the preceding molecular testing, PD-L1 testing can serve as a predictive marker of response to immunotherapy agents [43]. However, studies have also demonstrated the effectiveness of immunotherapy even in patients whose pathology demonstrates <1% PD-L1 positivity [44].

One of the benefits of immunotherapy has been the side effect profile and tolerability. Many patients with NSCLC have multiple comorbidities and decreased performance status. Immunotherapy can be very well tolerated, sometimes with minimal adverse effects. A small number of patients will experience adverse effects from the use of immunotherapy and will develop immune related toxicities, which can affect any organ system. The most commonly affected organ is the skin. Other affected organs can include the colon, endocrine organs (thyroid, adrenals, pituitary, pancreas), liver, and lung [45]. Close monitoring for these toxicities is essential, and when identified, they must be graded. The grade of the toxicity will help determine when to treat, how to treat, and whether immunotherapy can be resumed. Standard treatment for immunotherapy toxicity is high dose glucocorticoids, at a dose equivalent to prednisone 1–2 mg/kg [46]. Steroids must be weaned slowly to prevent rebound effects. For low grade toxicity and toxicity not involving vital organs such as endocrinopathies, one can consider rechallenging with immunotherapy. However, after a patient has experienced a grade 3 or 4 toxicity, or toxicity involving a vital organ, immunotherapy should be permanently discontinued. The use of immunotherapy in patients with known autoimmune disease, rheumatologic disease, and inflammatory bowel disease is controversial, and risks and benefits must be weighed.

In the metastatic setting, preferred first line regimens will include immunotherapy, either as monotherapy, in combination with chemotherapy, or in combination with a second immunotherapy agent. If not included in the first line regimen, then the preferred second line regimen is immunotherapy as monotherapy.

The different ways in which immunotherapy can be used depends on PD-L1 testing. For patients with >50% PD-L1 positivity, immunotherapy agents that target PD-1 or PD-L1 like pembrolizumab, atezolizumab, and cemiplimab can all be used as single agents in the first line [43, 47–49]. Pembrolizumab monotherapy can also be considered as first-line treatment in patients with PD-L1 expression of 1–49% who have poor performance status or have contraindications to chemotherapy [47]. Regardless of PD-L1 testing, immunotherapy can be combined with traditional chemotherapy in a variety of first-line regimens. For adenocarcinomas in patients with acceptable performance status, possible first-line regimens include: carboplatin/pemetrexed/pembrolizumab [44, 50]; carboplatin/paclitaxel/bevacizumab/atezolizumab [51]; and carboplatin/albumin-bound paclitaxel/atezolizumab [52]. Pemetrexed and bevacizumab are contraindicated in squamous cell carcinomas. Thus, for squamous cell carcinomas in patients with acceptable performance status, possible first-line regimens include: carboplatin/paclitaxel/pembrolizumab, and carboplatin/albumin-bound paclitaxel/pembrolizumab [53]. Additionally, dual agent immunotherapy, namely, the combination of ipilimumab (anti-CTLA4) and nivolumab (anti-PD1), has been proven effective, interestingly even in patients whose tumors do not express PD-L1 [54, 55]. Furthermore, this dual immunotherapy regimen can also be combined with chemotherapy, in a regimen of ipilimumab/nivolumab/carboplatin/pemetrexed for adenocarcinomas, and ipilimumab/nivolumab/carboplatin/paclitaxel for squamous cell carcinomas [55].

Choosing between these options can be challenging given limited data, so patient preferences, comorbidities, and potential toxicities must be taken into consideration. If there are no absolute contraindications to the use of immunotherapy, then immunotherapy should be included in a first-line regimen [56]. At the time of progression, if immunotherapy was included in the first-line regimen, then it should not be used again in the second-line regimen. Conversely, if immunotherapy was not included in the first-line regimen, then it should be used in the second-line regimen at the time of progression, provided there are no contraindications. If patients have contraindications to immunotherapy, either preexisting comorbidities, or due to prior immunotherapy toxicity, then there are a variety of regimens that can be used. In the first line, combination platinum doublet is preferred, with consideration for the addition of bevacizumab for adenocarcinoma [57]. As in the adjuvant setting for early-stage disease, pemetrexed is also the preferred second agent with platinum in the metastatic setting [58]. Gemcitabine-based doublet regimens can also be used in the first line [59, 60]. In second and subsequent lines, if unable to use immunotherapy, then a number of single agent chemotherapy regimens as well as combination ramucirumab/docetaxel can be used. As noted before, it is important to consider repeat biopsy to reassess for the development of driver mutations.

In addition to the preceding therapies, treatment targeting angiogenesis can be combined with chemotherapy or chemotherapy and immunotherapy. Bevacizumab is a monoclonal antibody directed against vascular endothelial growth factor (VEGF). Although an effective target for therapy, VEGF does not serve as a biomarker and is not measured. A modest improvement in OS was shown when used in combination with either platinum/paclitaxel or platinum/pemetrexed [52]. Building upon this observation, preclinical evidence of the effects of combining a VEGF inhibitor with immunotherapy, and data supporting the use of chemotherapy and immunotherapy, a four-drug regimen of carboplatin, paclitaxel, atezolizumab, and bevacizumab has now become one of several preferred first-line regimens for advanced non-squamous NSCLC [51]. A key caveat to the use of bevacizumab and other anti-VEGF therapies in NSCLC is the risk of bleeding, particularly in squamous histology tumors with central location [61]. Similarly, bevacizumab should be avoided or used with caution in patients at high risk for bleeding due to thrombocytopenia, hemoptysis, recent thromboembolism, and brain metastasis [62]. Bevacizumab can delay wound healing and cause wound dehiscence therefore it must also be held prior to and after surgery [63]. Although bevacizumab has been proven effective and can be safely used for many patients, these important contraindications and special considerations often limit its use [64]. Ramucirumab is a second monoclonal antibody agent in this class with activity against VEGFR2 which can be used in combination with docetaxel as second-line therapy following disease on a first-line regimen [65].

Overall, NSCLC remains a challenging disease to treat, but the number of treatment options has increased significantly. Though many patients with incurable metastatic disease previously had very poor prognosis, patients are now able to achieve OS on the order of years with personalized treatment regimens. There remains room for improvement, and hopefully with new targets and new drugs identified, we will continue to improve on these outcomes.

Small Cell Lung Cancer

An entity distinct from NSCLC, small cell lung cancer (SCLC) is a less common but more aggressive form of lung cancer. Though SCLC does have a traditional tumor, nodes, and metastasis (TNM) staging system, it is most often studied and discussed as limited stage and extensive stage, where limited stage disease is that which can be encompassed in a single radiation field, and extensive stage is when the extent of disease is too large for a single radiation field [66]. The vast majority of patients are diagnosed with advanced stage with metastatic involvement of the brain [67].

Unlike NSCLC, treatment options for SCLC are more limited. Targeted agents for identified targetable mutations in NSCLC are not used in SCLC. Additionally, while the role of immunotherapy in the treatment of SCLC is important, the number of options are more limited [68]. SCLC is a chemo-sensitive disease but with a high rate of recurrence and resistance.

For limited stage disease, there is a chance for cure with combined definitive chemoradiation, or adjuvant therapy if surgery is performed [69, 70]. In the setting of extensive stage disease, chemotherapy is the mainstay of treatment, though palliative radiation may also be used, often for the brain [71]. In either scenario, the preferred first-line regimen for SCLC is again platinum doublet, with either carboplatin or cisplatin as the platinum agent, and etoposide as the second. Given the performance status of these patients and most often palliative nature of the chemotherapy, carboplatin is preferred due to better tolerability [72, 73]. The first cycle of chemotherapy is often given urgently in the hospital as diagnosis is often made due to rapidly growing disease that has led to symptoms and hospitalization. Additional chemotherapeutic agents effective for SCLC include irinotecan [74] and topotecan [75, 76], as well as the newer agent lurbinectedin [77]. While all are effective, neither have drastically altered the disease course but remain options for the time of relapse.

One of the most important advances in the treatment of extensive stage SCLC was the addition of immunotherapy. The hallmark study looked at the addition of atezolizumab to standard chemotherapy, and a marked improvement in OS was seen, from approximately 10 months with chemotherapy alone, to 12 months with combined chemoimmunotherapy [78]. Although the prognosis remains poor, this improvement in OS was significant. Durvalumab has also been approved for the same indication [79]. Combined chemoimmunotherapy has become standard of care for patients with extensive stage disease, adequate performance status, and no contraindications to the use of immunotherapy, as reviewed earlier. There is an ongoing study examining the addition of atezolizumab to standard carboplatin plus etoposide for limited stage SCLC [80]. Additionally, immunotherapy agents like nivolumab [81] and pembrolizumab [82] can be used as second-line agents in relapsed SCLC.

Conclusions and Future Directions

The convergence of advances in basic science and clinical medicine have begun to change the prognosis of lung cancer. Advances in immunotherapy, molecular evaluation of targets, and development of new targeted agents continue to split lung cancer into subgroups that benefit from individualized approaches to treatment.

Between 2013 and 2016, incidence-based mortality for NSCLC decreased by 6.3% for men and 5.9% for women, compared to only 3.2% for men and 2.3% for women from 2008 to 2013 [83]. Similarly, lung cancer–specific survival for patients diagnosed with NSCLC improved from 26% in 2001 to 35% in 2014. When comparing PFS and OS between regimens, there are clear improvements when immunotherapy and targeted therapies can be incorporated into a patient's regimen. For example, as seen in Fig. 23.2, the PFS and OS for patients with metastatic NSCLC treated with platinum doublet alone was 4 months and 8 months, respectively. This compares to patients with metastatic non-squamous NSCLC treated with platinum,

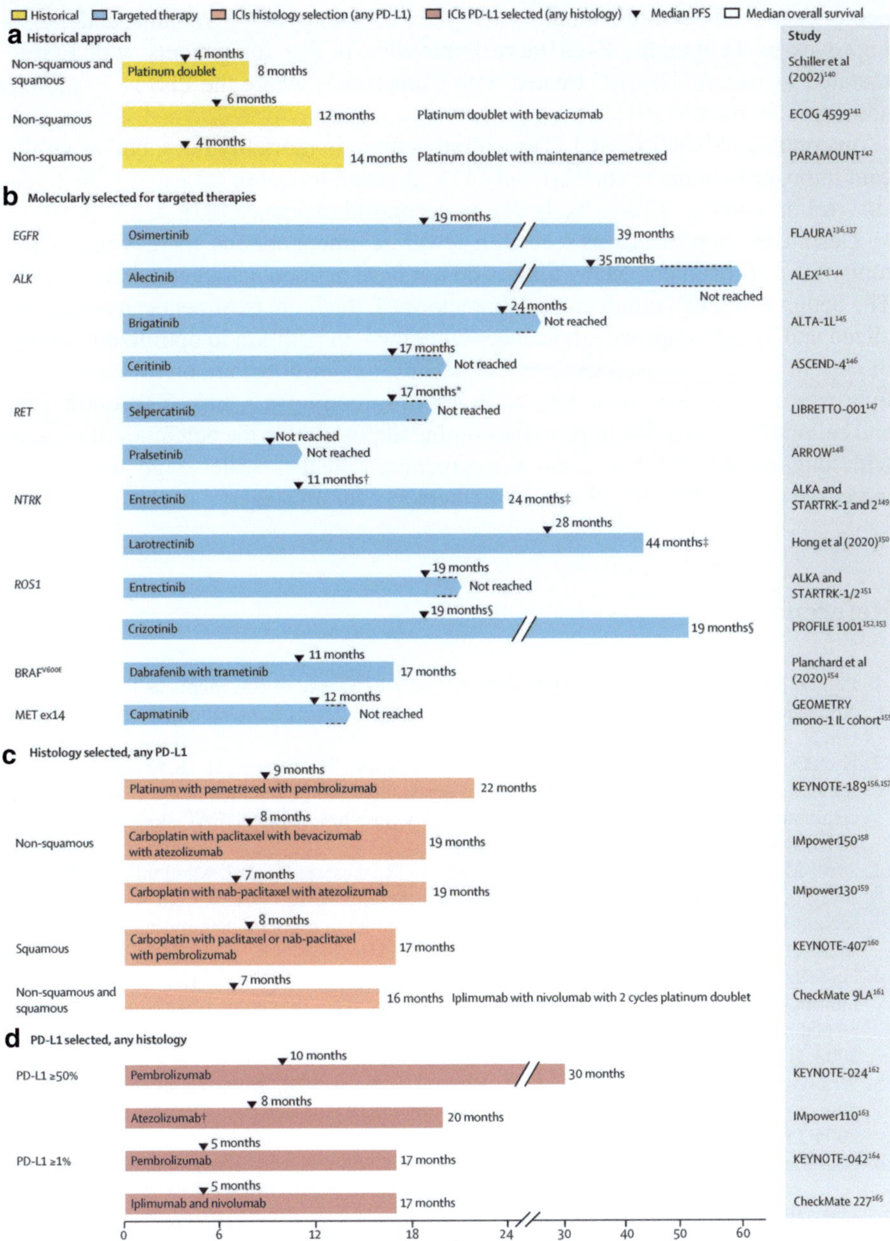

Fig. 23.2 Selected US Food and Drug Administration approved therapies for upfront treatment of patients with metastatic NSCLC. Historical approach (**a**), molecularly selected for targeted therapies (**b**), histology selected, any PD-L1 (**c**), and PD-L1 selected, any histology (**d**). (Used with permission from Thai et al. [84])

pemetrexed, and pembrolizumab, where the PFS improves to 9 months, and the OS improves to 22 months. Even more impressive is that for patients with EGFR-mutated metastatic NSCLC treated with osimertinib, where the PFS is 19 months and OS is 39 months [84].

In contrast to NSCLC, SCLC saw improvement in mortality rates, but no significant improvement in OS (in 2016 only 11% 2-year survival in men, and 17% 2-year survival in women). This is likely due to decreased incidence [83].

Despite the improvements seen with newer treatment options, there is still opportunity for improvement. Many tumors do not have actionable target mutations [84]. The better a patient's tumor can be characterized, the more treatment can be personalized and ideally improve lung cancer outcomes. In addition to optimizing our use of current treatments available, several new classes of drugs are on the horizon for lung cancer treatment, including antibody drug conjugates, bispecific antibodies, and cellular therapies. We hope to see continued progress in the outcomes of patients with lung cancer, with both increased screening to detect earlier stage disease, and increased availability of individualized therapies for all stages.

References

1. Pignon J-P, Tribodet H, Scagliotti GV, Douillard J-Y, Shepherd FA, Stephens RJ, et al. Lung adjuvant cisplatin evaluation: a pooled analysis by the LACE collaborative group. J Clin Oncol. 2008;26(21):3552–9.
2. Kreuter M, Vansteenkiste J, Fischer JR, Eberhardt W, Zabeck H, Kollmeier J, et al. Randomized phase 2 trial on refinement of early-stage NSCLC adjuvant chemotherapy with cisplatin and pemetrexed versus cisplatin and vinorelbine: the TREAT study. Ann Oncol. 2013;24(4):986–92.
3. Pérol M, Chouaid C, Pérol D, Barlési F, Gervais R, Westeel V, et al. Randomized, phase III study of gemcitabine or erlotinib maintenance therapy versus observation, with predefined second-line treatment, after cisplatin-gemcitabine induction chemotherapy in advanced non-small-cell lung cancer. J Clin Oncol. 2012;30(28):3516–24.
4. Fossella F, Pereira JR, von Pawel J, Pluzanska A, Gorbounova V, Kaukel E, et al. Randomized, multinational, phase III study of docetaxel plus platinum combinations versus vinorelbine plus cisplatin for advanced non-small-cell lung cancer: the TAX 326 study group. J Clin Oncol. 2003;21(16):3016–24.
5. Winton T, Livingston R, Johnson D, Rigas J, Johnston M, Butts C, et al. Vinorelbine plus cisplatin vs. observation in resected non-small-cell lung cancer. N Engl J Med. 2005;352(25):2589–97.
6. Non-Small Cell Lung Cancer Collaborative Group. Chemotherapy in non-small cell lung cancer: a meta-analysis using updated data on individual patients from 52 randomised clinical trials. BMJ. 1995;311(7010):899–909.
7. Douillard J-Y, Rosell R, De Lena M, Carpagnano F, Ramlau R, Gonzáles-Larriba JL, et al. Adjuvant vinorelbine plus cisplatin versus observation in patients with completely resected stage IB-IIIA non-small-cell lung cancer (adjuvant Navelbine international Trialist association [ANITA]): a randomised controlled trial. Lancet Oncol. 2006;7(9):719–27.
8. Arriagada R, Bergman B, Dunant A, Le Chevalier T, Pignon J-P, Vansteenkiste J, et al. Cisplatin-based adjuvant chemotherapy in patients with completely resected non-small-cell lung cancer. N Engl J Med. 2004;350(4):351–60.

9. Butts CA, Ding K, Seymour L, Twumasi-Ankrah P, Graham B, Gandara D, et al. Randomized phase III trial of vinorelbine plus cisplatin compared with observation in completely resected stage IB and II non-small-cell lung cancer: updated survival analysis of JBR-10. J Clin Oncol. 2010;28(1):29–34.

10. Strauss GM, Herndon JE, Maddaus MA, Johnstone DW, Johnson EA, Harpole DH, et al. Adjuvant paclitaxel plus carboplatin compared with observation in stage IB non-small-cell lung cancer: CALGB 9633 with the cancer and leukemia group B, radiation therapy oncology group, and north central cancer treatment group study groups. J Clin Oncol. 2008;26(31):5043–51.

11. Cuffe S, Booth CM, Peng Y, Darling GE, Li G, Kong W, et al. Adjuvant chemotherapy for non-small-cell lung cancer in the elderly: a population-based study in Ontario, Canada. J Clin Oncol. 2012;30(15):1813–21.

12. Felip E, Altorki N, Zhou C, Csőszi T, Vynnychenko I, Goloborodko O, et al. Adjuvant atezolizumab after adjuvant chemotherapy in resected stage IB-IIIA non-small-cell lung cancer (IMpower010): a randomised, multicentre, open-label, phase 3 trial. Lancet. 2021;398(10308):1344–57.

13. Wu Y-L, Tsuboi M, He J, John T, Grohe C, Majem M, et al. Osimertinib in resected EGFR-mutated non-small-cell lung cancer. N Engl J Med. 2020;383(18):1711–23.

14. Roth JA, Fossella F, Komaki R, Ryan MB, Putnam JB, Lee JS, et al. A randomized trial comparing perioperative chemotherapy and surgery with surgery alone in resectable stage IIIA non-small-cell lung cancer. J Natl Cancer Inst. 1994;86(9):673–80.

15. Jaklitsch MT, Herndon JE, DeCamp MM, Richards WG, Kumar P, Krasna MJ, et al. Nodal downstaging predicts survival following induction chemotherapy for stage IIIA (N2) non-small cell lung cancer in CALGB protocol #8935. J Surg Oncol. 2006;94(7):599–606.

16. Albain KS, Swann RS, Rusch VW, Turrisi AT, Shepherd FA, Smith C, et al. Radiotherapy plus chemotherapy with or without surgical resection for stage III non-small-cell lung cancer: a phase III randomised controlled trial. Lancet. 2009;374(9687):379–86.

17. Rusch VW, Giroux DJ, Kraut MJ, Crowley J, Hazuka M, Winton T, et al. Induction chemoradiation and surgical resection for superior sulcus non-small-cell lung carcinomas: long-term results of southwest oncology group trial 9416 (intergroup trial 0160). J Clin Oncol. 2007;25(3):313–8.

18. Shah AA, Berry MF, Tzao C, Gandhi M, Worni M, Pietrobon R, et al. Induction chemoradiation is not superior to induction chemotherapy alone in stage IIIA lung cancer. Ann Thorac Surg. 2012;93(6):1807–12.

19. Gaissert HA, Keum DY, Wright CD, Ancukiewicz M, Monroe E, Donahue DM, et al. POINT: Operative risk of pneumonectomy—influence of preoperative induction therapy. J Thorac Cardiovasc Surg. 2009;138(2):289–94.

20. Weder W, Collaud S, Eberhardt WEE, Hillinger S, Welter S, Stahel R, et al. Pneumonectomy is a valuable treatment option after neoadjuvant therapy for stage III non-small-cell lung cancer. J Thorac Cardiovasc Surg. 2010;139(6):1424–30.

21. Forde PM, Chaft JE, Smith KN, Anagnostou V, Cottrell TR, Hellmann MD, et al. Neoadjuvant PD-1 blockade in resectable lung cancer. N Engl J Med. 2018;378(21):1976–86.

22. Liang W, Cai K, Chen C, Chen H, Chen Q, Fu J, et al. Expert consensus on neoadjuvant immunotherapy for non-small cell lung cancer. Transl Lung Cancer Res. 2020;9(6):2696–715. https://tlcr.amegroups.com/article/view/47667. [cited 2022 Jan 30].

23. Xiong L, Li R, Sun J, Lou Y, Zhang W, Bai H, et al. Erlotinib as neoadjuvant therapy in stage IIIA (N2) EGFR mutation-positive non-small cell lung cancer: a prospective, single-arm, phase II study. Oncologist. 2019;24(2):157–e64.

24. Sun L, Guo Y-J, Song J, Wang Y-R, Zhang S-L, Huang L-T, et al. Neoadjuvant EGFR-TKI therapy for EGFR-mutant NSCLC: a systematic review and pooled analysis of five prospective clinical trials. Front Oncol. 2020;10:586596.

25. O'Rourke N, Figuls MRI, Farré Bernadó N, Macbeth F. Concurrent chemoradiotherapy in non-small cell lung cancer. Cochrane Database Syst Rev. 2010;(6):CD002140.

26. Choy H, Gerber DE, Bradley JD, Iyengar P, Monberg M, Treat J, et al. Concurrent pemetrexed and radiation therapy in the treatment of patients with inoperable stage III non-small cell lung cancer: a systematic review of completed and ongoing studies. Lung Cancer. 2015;87(3):232–40.

27. Senan S, Brade A, Wang L-H, Vansteenkiste J, Dakhil S, Biesma B, et al. PROCLAIM: randomized phase III trial of Pemetrexed-cisplatin or etoposide-cisplatin plus thoracic radiation therapy followed by consolidation chemotherapy in locally advanced nonsquamous non-small-cell lung cancer. J Clin Oncol. 2016;34(9):953–62.

28. Antonia SJ, Villegas A, Daniel D, Vicente D, Murakami S, Hui R, et al. Durvalumab after chemoradiotherapy in stage III non-small-cell lung cancer. N Engl J Med. 2017;377(20):1919–29.

29. Iyengar P, Wardak Z, Gerber DE, Tumati V, Ahn C, Hughes RS, et al. Consolidative radiotherapy for limited metastatic non-small-cell lung cancer: a phase 2 randomized clinical trial. JAMA Oncol. 2018;4(1):e173501.

30. Tartarone A, Lerose R, Tartarone M. Management of oligoprogression in non-small cell lung cancer patients. Med Oncol. 2022;39(5):56.

31. Weickhardt AJ, Scheier B, Burke JM, Gan G, Lu X, Bunn PA, et al. Local ablative therapy of oligoprogressive disease prolongs disease control by tyrosine kinase inhibitors in oncogene-addicted non-small-cell lung cancer. J Thorac Oncol. 2012;7(12):1807–14.

32. Rheinheimer S, Heussel C-P, Mayer P, Gaissmaier L, Bozorgmehr F, Winter H, et al. Oligoprogressive non-small-cell lung cancer under treatment with PD-(L)1 inhibitors. Cancers. 2020;12(4):E1046.

33. Aoki MN, Amarante MK, de Oliveira CEC, Watanabe MAE. Biomarkers in non-small cell lung cancer: perspectives of individualized targeted therapy. Anti Cancer Agents Med Chem. 2018;18(15):2070–7.

34. Campbell JD, Lathan C, Sholl L, Ducar M, Vega M, Sunkavalli A, et al. Comparison of prevalence and types of mutations in lung cancers among black and white populations. JAMA Oncol. 2017;3(6):801–9.

35. Tan AC, Tan DSW. Targeted therapies for lung cancer patients with oncogenic driver molecular alterations. J Clin Oncol. 2022;40(6):611–25.

36. Riudavets M, Sullivan I, Abdayem P, Planchard D. Targeting HER2 in non-small-cell lung cancer (NSCLC): a glimpse of hope? An updated review on therapeutic strategies in NSCLC harbouring HER2 alterations. ESMO Open. 2021;6(5):100260.

37. Harrison PT, Vyse S, Huang PH. Rare epidermal growth factor receptor (EGFR) mutations in non-small cell lung cancer. Semin Cancer Biol. 2020;61:167–79.

38. O'Leary CG, Andelkovic V, Ladwa R, Pavlakis N, Zhou C, Hirsch F, et al. Targeting BRAF mutations in non-small cell lung cancer. Transl Lung Cancer Res. 2019;8(6):1119–24.

39. Yang JC-H, Ahn M-J, Kim D-W, Ramalingam SS, Sequist LV, Su W-C, et al. Osimertinib in pretreated T790M-positive advanced non-small-cell lung cancer: AURA study phase II extension component. J Clin Oncol. 2017;35(12):1288–96.

40. Ramalingam SS, Yang JC-H, Lee CK, Kurata T, Kim D-W, John T, et al. Osimertinib as first-line treatment of EGFR mutation-positive advanced non-small-cell lung cancer. J Clin Oncol. 2018;36(9):841–9.

41. Ramalingam SS, Vansteenkiste J, Planchard D, Cho BC, Gray JE, Ohe Y, et al. Overall survival with Osimertinib in untreated, EGFR-mutated advanced NSCLC. N Engl J Med. 2020;382(1):41–50.

42. Liu Q, Yu S, Zhao W, Qin S, Chu Q, Wu K. EGFR-TKIs resistance via EGFR-independent signaling pathways. Mol Cancer. 2018;17(1):53.

43. Reck M, Rodríguez-Abreu D, Robinson AG, Hui R, Csőszi T, Fülöp A, et al. Pembrolizumab versus chemotherapy for PD-L1-positive non-small-cell lung cancer. N Engl J Med. 2016;375(19):1823–33.

44. Gandhi L, Rodríguez-Abreu D, Gadgeel S, Esteban E, Felip E, De Angelis F, et al. Pembrolizumab plus chemotherapy in metastatic non-small-cell lung cancer. N Engl J Med. 2018;378(22):2078–92.

45. Naidoo J, Page DB, Li BT, Connell LC, Schindler K, Lacouture ME, et al. Toxicities of the anti-PD-1 and anti-PD-L1 immune checkpoint antibodies. Ann Oncol. 2015;26(12):2375–91.
46. Brahmer JR, Lacchetti C, Schneider BJ, Atkins MB, Brassil KJ, Caterino JM, et al. Management of immune-related adverse events in patients treated with immune checkpoint inhibitor therapy: American Society of Clinical Oncology clinical practice guideline. J Clin Oncol. 2018;36(17):1714–68.
47. Mok TSK, Wu Y-L, Kudaba I, Kowalski DM, Cho BC, Turna HZ, et al. Pembrolizumab versus chemotherapy for previously untreated, PD-L1-expressing, locally advanced or metastatic non-small-cell lung cancer (KEYNOTE-042): a randomised, open-label, controlled, phase 3 trial. Lancet. 2019;393(10183):1819–30.
48. Herbst RS, Giaccone G, de Marinis F, Reinmuth N, Vergnenegre A, Barrios CH, et al. Atezolizumab for first-line treatment of PD-L1-selected patients with NSCLC. N Engl J Med. 2020;383(14):1328–39.
49. Sezer A, Kilickap S, Gümüş M, Bondarenko I, Özgüroğlu M, Gogishvili M, et al. Cemiplimab monotherapy for first-line treatment of advanced non-small-cell lung cancer with PD-L1 of at least 50%: a multicentre, open-label, global, phase 3, randomised, controlled trial. Lancet. 2021;397(10274):592–604.
50. Langer CJ, Gadgeel SM, Borghaei H, Papadimitrakopoulou VA, Patnaik A, Powell SF, et al. Carboplatin and pemetrexed with or without pembrolizumab for advanced, non-squamous non-small-cell lung cancer: a randomised, phase 2 cohort of the open-label KEYNOTE-021 study. Lancet Oncol. 2016;17(11):1497–508.
51. Socinski MA, Jotte RM, Cappuzzo F, Orlandi F, Stroyakovskiy D, Nogami N, et al. Atezolizumab for first-line treatment of metastatic nonsquamous NSCLC. N Engl J Med. 2018;378(24):2288–301.
52. Sandler A, Gray R, Perry MC, Brahmer J, Schiller JH, Dowlati A, et al. Paclitaxel-carboplatin alone or with bevacizumab for non-small-cell lung cancer. N Engl J Med. 2006;355(24):2542–50.
53. Paz-Ares L, Luft A, Vicente D, Tafreshi A, Gümüş M, Mazières J, et al. Pembrolizumab plus chemotherapy for squamous non-small-cell lung cancer. N Engl J Med. 2018;379(21):2040–51.
54. Reck M, Schenker M, Lee KH, Provencio M, Nishio M, Lesniewski-Kmak K, et al. Nivolumab plus ipilimumab versus chemotherapy as first-line treatment in advanced non-small-cell lung cancer with high tumour mutational burden: patient-reported outcomes results from the randomised, open-label, phase III CheckMate 227 trial. Eur J Cancer. 2019;1990(116):137–47.
55. Paz-Ares L, Ciuleanu T-E, Cobo M, Schenker M, Zurawski B, Menezes J, et al. First-line nivolumab plus ipilimumab combined with two cycles of chemotherapy in patients with non-small-cell lung cancer (CheckMate 9LA): an international, randomised, open-label, phase 3 trial. Lancet Oncol. 2021;22(2):198–211.
56. Bodor JN, Kasireddy V, Borghaei H. First-line therapies for metastatic lung adenocarcinoma without a driver mutation. J Oncol Pract. 2018;14(9):529–35.
57. Schiller JH, Harrington D, Belani CP, Langer C, Sandler A, Krook J, et al. Comparison of four chemotherapy regimens for advanced non-small-cell lung cancer. N Engl J Med. 2002;346(2):92–8.
58. Scagliotti GV, Parikh P, von Pawel J, Biesma B, Vansteenkiste J, Manegold C, et al. Phase III study comparing cisplatin plus gemcitabine with cisplatin plus pemetrexed in chemotherapy-naive patients with advanced-stage non-small-cell lung cancer. J Clin Oncol. 2008;26(21):3543–51.
59. Pujol J-L, Breton J-L, Gervais R, Rebattu P, Depierre A, Morère J-F, et al. Gemcitabine-docetaxel versus cisplatin-vinorelbine in advanced or metastatic non-small-cell lung cancer: a phase III study addressing the case for cisplatin. Ann Oncol. 2005;16(4):602–10.
60. Tan EH, Szczesna A, Krzakowski M, Macha HN, Gatzemeier U, Mattson K, et al. Randomized study of vinorelbine—gemcitabine versus vinorelbine--carboplatin in patients with advanced non-small cell lung cancer. Lung Cancer. 2005;49(2):233–40.

61. Johnson DH, Fehrenbacher L, Novotny WF, Herbst RS, Nemunaitis JJ, Jablons DM, et al. Randomized phase II trial comparing bevacizumab plus carboplatin and paclitaxel with carboplatin and paclitaxel alone in previously untreated locally advanced or metastatic non-small-cell lung cancer. J Clin Oncol. 2004;22(11):2184–91.

62. Garcia J, Hurwitz HI, Sandler AB, Miles D, Coleman RL, Deurloo R, et al. Bevacizumab (Avastin®) in cancer treatment: a review of 15 years of clinical experience and future outlook. Cancer Treat Rev. 2020;86:102017.

63. Gordon CR, Rojavin Y, Patel M, Zins JE, Grana G, Kann B, et al. A review on bevacizumab and surgical wound healing: an important warning to all surgeons. Ann Plast Surg. 2009;62(6):707–9.

64. Crinò L, Dansin E, Garrido P, Griesinger F, Laskin J, Pavlakis N, et al. Safety and efficacy of first-line bevacizumab-based therapy in advanced non-squamous non-small-cell lung cancer (SAiL, MO19390): a phase 4 study. Lancet Oncol. 2010;11(8):733–40.

65. Garon EB, Ciuleanu T-E, Arrieta O, Prabhash K, Syrigos KN, Goksel T, et al. Ramucirumab plus docetaxel versus placebo plus docetaxel for second-line treatment of stage IV non-small-cell lung cancer after disease progression on platinum-based therapy (REVEL): a multicentre, double-blind, randomised phase 3 trial. Lancet. 2014;384(9944):665–73.

66. Vallières E, Shepherd FA, Crowley J, Van Houtte P, Postmus PE, Carney D, et al. The IASLC lung cancer staging project: proposals regarding the relevance of TNM in the pathologic staging of small cell lung cancer in the forthcoming (seventh) edition of the TNM classification for lung cancer. J Thorac Oncol. 2009;4(9):1049–59.

67. Wang S, Zimmermann S, Parikh K, Mansfield AS, Adjei AA. Current diagnosis and management of small-cell lung cancer. Mayo Clin Proc. 2019;94(8):1599–622.

68. Rudin CM, Brambilla E, Faivre-Finn C, Sage J. Small-cell lung cancer. Nat Rev Dis Primers. 2021;7(1):3.

69. Stinchcombe TE, Gore EM. Limited-stage small cell lung cancer: current chemoradiotherapy treatment paradigms. Oncologist. 2010;15(2):187–95.

70. Faivre-Finn C, Snee M, Ashcroft L, Appel W, Barlesi F, Bhatnagar A, et al. Concurrent once-daily versus twice-daily chemoradiotherapy in patients with limited-stage small-cell lung cancer (CONVERT): an open-label, phase 3, randomised, superiority trial. Lancet Oncol. 2017;18(8):1116–25.

71. Demedts IK, Vermaelen KY, van Meerbeeck JP. Treatment of extensive-stage small cell lung carcinoma: current status and future prospects. Eur Respir J. 2010;35(1):202–15.

72. Griesinger F, Korol EE, Kayaniyil S, Varol N, Ebner T, Goring SM. Efficacy and safety of first-line carboplatin-versus cisplatin-based chemotherapy for non-small cell lung cancer: a meta-analysis. Lung Cancer. 2019;135:196–204.

73. Hatfield LA, Huskamp HA, Lamont EB. Survival and toxicity after cisplatin plus etoposide versus carboplatin plus etoposide for extensive-stage small-cell lung cancer in elderly patients. J Oncol Pract. 2016;12(7):666–73.

74. Noda K, Nishiwaki Y, Kawahara M, Negoro S, Sugiura T, Yokoyama A, et al. Irinotecan plus cisplatin compared with etoposide plus cisplatin for extensive small-cell lung cancer. N Engl J Med. 2002;346(2):85–91.

75. von Pawel J, Schiller JH, Shepherd FA, Fields SZ, Kleisbauer JP, Chrysson NG, et al. Topotecan versus cyclophosphamide, doxorubicin, and vincristine for the treatment of recurrent small-cell lung cancer. J Clin Oncol. 1999;17(2):658–67.

76. O'Brien MER, Ciuleanu T-E, Tsekov H, Shparyk Y, Cuceviá B, Juhasz G, et al. Phase III trial comparing supportive care alone with supportive care with oral topotecan in patients with relapsed small-cell lung cancer. J Clin Oncol. 2006;24(34):5441–7.

77. Trigo J, Subbiah V, Besse B, Moreno V, López R, Sala MA, et al. Lurbinectedin as second-line treatment for patients with small-cell lung cancer: a single-arm, open-label, phase 2 basket trial. Lancet Oncol. 2020;21(5):645–54.

78. Horn L, Mansfield AS, Szczęsna A, Havel L, Krzakowski M, Hochmair MJ, et al. First-line Atezolizumab plus chemotherapy in extensive-stage small-cell lung cancer. N Engl J Med. 2018;379(23):2220–9.

79. Paz-Ares L, Dvorkin M, Chen Y, Reinmuth N, Hotta K, Trukhin D, et al. Durvalumab plus platinum-etoposide versus platinum-etoposide in first-line treatment of extensive-stage small-cell lung cancer (CASPIAN): a randomised, controlled, open-label, phase 3 trial. Lancet. 2019;394(10212):1929–39.
80. Higgins KA, Hu C, Stinchcombe TE, Jabbour SK, Kozono DE, Owonikoko TK, et al. NRG oncology/alliance LU005: a phase II/III randomized study of Chemoradiation vs. Chemoradiation plus Atezolizumab in limited stage small cell lung cancer. Int J Radiat Oncol Biol Phys. 2021;111(3):e470–1.
81. Antonia SJ, López-Martin JA, Bendell J, Ott PA, Taylor M, Eder JP, et al. Nivolumab alone and nivolumab plus ipilimumab in recurrent small-cell lung cancer (CheckMate 032): a multicentre, open-label, phase 1/2 trial. Lancet Oncol. 2016;17(7):883–95.
82. Chung HC, Piha-Paul SA, Lopez-Martin J, Schellens JHM, Kao S, Miller WH, et al. Pembrolizumab after two or more lines of previous therapy in patients with recurrent or metastatic SCLC: results from the KEYNOTE-028 and KEYNOTE-158 studies. J Thorac Oncol. 2020;15(4):618–27.
83. Howlader N, Forjaz G, Mooradian MJ, Meza R, Kong CY, Cronin KA, et al. The effect of advances in lung-cancer treatment on population mortality. N Engl J Med. 2020;383(7):640–9.
84. Thai AA, Solomon BJ, Sequist LV, Gainor JF, Heist RS. Lung cancer. Lancet. 2021;398(10299):535–54.

Part V
Engaging the Community

Chapter 24
Lung Cancer and Social Justice: What Do I Need to Know?

Gregory C. Kane and Nathaniel R. Evans III

> *The ultimate measure of a man is not where he stands in moments of comfort and convenience, but where he stands at times of challenge and controversy.*
>
> —Martin Luther King, Jr., 1963

Dr. David Leach joined the Accreditation Council on Graduate Medical Education (ACGME) in 1997 from the Henry Ford Hospital and implemented the "Outcomes Project," which led to seismic shifts in medical education from an apprentice model to a competency or outcomes-driven model [1]. The impact was immediate and by 1999, the six clinical competencies were developed and implemented, forever committing organized medical education in the United States to a competency-based approach anchored to the achievement of specific skills and habits by the learner. These competencies could then be objectively observed and documented. The competencies were expanded as part of the Milestones Project in medical education and these have served us well in delineating the specific skills and milestones medical trainees must acquire in their preparation for independent practice [2–4]. Indeed, the Milestones provide a framework for social justice education through the System-Based Practice Milestone outlined in the most recently published version of the Internal Medicine Milestone which identify a specific expectation for trainees to "demonstrate knowledge of population and community health needs and disparities" with the aspirational goal that the trainee "leads innovations and advocates for populations and communities with health care inequities." Moreover, as faculty members in an ACGME training environment, these authors completed questions

G. C. Kane (✉)
Department of Medicine, Thomas Jefferson University, Philadelphia, PA, USA
e-mail: Gregory.Kane@Jefferson.edu

N. R. Evans III
Department of Surgery, Thomas Jefferson University, Philadelphia, PA, USA
e-mail: Nathaniel.Evans@Jefferson.edu

through their most recent ACGME questionnaire (being administered through April 17, 2022) about recruiting diverse students, residents, and fellows. There were, however, no specific questions about developing knowledge about social justice. Necessary to this end, the trainee must be well versed in social justice. But, how is it that the trainee, or the established physician or nurse, will acquire this knowledge or awareness?

Lung cancer care is challenged by a number of disparities, the most basic and important of which are the undisputable facts of mortality. Black men are more likely to die from lung cancer than white men, and black women are more likely to die from lung cancer than white women [5]. This disparity is evident in the most recently published cancer statistics, which show 15–17% higher mortality among black persons compared to white persons. Even when diagnosed at early stage, black patients are less likely to be offered or to proceed with surgical resection [6–9].

While this basic difference suggests that we have much work to do in health care delivery to address this disparity, recent literature has helped us focus on specific iterative steps that we might take. It is important to also acknowledge that the key literature establishing the role of screening with low dose CT in smokers and former smokers 55 years and older with the requisite tobacco exposure only included less than 5% blacks – far less representative than the general US population [10]. Moreover, the expansion of the criteria to smokers with lower pack-years (just 20 pack-years) and as young as age 50 only occurred in 2021. Shockingly, disparities are evident from the earliest stages of prevention and early intervention [7]. Lake and colleagues identified that black patients referred for lung cancer screening were less likely to actually undergo the T0 or initial scan. In underscoring the specific and granular differences of missed exams, poor adherence, and delayed follow-up when referred for lung cancer screening, Lake and colleagues challenge us to address the specific barriers of these disparities at the earliest interactions with eligible patients [11]. Even though lung cancer screening is a new service, there is evidence from a social justice perspective that inequity already exists despite this early stage of its implementation. Despite wide acceptance and support for screening currently, lung cancer screening is still not measured as part of the Health Education Database Information Set (HEDIS) Measures established and updated by the National Committee for Quality Assurance (NCQA).

What is essential, then, to understand such barriers? First, it is the recognition that inequity exists already in lung cancer screening, but also that some investigators are already taking steps to address this issue [12, 13]. More broadly, it is the awareness of social justice, past harms and experiences, related to specific populations, and the history of disparate care throughout the troubled past of American Medicine in general that is essential. This experience and understating can and should be acquired by healthcare professionals, but especially physicians, nurses, and public health professionals through multiple sources. Such sources can be divided into important books and articles that are part of the canon of social justice in healthcare, or through representative productions addressing social justice from theatre, plays, and other arts – especially when coupled with reflection, and, finally, empathic listening by clinicians encountering diverse populations of patients. In this chapter, we will focus on books, which the reader might consider adding to their reading list (a comprehensive list of articles and artistic productions would simply be beyond the scope of this effort). If the reader chooses to do so, he/she might find greater understanding of the complex worlds we live in and our troubled past. More importantly, the result might be elevating rather than demoralizing. In confronting the sins of our past, we have a chance to move forward with a greater sense of purpose and awareness. These sins belong to all of us, white and black, male and female, god-fearing or atheist, immigrant or Native American. Transparency and awareness can help inform the healthcare professional so that he/she/they can address inequities in their work.

The scope of this chapter does not permit a comprehensive discussion of every published work of the last half century since the Civil Rights movement of the 1960s, but the idea that there is indeed a "canon" of essential readings should be clearly accepted and these authors believed that such an attempt, despite limitations and criticisms, should be put forth. We acknowledge that others might suggest that this list be expanded to make it even more comprehensive. Not only is this canon selected because of the topics addressed, but because of the diversity of authors and voices selected to bring about greater understanding. Examples of such a proposed canon are outlined in the Table 24.1.

Table 24.1 A suggested modern canon of social justice reading (This is just a suggested list and the reader may wish to add or subtract titles)

Reference	Author	Title	Comment
[14]	Harriet Washington, MA	Medical Apartheid	Essential reading for every healthcare professional and especially those conducting clinical research
[15]	Isabel Wilkerson	Caste	In describing slavery and racial tension from the perspective of caste, Wilkerson helps us all find a path forward to a more equitable society
[16]	Clint Smith, PhD	How the Word Is Passed	Many of the focal points of our nation's racial inequities are in plain view. Not only does Clint Smith describe the significance of these places, but he engages ordinary Americans in crucial conversations to help us better understand the current tensions in our society
[17]	Dorothy Roberts, JD	Fatal Invention	This extensively researched work exploring the biological basis of race dispels any basis of race in science and genetics. In doing so Roberts establishes that the concept of race is a myth and that its perpetuation continues to harm our communities
[18]	John Lewis	Across That Bridge	Every student of civil rights should read John Lewis' lyrical memoir. And in doing so, you will be transported across that bridge and toward more equitable future

(continued)

Table 24.1 (continued)

Reference	Author	Title	Comment
[19]	Susan Kamei, JD	When Can We Go Back to America?	The tensions that immigrants experience in our country are clearly evident in this travesty in which US citizens were imprisoned in work camps during WWII. In a land built by immigrants, it is hard to fathom that this could have happened. The reader will be forced to acknowledge the hypocrisy of our xenophobia
[20]	Greg Boyle, MA, MDiv, STM	Tattoos on the Heart	Disparities which deprive Hispanic youths in Los Angeles from finding a path in life can be addressed, if we only have the courage
[21]	Mona Hanna-Attisha, MD, MPH,	What Seethe Eyes Don't See	Dr. Hanna-Attisha addresses stark disparities at a neighborhood level which have left America's poor and disadvantaged with a failing infrastructure
[22]	Filipe Fernandez-Armesto, D. Phil	Our America: A Hispanic History of the United States	Hispanic Americans are often viewed as immigrants to the United States, while in truth, many have been in the Americas long before northern European immigrants arrived
[23]	Jerry Ellis	Walking the Trail: One Man's Journey Along the Cherokee Trail of Tears	This modern account of a walk across the trail of tears from the rural south to Oklahoma is recounted by a descendent of the Cherokee tribe reminding Americans that we were not the first to inhabit this land and that we violated numerous treaties signed both before and after the US constitution
[24]	C. Riley Snorton, PhD	Black on Both Sides: A Racial History of Trans Identity	This story of being trans in America takes us back to early narratives of Christine Jorgenson, who transitioned after returning from military service in WWII and became a strong advocate for transgender individuals becoming a celebrity in the process
[25]	Dina Gilio-Whitaker, MA	As Long as Grass Grows	A compelling reminder to all environmentalists that our indigenous peoples in the Americas have an important stake in preserving the beauty of forests, fields, and streams
[26]	NA	The Gold Humanism Society Offers Annual Collections of "Summer Reading" for the Compassionate Clinician	See reference for details for the gold humanism society website

What follows is a more extended synopsis of each of these books to help the reader prioritize their reading and prepare for the important perspective cyst to be learned.

Medical Apartheid, by Harriet Washington, MA

With clarity of voice Washington describes in remarkable prose how Dr. J. Marion Sims used "enslaved experimental subjects as the ultimate controllable patient" and administered morphine only after surgery while forcing his patients to undergo his experimental surgical technique for repair of vesico-vaginal fistulae without any use of available anesthetics. The extraordinary detail by Ms. Washington and the insight and depth of her research and writing leads to a stark understanding of the horrors of Sims surgical experimentation. It is simply mandatory that every physician know this story and understand how it still impacts the perspective of African Americans today more than 150 years hence.

Caste, by Isabel Wilkerson

The power of Wilkerson's Pulitzer Prize winning book is not only in its detailed discussion of slavery and the caste system, but in its call to repair our relationships and the challenge to no longer ignore the stain of slavery upon our past but to reconcile and remedy it to secure our future. While some might like to conclude that the sins of slavery are fully in the past, Wilkerson uses a powerful analogy of a faulty foundation in one's own home. To secure the structure into the future, the foundation must be repaired. The question is whether we have the courage to acknowledge a painful past.

How the Word Is Passed, by Clint Smith, PhD

Smith leads us on an uncomfortable tour through the historical map of slavery in a book that, while essential reading for all healthcare professionals, does not comment upon the historical wrongs of organized medicine. While not written for the medical professionals, the roots of our forest of discontent are planted within this important work. These roots described the "national problem" of slavery, tracing it from before the founding of our nation through Monticello of Virginia and the Whitney Plantation of Louisiana and on through to Angola Prison in central Louisiana. Along this journey, Smith explores the crevices of social justice by engaging ordinary Americans and exploring their perspective to see how far we have come or how far we have to go.

Fatal Invention, by Dorothy Roberts, JD

Roberts succeeds in proving her assertion that race was invented by white people to subjugate blacks; that race has no basis, whatsoever, in biology. She also highlights that skin tone is an imperfect substitute for these characterizations. Her arguments are supported by troves of medical and sociological literature leaving no doubt for the reader that separation into racial groups lacking in biological basis should be rejected in every way.

Across that Bridge, by John Lewis

After reading John Lewis' vision for change and the future of United States, you will feel as if you were with him when he walked across the Edmund Pettus Bridge – a bridge named for a member of the Ku Klux Klan – a name that is so hard to write that you will be transported to the Edmund Pettus bridge and you most certainly will find yourself joining hands with John Lewis in one final trip across the Alabama River on a journey toward a more equitable future for us all.

When Can We Go Back to America?, by Susan Kamei, JD

Susan Kamei reminds us of a painful part of our World War II history during which we placed Japanese Americans in internment camps. This work captures our xenophobia and challenges us to make amends for the mistreatment of Japanese American immigrants. This story also reminds us that we are all immigrants and mistreatment of any one immigrant group is tantamount to mistreatment of all immigrant groups. This painful story for our shared past forces us to come to grips with our own shared humanity.

Tattoos on the Heart, by Greg Boyle, MA, MDiv, STM

Boyle helps address the issues of poverty, hopelessness, and fatalism in one of the toughest and most violent neighborhoods of Los Angeles. He shows that love can help address the difficult problems of homelessness, gangs, and social disenfranchisement, but only when coupled with being present in the lives of those afflicted and offer solutions that are not so much handouts but rather an offer for a hand up toward opportunity and engagement. Addressing the lives of young men engaged in gangs may have seemed impossible, until Greg Boyle looked at new ways and new approaches.

What the Eyes Can't See, by Mona Hanna-Attisha, MD, MPH

Dr. Hanna-Attisha, an Iraqi-American, is the first to recognize lead poisoning in her patients and also uncovers the impact of a recent change in the water supply that has disturbed the passivation layer of the water infrastructure leading to release of harmful concentrations of lead in the water in Flint Michigan. Her magnificent book tells the story of her determination to uncover the truth and protect local residents from the harms in their water supply while battling the local and state authorities who should have been her allies. A hero in every sense of the word, Hanna-Attisha shows how one doctor's advocacy can change a city and the world.

Our America: A Hispanic History of the United States, by Filipe Fernandez-Armesto, D Phil

This important story highlights that Hispanic populations arrived in the Americas before Anglo populations from northern European countries dominated North America. This is an important aspect of history to acknowlegde. Fernandez-Armesto provides clarity of this background in his landmark treatise.

Walking the Trail: One Man's Journey Along the Cherokee Trail of Tears, by Jerry Ellis

If you do not know the story of the Trail of Tears, Ellis's personal memoir will provide reflections on his path retracing the route of the Trail of Tears which moved settled and peaceful Native Americans of Cherokee Tribes from lands they had legal ownership of through signed treaties with the US Government. The treaties were not honored, and in March 1830, the Indian Relocation Act displaced more than 46,000 Cherokee Indian natives on a forced relocation march that led to as many as 4000 deaths from starvation, exposure to the elements, and disease.

Black on Both Sides: A Racial History of Trans Identity, by C. Riley Snorton, PhD

Currently, trans rights are being challenged in state houses across the country as culture wars rage and trans persons and their families face even greater persecution. It is important to emphasize that transgender or non-binary persons are only asking to be treated the same as everyone else. Snorton, through his award winning book, reminds as that being trans is not a new issue as, historically, many brave trans persons have courageously considered or pursued living their true lives and true gender identities over the last century. Perhaps this historical reflection will help health care providers offer even greater advocacy for transitioning, trans, non-binary, and gender fluid persons with dignity and professionalism.

As Long as Grass Grows, by Dina Gilio-Whitaker, MA

Gilio-Whitaker reminds us that with regard to environmental justice, no group has a stronger claim to our sacred outdoor spaces in the Americas than indigenous peoples who have a connection to this land predating any European settlers and whose culture is tied to sustainable living off the resources of the land. Gilio-Whitaker also dispels the myth of the "vanishing Indians" of the west, reminding us that so many perished through genocide or forced relocation. Her refreshing perspective and narrative of recent controversies including that of water rights in the Dakotas will cause immigrants to reconsider everything.

This proposed canon is perhaps a tall order and may not be practicable for many. Given this reality, one must consider alternate paths to a greater understanding of inequities in the United States, inequities in medicine, and the challenges of addressing these in medicine. An alternative approach is to listen and learn – to learn from our patients. Remarkably, their rich histories, shared in the privacy of the examination room or at the bedside, can only allow us to be better healers and come to a greater understanding. What follows is a discussion of listening techniques that may inform our learning and understanding.

Empathic Listening as a Tool to Understand Our Patients

Active listening was coined in the 1950s and relies on the attentiveness and genuine interest of the listener, which can be conveyed through appropriate questions [27]. Even for healthcare professionals who are not well versed in the "Canon of Social Justice," active listening when caring for any patient who has suffered from injustice can inform the healthcare professional regarding suffering and the human condition and allow the healthcare professional to provide culturally competent and humanistic care. Beyond active listening, *empathic listening* is a structured listening and questioning technique that can permit the healthcare professional to achieve equitable and more therapeutic relationships with patients who have experienced suffering or social injustice in their previous healthcare encounters [28]. As such, empathic listening, through which the healthcare professional places themselves in the "shoes of the subject" takes active listening techniques to another level, allowing the physician or nurse to come to a greater understanding even if the past wrong cannot be fixed. That awareness permits all of us to be in touch with our own shared humanity and be more effective healers.

The purpose of this is two-fold. First, the authors wish to remind the reader that lung cancer care is inequitable, but we can and must do better. If one accepts this and wishes to commit to this journey, it is essential to do so informed on social justice as they impact our patients. Fortunately, these topics are being addressed in our society and authors suggest a "canon of social justice" so that the reader might be able to broaden their knowledge and understanding of social justice issues as they might affect their patients. This is just a suggested list and others might add or subtract from this collection. In addition, we all have a chance to deepen our understanding in every patient encounter through active and empathic listening. The results can be extraordinary and lead to a greater understanding of your patients and society. Another way of saying this comes from the former acting Secretary of Health and Human Services (HHS), Donald Berwick, MD, who gave the Yale School of Medicine Commencement Speech in 2010. His address is excerpted in the following text:

> "But, now I will tell you a secret – a mystery. Those who suffer need you to be something more than a doctor; they need you to be a healer. And, to become a healer, you must do something even more difficult than putting your white coat on. You must take your white coat off. You must recover, embrace, and treasure the memory of your shared, frail humanity – of the dignity in each and every soul. When you take off that white coat in the sacred presence of those for whom you will care – in the sacred presence of people just like you – when you take off that white coat, and, tower not over them, but join those you serve, you become a healer in a world of fear and fragmentation, an "aching" world, as your Chaplain put it this morning, that has never needed healing more" [29].

References

1. Leach DC. Changing education to improve patient care. Qual Health Care. 2001;10(Suppl 2):ii54–8.
2. Nasca TJ, Philibert I, Brigham T, Flynn TC. The next accreditation system- rationale and benefits. N Engl J Med. 2012;366:1051–6.
3. Caverzagie KJ, Iobst WF, Aagaard EM, Hood S, Chick DA, Kane GC, Brigham TP, Swing SR, Meade LB, Bazari H, Bush RW, Kirk LM, Green ML, Hinchey KT, Smith CD. The internal medicine reporting milestones and the next accreditation system. Ann Intern Med. 2013;158(7):557–9. https://doi.org/10.7326/0003-4819-158-7-201304020-00593.
4. www.acgme.org/globalassets/PDFs/Milestones/InternalMedicineMilestones.pdf.0 Accessed 12 Feb 2022.
5. Siegel RL, Miller KD, Fuchs HE, Jemal A. Cancer statistics 2022. Cancer J Clin. 2022;72:7.

 6. Taioli E, Wolf AS, Camacho-Rivera M, Kaufman A, Lee D, Bhora F, et al. Racial disparities in esophageal cancer survival after surgery. J Surg Oncol. 2016;113(6):659–64.
 7. Merritt RE, Abdel-Rasoul M, D'Souza DM, Kneuertz PJ. Racial disparities in overall survival and surgical treatment for early stage lung cancer by facility type. Clin Lung Cancer. 2021;22(5):e691–8.
 8. Savitch SL, Grenda TR, Scott W, Cowan SW, Posey J, Mitchell EP, et al. Racial disparities in rates of surgery for esophageal cancer: a study from the National cancer database. J Gastrointest Surg. 2021;25(3):581–92.
 9. Evans NR, Grenda T, Alvarez NH, Okusanya OT. Narrative review of socioeconomic and racial disparities in the treatment of early stage lung cancer. J Thorac Dis. 2021;13(6):3758–63.
10. The National Lung Cancer Screening Research Team. Reduced lung-cancer mortality with low-dose computed tomographic screening. N Engl J Med. 2011;365(5):395–409.
11. Lake M, Shusted CS, Juon HS, et al. Black patients referred to a lung cancer screening program experience lower rates of screening and longer time to follow-up. BMC Cancer. 2020;20:561.
12. Shusted CS, Evans NR, Juon HS, Kane GC, Barta JA. Association of race with lung cancer risk among adults undergoing lung cancer screening. JAMA Netw Open. 2021;4(4):e214509. https://doi.org/10.1001/jamanetworkopen.2021.4509. PMID: 33822072; PMCID: PMC8025120.
13. Tanner NT, Brasher PB, Wojciechowski B, Ward R, Slatore C, Gebregziabher M, Silvestri GA. Screening adherence in the veterans administration lung cancer screening demonstration project. Chest. 2020;158(4):1742–52. https://doi.org/10.1016/j.chest.2020.04.063. Epub 2020 May 19
14. Washington H. Medical Apartheid: the dark history of medical experimentation on black Americans from colonial times to the present. New York, NY: Harlem Moon, Broadway Books; 2006.
15. Wilkerson I. Caste: the origins of our discontents. New York, NY: Random House; 2020.
16. Smith C. How the word is passed. A reckoning with the history of slavery across America. Botson, MA: Little Brown and Company; 2021.
17. Dorothy R. Fatal invention: how science, politics, and big business re-create race in the twenty-first century. New York: New Press/ORIM; 2011.
18. Lewis J. Across that bridge: life lessons and a vision for change. Botson, MA: Legacy Lit; 2012.
19. Kamei SH. When can we go Back to America? Simon and Shuster Books; 2021.
20. Boyle G. Tattoos on the heart: the power of boundless compassion. New York: Simon and Schuster; 2011.
21. Fernández-Armesto F. Our America: a Hispanic history of the United States. New York, NY: WW Norton & Company; 2014.
22. Hanna-Attisha M. What the eyes don't see: a story of crisis, resistance, and hope in an American city. One World; 2019.
23. Jerry E. Walking the trail: one man's journey along the Cherokee trail of tears. Lincoln, NE: University of Nebraska Press; 2001.
24. Snorton CR. Black on both sides: a racial history of trans identity. Minneapolis, MN: University of Minnesota Press; 2017.
25. Gilio-Whitaker D. As long as grass grows: the indigenous fight for environmental justice, from colonization to standing rock. Boston, MA: Beacon Press; 2019.
26. https://www.gold-foundation.org/newsroom/blog/2021-summer-reading-list/. Accessed March 3, 2022.
27. Levitt DH. Active listening and counselor self-efficacy: Emphasis on one microskill in the beginning counselor training. Clin Superv. 2001;20(2):101–15.
28. Gearhart CC, Bodie GD. Active-empathic listening as a general social skill: evidence from bivariate and canonical correlations. Commun Rep. 2011;24(2):86–98.
29. https://www.denisesilber.com/files/berwickyalemedicalschoolgraduationaddressmay10.pdf. Accessed 2 Feb 2022.

Chapter 25
Reaching Vulnerable Populations and Areas of Need

Kristine Pham and Rickie Brawer

Background

Approximately 36% of adults in the United States have low health literacy, especially among those who are elderly, have low socioeconomic status (SES), have limited English proficiency (LEP), and are eligible for Medicaid. Adults with low health literacy also tend to have four times higher health care costs, 6% more hospital visits, and longer hospital stays compared to those with proficient health literacy [1, 2]. The meaning of health literacy was recently updated with the release of the government's *Healthy People 2030* plan and currently includes two separate definitions:

- Personal health literacy—"the degree to which individuals have the ability to find, understand, and use information and services to inform health-related decisions and actions for themselves and others"
- Organizational health literacy—"the degree to which organizations equitably enable individuals to find, understand, and use information and services to inform health-related decisions and actions for themselves and others"

This revision places emphasis on people's ability to both use and understand health information, focuses on the ability to make informed decisions, recognizes that organizations have a responsibility to address health literacy, and integrates a public health perspective by connecting literacy with health equity [3].

K. Pham (✉) · R. Brawer
Department of Medical Oncology, Thomas Jefferson University, Philadelphia, PA, USA
e-mail: kristine.pham@jefferson.edu; rickie.brawer@jefferson.edu

Solutions for addressing this disparity are multifaceted and require interdisciplinary approaches that rely on patients, providers, health care systems, educational institutions, community organizations, and others to work together. The Lung Cancer Learning Community (LC2), a multidisciplinary group of diverse stakeholders was created to address lung cancer screening disparities among several underserved populations affected by high rates of smoking and lung cancer mortality. While the LC2 consists of various committees that each have a specific focus in relation to lung cancer screening, we collectively recognized that health literacy plays a major part in low screening uptake and pursued efforts that address health literacy from both patient and provider perspectives.

One of the major keys to improving health outcomes is to ensure that information about health-related matters is presented to the patient and the community at large through modalities that are easy to understand and digest. It is important to engage patients in a way that allows them to make informed and educated decisions about their health and empower them to advocate for themselves as well. The LC2 Initiative applied several health literacy and community-oriented principles to our work with vulnerable populations in an urban setting[1]. These evidence-based frameworks have been widely recognized as tools to consider and incorporate into any initiative that seeks to improve health outcomes and include the Health Literate Care Model, National Institutes of Health (NIH) *Clear & Simple* strategy, and community-based participatory research (CBPR).

Health Literate Care Model

The Health Literate Care Model was first proposed in 2013 to improve patient engagement in health care, combining health literacy concepts into the widely accepted Care Model (formerly Chronic Care Model). Numerous organizations have employed the Care Model as a system to increase quality of care due to its effectiveness on health outcomes [4]. It encourages health care systems to incorporate the following six elements to improve high-quality chronic disease care: community resources, health system, self-management support, delivery system design, shared-decision making support, and clinical information systems [5].

Although the Care Model has been shown to make a difference in health outcomes, it does not explicitly address the issue of health literacy. Therefore, to close this gap, the Health Literate Care Model incorporates health literacy from both the patient and healthcare provider perspective into the preexisting Care Model. Initially, it calls for approaching the patient with the assumption that they are at risk of not understanding their health conditions or how to deal with them and then confirming and ensuring their understanding. Secondly, for health care organizations,

---

[1] Refer to Chap. 21 titled, *Engaging Patients from Diverse Backgrounds in Lung Cancer Screening,* for more detailed information about other health communication strategies not discussed here.

health literacy becomes an organizational value and quality measure infused into all processes of planning and operation such as the six elements previously mentioned [4].

The LC2 Initiative is a multidisciplinary approach that seeks to increase lung cancer screening rates from a variety of perspectives and adheres to several fundamentals of the Health Literate Care Model. Though there is overlap, our clinicians and centralized lung cancer screening program primarily addresses screening from the health system, delivery system design, clinical information systems, and self-management support standpoints, while our population science and public health team work to connect patients with community resources. Connecting patients with local community resources is critical to our work with vulnerable populations.

National Institutes of Health (NIH) *Clear & Simple* Strategy and Community-Based Participatory Research

The *Clear & Simple* strategic guide developed by the NIH outlines five basic steps for developing health information for all populations, with particular emphasis on reaching those with lower health literacy: define the intended audience (population of interest), conduct the research, develop a concept for the product, develop content and visual design of materials, pretest and revise material [6].

Step One: Define the Intended Audience

Health disparities can occur across and within different populations. Populations of interest can be defined by age, gender, educational level, income level, religion, race, ethnicity, language, geographic location, health-related attitudes and behaviors, and combinations of these and other characteristics. The intended/target audience is the group of individuals that the key message(s) should reach [6]. The LC2 Initiative identified four disproportionately affected populations of interest based on national and local data on lung cancer mortality and smoking rates: Black/African Americans, veterans, LGBTQ+ community, and the Asian immigrant community, including those who lack English proficiency.

Step Two: Conduct Research

After identifying the appropriate audience, the next step is to conduct research alongside these communities to better understand all of the possible influences that may affect someone's decision regarding a certain health decision, such as lung cancer screening. These factors may include physical, behavioral, demographic, and psychographic characteristics. By exploring these factors, it allows researchers to comprehend how receptive the audience may be to the topic at hand [6]. It is important to understand what the target audience may already know about the topic, what common misconceptions there are regarding it, how people may feel toward the subject, and what potential information gaps need to be filled so that the "product" or intervention that is to be developed by the team is well-informed, meaning it is tailored to be culturally relevant and linguistically appropriate.

Community-based participatory research (CBPR) methodology can be used to conduct this type of research. The W.K. Kellogg Foundation Community Health Scholars Program defines CBPR as collaborative strategies that equitably engage researchers and community members in developing and conducting research and interventions that aim to improve community health and eliminate health disparities [7]. The process may entail elements such as an initial needs assessment, planning, research intervention design, implementation, evaluation, and dissemination [8]. The CBPR framework is an evidence-based practice that has resulted in successful community level interventions, due to the early establishment of a relationship between the researchers and the community/intended audience they are hoping to target. This is extremely vital to the foundation of CBPR and community outreach, especially with underserved populations who may already be wary of the health-care system.

We engaged the community by convening advisory groups to provide guidance during the development, implementation, and dissemination of the research. Two advisory groups were formed, one focused on health care providers, and the other on the populations of interest and was comprised of patients from the intended audiences and community organizations serving those populations. Engaging patients and community organizations as equal partners in the research encourages ownership in the process, results, and communication strategies (materials, programs, services, etc.) that are developed based on the findings. Involving these key players also ensures that the product(s) will meet the needs of the intended audience.

Research Methods

Guided by behavioral health theories such as the Health Belief Model [9] and Integrated Behavioral Model [10], research plans were developed and presented to the advisory groups for discussion to ensure the information to be gathered was relevant, and that proposed methods were appropriate for each of the intended audiences. As discussed earlier, it is important to understand what the intended audiences may already know about lung cancer, what myths and misinformation may be prevalent, and attitudes and beliefs about lung cancer, such as cultural preferences and sensitivities, barriers to lung cancer screening, and motivations for lung cancer screening uptake, and our advisory boards were able to assist with the creation of the discussion guides that were utilized in the needs assessment. This information combined with a review of the literature informed the research methods that were used (surveys, focus groups, key informant interviews) and questionnaire content for the intended audiences to inform the development of communication strategies and materials.

Table 25.1 provides examples of potential research constructs and related questions to consider and Table 25.2 provides a brief summary of the top findings from our focus groups and interviews with individuals across all the populations of interest. Participants included individuals who have been screened, who have not been screened, and/or are knowledgeable about the intended audiences. With the assistance of our advisory board and preexisting community partners, the research team identified initial interview/focus group participants and utilized "snowball sampling" to reach a larger network of individuals who were representative of and/or serve the intended audiences such as church leaders, neighborhood block captains, local community leaders, salon owners, etc., depending on the population [11]. It is important to ask those directly in the community who they believe should be engaged.

We also conducted a needs assessment with healthcare providers (Family and Community Medicine and Internal Medicine clinicians) to better understand low lung cancer screening rates from their perspective, as this is a multifaceted issue that should be addressed holistically. We conducted interviews and distributed an online survey to obtain their insight on knowledge, attitudes, beliefs, and barriers to lung cancer screening referrals. The main barriers that were the most salient for providers when it came to recommending lung cancer screening included a "lack of time to counsel patients" and a "lack of training in shared-decision making."[2]

Table 25.1 Potential research constructs and related guided questions

Theoretical construct	Focus of guided questions
Perceived susceptibility and severity	Does the individual believe he/she is at risk of lung cancer and what could happen as a result of the diagnosis?
Self-efficacy	Individual's knowledge about lung cancer and screening, and confidence about being able to get screened
Perceived benefits to screening	What are the benefits of lung cancer screening?
Perceived barriers to screening	What barriers exist to screening such as cost, transportation, time off from work, convenience of appointments, stigma?
Cues to action	What motivations exist for screening uptake such knowing someone diagnosed with or dying from lung cancer; health care provider recommendation?
Individual attitudes/beliefs toward screening	Does the individual have a positive or negative attitude toward lung cancer screening?
Normative beliefs of other influencers toward screening	Do family members and others support lung cancer screening? Is screening supported by faith and cultural influencers?

---

[2] Refer to Chap. 4 titled, *Training in Shared Decision Making About Lung Cancer Screening: Patient Eligibility Assessment, Education, and Decision Counseling* for more information regarding a training program that was developed by the LC2 Initiative to educate providers on shared-decision making.

Table 25.2 Common key findings from LC2 community/patient needs assessment

Theme	Subtheme
Knowledge	Lack of knowledge about lung cancer/screening
Attitudes and beliefs	Fear
	Religion
	Stigma
	Fatalism[a]
Access barriers	Cost
	Insurance
	Transportation/location
	Family/work-related barriers
	Patient navigation (i.e., interpretation services)
	Immigration status[a]

[a]Specific to the Asian immigrant community

Step Three: Develop a Concept for the Product

Once needs assessment data collection has concluded, the next step involves using the assessment findings to guide the objectives, style, format, and approach of the product(s) that will promote the desired message(s). Defining behavioral objectives of the material informs the messages and actions needed to achieve behavioral changes, selection of the most fitting presentation method(s), appropriate reading level, and logical organization of topics [6].

An overall lack of knowledge regarding lung cancer and lung cancer screening across all groups was observed. Participants were asked at the conclusion of the interviews/focus groups for their preferences regarding educational materials and strategies. Most expressed the preference for in-person, educational classes or seminars that are co-led by a healthcare provider and trusted community leader/member (with lived experience if possible). Based on this, we chose to create an interactive presentation that was tailored for each specific target population, a worksheet/checklist, and two infographics. Our goal was for these materials to serve as "cues to action," a central construct in the Health Belief Model [9]. The worksheet/checklist especially exemplifies this component, as it allows patients to complete a personal action plan to identify next steps in their lung cancer screening journey.

Step Four: Develop Content and Visuals

Key elements to keep in mind during the content and visual development phase are content/style, layout, visuals, and readability [6]. Patient interaction encourages empowerment and self-efficacy. The content/style of the materials should be interactive and involve patients or the intended audience, utilizing familiar and simple terms and sentences. If technical terms need to be used, there should be a brief explanation/definition/visual to accompany the term [6]. In order to achieve this, medical terms such as "LDCT" and "false-positive" were clearly explained in the presentation. "Smoking cessation" was commonly identified during interviews and focus groups as an unfamiliar term. Instead, "quit smoking" was used wherever applicable.

All materials (Prezi presentations, "Next Steps" checklist, "Lung Cancer Screening Basics" infographic (Fig. 25.1), and "Questions to Ask your Healthcare Provider" infographic (Fig. 25.2)) were created on a fifth-grade reading level, as required by Centers for Medicare & Medicaid Services (CMS) for organizations receiving federal funding (Plain Writing Act of 2010) [12]. There are several tools that can determine the reading level of a printed material such as the SMOG Readability Calculator and Flesch Kincaid Grade Level [6, 13].

The layout of information in the materials is vital when developing health literate resources. It is important to consider the use of headings and labeling, the ratio of white space to words and images, and font selection (sharp contrast between text and background; 12 point or larger) which may vary depending on the audience [6].

We also tailored and are continuing to tailor our materials to meet the needs of our vulnerable populations and make it easier for them to digest key messages. For example, the presentations for veterans and LGBTQ+ individuals contain specific content regarding smoking, risks, and beliefs related to that group to emphasize the importance of screening. Our materials have also been translated and back-translated into Chinese, Korean, and Vietnamese as a starting point for the Asian immigrant community and we will continue to translate as needed into other languages. Back-translation is a quality measure and occurs when another person translates what was originally translated back into English. Due to the varying nuances of language dependent on jargon, idioms, and culture, back-translation can help improve a translation's validity, accuracy, and readability [14]. It can pinpoint any discrepancies that may have occurred during the initial translation process of the material and ensures the terms and words that are translated are commonly understood and utilized by the specified population.

Content creation was primarily done by the research team in a remote setting during the onset of the COVID-19 pandemic (2020), as most non-essential organizations and workplaces ceased in-person services. While the team was able to seamlessly pivot to a virtual work environment, the pandemic made it more difficult to work directly with the community. Pre-COVID, many of the clients that the community partners served heavily relied on obtaining resources, information, and aid in-person, which allowed the team to easily convene focus groups and interviews. However, the COVID-19 pandemic proved to be a major barrier that delayed progress due to the inability to reach community members, as the intended audiences for the project were older adults who may have lacked access or were unable to use technology such as Zoom (i.e., smartphone, computer, laptop, Internet, etc.). Therefore, during this time period, we primarily depended on our advisory boards and community organization partners for feedback and input on the educational materials through teleconferencing. It is interesting to note that lung cancer screening rates during this time frame also experienced a pause in growth activity, falling slightly from 6.6% nationally in 2019, to 6.5% in 2020 [15].

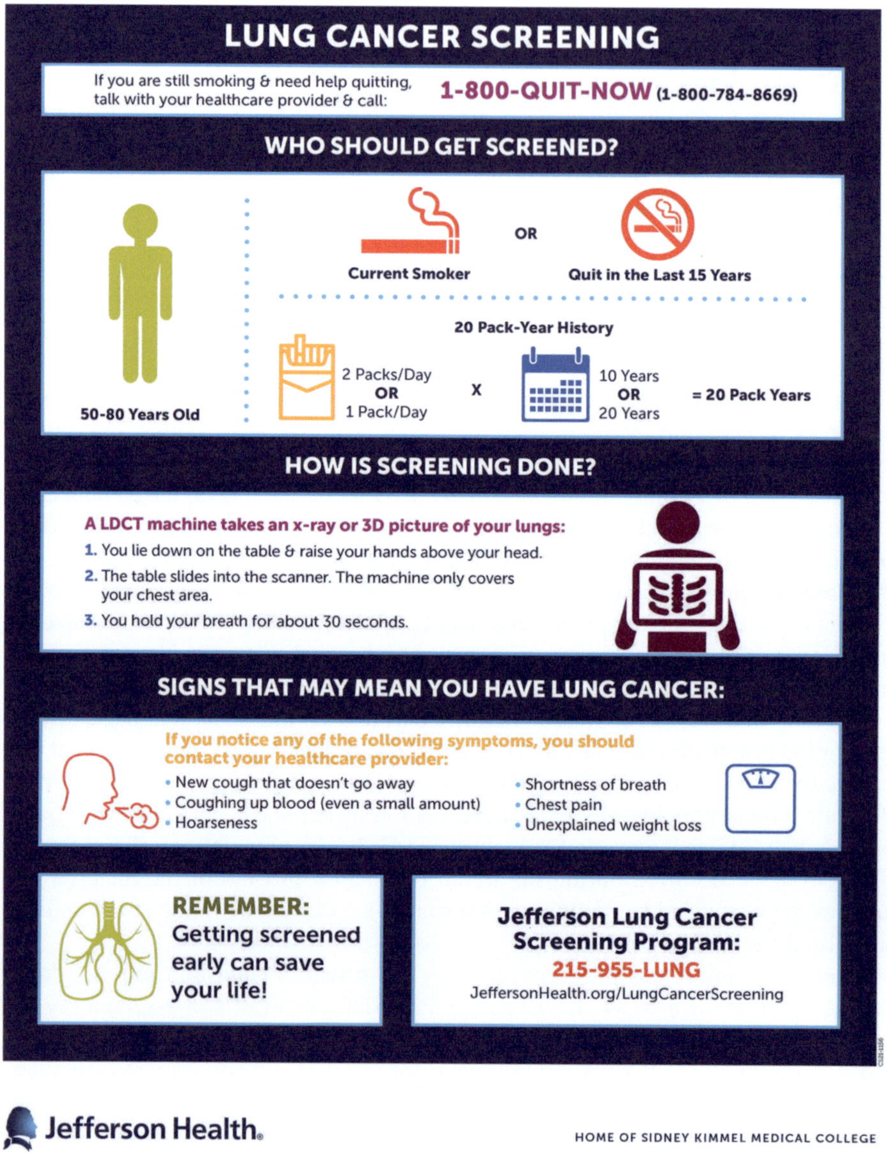
LUNG CANCER SCREENING
If you are still smoking & need help quitting, talk with your healthcare provider & call:
1-800-QUIT-NOW (1-800-784-8669)
WHO SHOULD GET SCREENED?
50-80 Years Old
Current Smoker
OR
Quit in the Last 15 Years
20 Pack-Year History
2 Packs/Day
OR
1 Pack/Day
X
10 Years
OR
20 Years
= 20 Pack Years
HOW IS SCREENING DONE?
A LDCT machine takes an x-ray or 3D picture of your lungs:
1. You lie down on the table & raise your hands above your head.
2. The table slides into the scanner. The machine only covers your chest area.
3. You hold your breath for about 30 seconds.
SIGNS THAT MAY MEAN YOU HAVE LUNG CANCER:
If you notice any of the following symptoms, you should contact your healthcare provider:
• New cough that doesn't go away
• Coughing up blood (even a small amount)
• Hoarseness
• Shortness of breath
• Chest pain
• Unexplained weight loss
REMEMBER:
Getting screened early can save your life!
Jefferson Lung Cancer Screening Program:
215-955-LUNG
JeffersonHealth.org/LungCancerScreening
Jefferson Health.
HOME OF SIDNEY KIMMEL MEDICAL COLLEGE

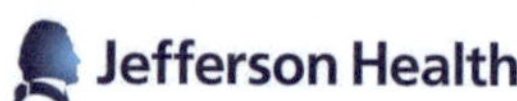

Fig. 25.1 "Lung Cancer Screening Basics" infographic

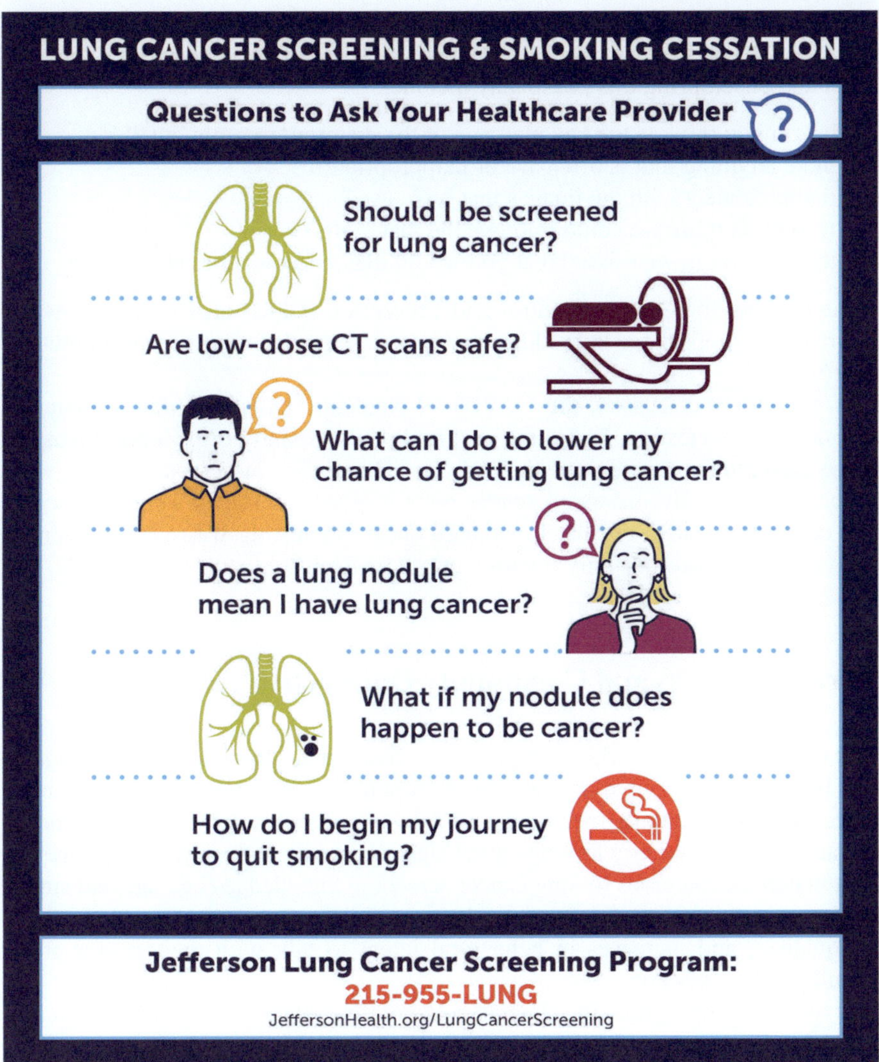

Fig. 25.2 "Questions to Ask Your Healthcare Provider" infographic

Step Five: Pretest and Revise

The final step in the *Clear & Simple* strategy is to pretest and revise materials as necessary. This is essential because audience understanding and acceptance necessitates that the materials are culturally relevant and meet the needs or concerns of the intended audience. Three main components that should be tested include comprehension, attractiveness, and acceptability [6]. Questions to consider asking the pretest audience during this phase may include:

- What do you think is the key message of the material/program/etc.?
- Is there anything that is offensive or inappropriate?
- Did you connect with the images that were used?
- How do you think we could improve the material(s)?
- Is there anything we missed that you would like to know more about?

The Centers for Disease Control and Prevention (CDC) also provides several resources and toolkits for individuals to apply during educational material pretesting [16].

As previously discussed, the COVID-19 pandemic halted community interactions, delaying pretesting. Pretesting occurred predominantly over Zoom if feasible for the community partner and their clients. Otherwise, in-person sessions were conducted in socially distanced spaces once in-person services were resumed at these community sites. Feedback gathered during pretesting was overwhelmingly positive and the materials only required minor revisions.

Current Progress and Community Outreach

The LC2 is currently working to pilot and disseminate the educational program more broadly across our four main target populations. Overall, piloting has been successful and community members were fully engaged throughout the educational programming. Preliminary findings show high receptivity and interest in the presentation/materials, increases in lung cancer screening knowledge (i.e., age and smoking history requirement), increases in behavioral intent to get screened (fo those who qualify), and increases in behavioral intent to talk with their doctor about screening going forward.

As reiterated throughout the chapter, collaborative relationships with community partners and community-based organizations are crucial to reaching the intended audience, especially when the intent is to work with vulnerable populations. Many of these leaders are trusted because they have worked extensively within these neighborhoods and understand the barriers that these underserved groups face. Therefore, maintaining these connections in the community is crucial, because as trusted messengers, they can reach members of the intended audiences and give credibility to the health system's lung cancer screening program.

Locations for community outreach will vary depending on the intended audience and goals of the intervention or project. Input from community partners and advisory board and the research will help determine which locations are best for which populations. For example, places of worship may be more prevalent in one culture but not in another. Some religious leaders may have strong vested interest in health matters but others may not. For the LC2 Initiative, we focus on these main sites to reach community members who may meet lung cancer screening guidelines:

- Places of worship (i.e., African American churches, Chinese churches, Korean churches, temples)
- Social service organizations (i.e., Veteran-specific, Asian immigrant specific)
- Adult day cares
- Senior centers
- Community development corporations
- Immigrant/refugee driven organizations
- Federally qualified health centers (FQHCs)
- Pharmacies
- Libraries
- Homeless shelters
- Community centers (i.e., LGBTQ+ specific)
- Other health clinics/systems (i.e., city health clinics, the VA hospital)

Next Steps

The LC2 Initiative continues to pilot test and work to disseminate the materials more broadly across both Jefferson Health system and the surrounding community. In addition, programming and materials are being made available to providers at Jefferson, neighboring health systems, city health centers, and FQHCs for their patients. As part of this endeavor, these materials are being made available digitally on Jefferson Health website. Providing translated and recorded program sessions online allows individuals to access the educational materials at their own convenience. Development of an evaluation system to track external/community referrals to Jefferson's lung cancer screening program is underway to determine the extent of our educational outreach. This data collection will include the numbers of individuals reached, self-referrals, and people who screen/complete appointments.

Lastly, a training toolkit that will educate trusted messengers from the intended audiences on how to lead the educational program and raise awareness about lung cancer screening in their own communities and neighborhoods is being developed. Other individuals who will be trained as "lung cancer screening community advocates" include community health workers (CHWs), home health aides, social workers, and case managers. Expansion of our reach to other communities who were not initially included in our intended audiences, such as the Latino community, is being considered.

Reaching vulnerable communities is a challenging endeavor and cannot be attained without the assistance and partnership of the communities themselves. The LC2 Initiative is a clear example of how community-based participatory research can aid in bridging the connection between health systems and underserved populations surrounding them to create lasting, sustainable relationships that aim to improve community health and reduce health disparities for those who need it most.

References

1. Health Literacy Fact Sheets—Center for Health Care Strategies [Internet]. [cited 2022 Mar 13]. https://www.chcs.org/resource/health-literacy-fact-sheets/.
2. Center for Health Care Strategies. What is Health Literacy? 2013. [cited 2022 Mar 11]. https://www.chcs.org/media/What_is_Health_Literacy.pdf.
3. What Is Health Literacy?|Health Literacy|CDC [Internet]. [cited 2022 Mar 14]. https://www.cdc.gov/healthliteracy/learn/index.html.
4. Koh HK, Brach C, Harris LM, Parchman ML. A proposed "health literate care model" would constitute a systems approach to improving patients' engagement in care. Health Aff (Millwood). 2013;32:357–67.
5. Integrating Chronic Care and Business Strategies in the Safety Net Toolkit [Internet]. [cited 2022 Mar 13]. https://www.ahrq.gov/ncepcr/care/chronic-tool/intro.html.
6. 9. Clear & Simple|National Institutes of Health (NIH) [Internet]. [cited 2022 Mar 14]. https://www.nih.gov/institutes-nih/nih-office-director/office-communications-public-liaison/clear-communication/clear-simple.
7. Faridi Z, Grunbaum JA, Gray BS, Franks A, Simoes E. Community-based participatory research: necessary next steps. Prev Chronic Dis. 2007;4:A70.
8. Community-Based Participatory Research Program (CBPR) [Internet]. [cited 2022 Mar 14]. https://www.nimhd.nih.gov/programs/extramural/community-based-participatory.html.
9. Boston University School of Public Health. The Health Belief Model [Internet]. [cited 2022 Mar 15]. https://sphweb.bumc.bu.edu/otlt/mph-modules/sb/behavioralchangetheories/behavioralchangetheories2.html.
10. Yzer M. Designing Messages for Health Communication Campaigns: Theory and Practice [Internet]. 2012 [cited 2022 Mar 15]. https://www.sagepub.com/sites/default/files/upm-binaries/43568_2.pdf.
11. Foundations—SAGE Research Methods [Internet]. [cited 2022 Mar 14]. https://methods.sagepub.com/foundations/snowball-sampling.
12. Law and requirements|plainlanguage.gov [Internet]. [cited 2022 Mar 15]. https://www.plain-language.gov/law/.
13. Flesch Reading Ease and the Flesch Kincaid Grade Level—Readable [Internet]. [cited 2022 Mar 14]. https://readable.com/readability/flesch-reading-ease-flesch-kincaid-grade-level/.
14. What is Back Translation and Why is it Necessary? [Internet]. [cited 2022 Mar 14]. https://www.daytranslations.com/blog/what-is-back-translation/.
15. Fedewa SA, Bandi P, Smith RA, Silvestri GA, Jemal A. Lung cancer screening rates during the COVID-19 pandemic. Chest. 2022;161:586–9.
16. Testing|Health Literacy|CDC [Internet]. [cited 2022 Mar 15]. https://www.cdc.gov/healthliteracy/developmaterials/testing-messages-materials.html.

Chapter 26
Lung Cancer Myths and How Do I Address Them?

Brian M. Till, Kathleen Jarrell, and Nathaniel R. Evans III

Background

It is important to recognize the common misperceptions described in this chapter, which may be common among lung cancer screening-eligible populations. Whether these concerns or beliefs are outwardly expressed has little to do with their prevalence, and creating an environment conducive to addressing these myths is critical. Next, after recognizing the problem posed by myths and misperceptions, it is important that clinicians dedicate time and energy to developing a strategy to address them. Here we describe eight common myths and detail relevant evidence that can be used to combat them. In addition, we describe six key elements of an approach for effectively addressing myths and misperceptions within a target lung cancer screening program (LCSP) population.

The Myths

Myth One: "Only Smokers Get Lung Cancer"

While smoking has been identified as the strongest, single risk factor for the development of lung cancer, a significant number of patients with no smoking history or minimal smoking history are diagnosed with lung cancer each year. In the United

B. M. Till · K. Jarrell
Department of Surgery, Thomas Jefferson University Hospital, Philadelphia, PA, USA
e-mail: Brian.Till@jefferson.edu; Kathleen.Jarrell@jefferson.edu

N. R. Evans III (✉)
Department of Surgery, Thomas Jefferson University, Philadelphia, PA, USA
e-mail: Nathaniel.Evans@Jefferson.edu

States, it is believed that between 10% and 20% of those diagnosed with lung cancer have never smoked or are people who have smoked less than 100 cigarettes in their lives, comprising between 20,000 and 40,000 individuals each year [1]. Worldwide, it is estimated that 25% of lung cancers occur in never smokers, with the majority of these cases seen in women and younger patients [2, 3]. Risk factors for non-smokers who develop lung cancer include secondhand smoke, radon exposure, air pollution, work-related carcinogens such as asbestos, heavy metals, and diesel exhaust. Thus, while most of those diagnosed with lung cancer each year have significant smoking histories, there are tens of thousands of non-smokers who are similarly diagnosed with lung cancer each year.

Myth Two: "Vaping Is a Safe Alternative to Smoking"

While there is minimal evidence on the relationship between e-cigarettes or vaporizers and lung cancer, existing evidence suggests that physicians and the general public should be wary of the risks posed by these novel smoking devices. This paucity of evidence is primarily due to the recent advent of these devices and the long latency period between smoking and development of lung cancer. Nonetheless, existing studies demonstrate that many of the same carcinogens found in conventional tobacco smoke are also found in e-cigarette smoke, including nicotine derivatives (such as nitrosnornicotine and nitrosamine ketone), polycyclic aromatic hydroxycarbons, heavy metals, and aldehydes [4]. Experiments in animal models have demonstrated comparable and in some cases higher concentrations of these molecules accumulating in airways and lung parenchyma with exposure to e-cigarette smoke as compared to cigarette smoke, and has also demonstrated comparable corresponding DNA-level changes [4–7]. Thus, while the exact relationship between lung cancer and e-cigarettes has not been established, there is ample reason to suspect usage may confer significant risk for the future development of lung cancer.

Myth Three: "If You Get Lung Cancer From Smoking, It Is Your Own Fault"

Developing cancer is recognized as a complex interaction of behavioral risk factors, environmental risk factors, and underlying genetic susceptibility. While smoking is understood to be the primary risk factor for the development of lung cancer, it is important to acknowledge that the majority of smokers do not develop lung cancer, thus suggesting factors beyond an individual's choice to smoke significantly impacts likelihood of developing lung cancer.

Myth Four: "There's No Way To Detect Lung Cancer Early"

Historically, the early detection of lung cancer was difficult owing to poor sensitivity of X-ray in the identification of cancers [8, 9]. More recently, the use of low-dose radiation computer tomography (CT) scans has changed this, and this screening modality is associated with a sensitivity of 88.9% [10]. Large randomized controlled trials have demonstrated significant lung cancer mortality benefit with annual low-dose computed tomography (LDCT) for high-risk individuals [11]. In fact, the editorial accompanying publication of the NELSON trial stated, "There can no longer be any doubt as to the efficacy of periodic low-dose CT screening in reducing mortality from lung cancer" [12].

Myth Five: "If I Am in a Screening Program, There Is No Reason to Stop Smoking"

The literature shows that close to half of current smokers enrolled in LCS Programs report decreased interest in smoking cessation due to enrollment [13], owing to perceived protection offered by screening programs. It is thus critical that LCS Programs explain to patients that screening does not protect against cancer, but rather offers approximately a 20% risk reduction for mortality [11]. All LCS patients would thus benefit from smoking cessation for a range of reasons, not least of which being reduction in risk of development of all histologic subtypes of lung cancer [14].

Myth Six: "If You Already Have Lung Cancer, There Is No Reason To Stop Smoking"

There is a large body of evidence showing the benefit of smoking cessation among those who have been diagnosed with lung cancer. These studies show benefit with regard to likelihood of achieving treatment response, overall survival, and general well-being. For patients undergoing surgical resection, continued smoking has been linked to inferior outcomes, including more frequent wound infections, higher complication rates, and longer hospital stays [15]. Continued smoking has been linked to worse survival both in the immediate postoperative period [16] and in the 5 years following surgery [17]. For patients undergoing radiation treatment, there is evidence that continued smoking is linked to worse survival [18] and may increase the risk of developing radiation pneumonitis [19]. And for patients treated with chemotherapy, continued smoking may limit the effectiveness of these therapies [20, 21] while worsening side effect profiles by altering metabolism of these agents [22, 23]. Finally, continued smoking after lung cancer diagnosis has been linked to decreased quality of life, with continued smokers demonstrating less activity tolerance; increased coughing, dyspnea, and fatigue; increased pain; and worse overall quality of life [24–26].

Myth Seven: "Surgery Causes Lung Cancer To Spread"

As many as 38% of patients seen in Pulmonary Nodule Clinics may believe that lung cancer will spread secondary to exposure to open air that occurs during surgery [27], and as many as 19% of Black patients and 5% of White patients may avoid undergoing resection for this reason. There is no evidence that lung cancer progression is altered by surgical intervention, and it is unclear how this myth developed and gained traction. It has been hypothesized that the discovery of metastatic disease at the time of surgery has been conflated with cause rather than discovery of disease spread among the lay population, but further study is needed to understand the etiology of this myth's prevalence.

Myth Eight: "Surgery for Lung Cancer Requires a Long Recovery Period"

In recent years, two major advances have substantially improved patient recovery following lung cancer surgery. Generally speaking, patients undergoing an uncomplicated, minimally invasive lobar or sub-lobar resection can expect a hospital stay of 1–2 days [28, 29], and the majority of patients can expect a return to work in approximately 2 weeks if treated with robotic resection and 6 weeks if treated with traditional video-assisted thoracoscopic surgery (VATS) [30]. These drastic improvements are attributed to two factors: First, the adoption of minimally invasive surgical approaches, and, second, adoption of enhanced recovery after surgery (ERAS) pathways in the immediate postoperative period. Patients undergoing minimally invasive thoracic surgery have shorter lengths of hospital stay and fewer major postoperative complications such as pneumonia and arrhythmias [31] compared to those treated via thoracotomy. These patients have also demonstrated decreased postoperative pain, less sleep-interference, improved ambulation postoperatively [32], and higher quality of life [33]. ERAS protocols have focused clinician attention on optimizing care in the immediate postoperative period by emphasizing patient education, early mobilization and feeding, and expedient removal of arterial lines, Foley catheters, and chest tubes. Use of these pathways has been linked to shorter hospital stays [34–36], decreased analgesic requirements [36], lower rates of complications [34, 37], and decreased readmissions [38].

Myth Nine: "I Am Too Old to Benefit from Treatment for Lung Cancer"

It is critical to discuss several issues related to age and lung cancer with potential LCS patients. First, there is evidence that lung cancer is more treatable for older patients, given that stage I disease is found in 87% of those over diagnosed after the age of 75 as compared to 79% of those diagnosed under 65 years [39]. Second, there are a range of treatment options available for elderly patients diagnosed with lung cancer [40] including surgical resection [41, 42], radiation therapy [43, 44], chemotherapy [45], combined chemotherapy and radiation [39, 46], and immunotherapy [47], all of which have shown survival benefit for those of advanced age. It is thus critical for providers and patients to discuss which treatment option is most consistent with a patient's goals and priorities.

Surgical resection remains the standard of care for those with early-stage disease, and it is critical that elderly patients understand that minimally invasive techniques have substantially reduced morbidity and mortality associated with surgical treatment as discussed in the preceding text. Of note, a comprehensive review of evidence on the resection of early lung cancers in the elderly found no difference, mortality, and quality for those over 70 compared to younger patients [48]. Thus, for both surgically fit and unfit elderly patients, there are a range of therapeutic options available that have demonstrated both survival benefit and acceptable risk profiles.

Myth Ten: "Lung Cancer Is a Death Sentence"

Lung cancer, while historically linked to poor survival rates, has seen a substantial improvement in survivorship in recent years. For those treated with surgical resection, recent studies have shown 5-year survival rates ranging from 83% [49] to 91% [50]. For patients with screening detected nodules who undergo surgical resection within 1 month of diagnosis, there is some evidence that 10-year survivorship may be as high as 92% [51]. For those who are too frail for surgery, radiation therapy offers survival rates between 73% and 92% for early-stage disease [52]. Even in later stage disease, current and emerging therapies have shown impressive ability to allow long-term survival in patients in whom this was not previously possible [53–55].

Addressing Lung Cancer Myths

Step One: Have a Forward-Leaning Posture Related to Misperceptions and Myths

We advocate for developing patient education tools specifically designed to confront myths that can be used in conjunction with outreach events and initiating conversations regarding these issues early with target groups. Rather than waiting for patients to bring forward misperceptions, a well-designed strategy can address these common concerns and misunderstandings preemptively.

Step Two: Fully Appreciate the Complexity of Physician–Patient Communication

Studies have repeatedly demonstrated poor provider patient communication across a variety of domains, including patient understanding of abnormal radiologic findings [53, 54]. Further, the literature has demonstrated that patients are frequently unable to recognize the limits of their comprehension when engaging medical providers [55, 56]. Because of this, it is imperative that physicians and LCS Programs undertake discussion about lung cancer myths and misperceptions with awareness of the chasm that can exist between patients and providers. We recommend strategies for engagement which minimize medical jargon, focus on conveying a few key points, and utilize "teach back" tactics, whereby patients explain back to a provider what they have learned from a conversation [57, 58].

Step Three: Ensure Available Information Is Properly Designed for Your Target Population

Analyses of lung cancer–related patient education tools frequently demonstrate that materials are written beyond the eighth-grade reading level, thus making them inaccessible to 51% of the adult US population [59]. Further, as the US population becomes more diverse, it is important that materials and providers are able to accommodate a range of non-English language speakers that may represent their target LCS-eligible population. Outreach utilizing native speakers and development of informative materials in the appropriate languages is key.

Step Four: Build a Team That Is Culturally Accessible to a Diverse Patient Population

A large and growing body of evidence has shown that minority patients report lower patient–physician communication quality and satisfaction, notably including less information-giving, less partnership building, and less participatory decision making [60, 61]. Approximately one-fifth of people in the United States speak a language other than English while at home, and at least 25 million people in the United States are recognized as having limited proficiency in English [62]. These patients may be less likely to receive preventative care or be enrolled in cancer screening programs [63]. Thus, those developing LCS Programs should seek to build an inclusive and representative team, capable of effectively engaging with the community it has set out to serve.

Step Five: Make Space for Patients to Ask Questions About Myths and Misperceptions That They Feel Otherwise Feel Uncomfortable Raising

Because of a well-defined power differential between patients and providers, a large proportion of patients may feel uncomfortable asking questions of their medical team members [64]. It is thus critical to create an atmosphere conducive to raising concerns about commonly held myths or misperceptions. We suggest language such as:

> A lot of patients we meet have heard or read things about lung cancer that they're not sure whether to believe or not. Are there things like this that you're concerned about that we could discuss?

Step Six: Continue the Conversation

Some patients may be assuaged by a discussion with their physician or medical team about inaccurate information, but others may not. Be ready to offer additional resources to patients from your institution or other institutions, and be willing to take time to discuss existing evidence with them. Re-engage with the issue in subsequent visits or via patient portals in the electronic health records.

References

1. Lung Cancer Among People Who Never Smoked: Center for Disease Control and Prevention; 2021. https://www.cdc.gov/cancer/lung/nonsmokers/index.htm. Accessed 18 Aug 2021.
2. Okazaki I, Ishikawa S, Ando W, Sohara Y. Lung adenocarcinoma in never smokers: problems of primary prevention from aspects of susceptible genes and carcinogens. Anticancer Res. 2016;36(12):6207–24.
3. Saito N, Mine N, Kufe DW, Von Hoff DD, Kawabe T. CBP501 inhibits EGF-dependent cell migration, invasion and epithelial-to-mesenchymal transition of non-small cell lung cancer cells by blocking KRas to calmodulin binding. Oncotarget. 2017;8(43):74006–18.
4. Bracken-Clarke D, Kapoor D, Baird AM, Buchanan PJ, Gately K, Cuffe S, et al. Vaping and lung cancer - a review of current data and recommendations. Lung Cancer. 2021;153:11–20.
5. Floyd EL, Queimado L, Wang J, Regens JL, Johnson DL. Electronic cigarette power affects count concentration and particle size distribution of vaping aerosol. PLoS One. 2018;13(12):e0210147.

6. Lee HW, Park SH, Weng MW, Wang HT, Huang WC, Lepor H, et al. E-cigarette smoke damages DNA and reduces repair activity in mouse lung, heart, and bladder as well as in human lung and bladder cells. Proc Natl Acad Sci U S A. 2018;115(7):E1560–E9.

7. Shahab L, Goniewicz ML, Blount BC, Brown J, McNeill A, Alwis KU, et al. Nicotine, carcinogen, and toxin exposure in long-term E-cigarette and nicotine replacement therapy users: a cross-sectional study. Ann Intern Med. 2017;166(6):390–400.

8. Gavelli G, Giampalma E. Sensitivity and specificity of chest X-ray screening for lung cancer: review article. Cancer. 2000;89(11 Suppl):2453–6.

9. Bradley SH, Abraham S, Callister ME, Grice A, Hamilton WT, Lopez RR, et al. Sensitivity of chest X-ray for detecting lung cancer in people presenting with symptoms: a systematic review. Br J Gen Pract. 2019;69(689):e827–e35.

10. Toyoda Y, Nakayama T, Kusunoki Y, Iso H, Suzuki T. Sensitivity and specificity of lung cancer screening using chest low-dose computed tomography. Br J Cancer. 2008;98(10):1602–7.

11. National Lung Screening Trial Research T, Aberle DR, Adams AM, Berg CD, Black WC, Clapp JD, et al. Reduced lung-cancer mortality with low-dose computed tomographic screening. N Engl J Med. 2011;365(5):395–409.

12. Duffy SW, Field JK. Mortality reduction with low-dose CT screening for lung cancer. N Engl J Med. 2020;382:572–3.

13. Zeliadt SB, Heffner JL, Sayre G, Klein DE, Simons C, Williams J, et al. Attitudes and perceptions about smoking cessation in the context of lung cancer screening. JAMA Intern Med. 2015;175(9):1530–7.

14. Khuder SA, Mutgi AB. Effect of smoking cessation on major histologic types of lung cancer. Chest. 2001;120(5):1577–83.

15. Moller AM, Villebro N, Pedersen T, Tonnesen H. Effect of preoperative smoking intervention on postoperative complications: a randomised clinical trial. Lancet. 2002;359(9301):114–7.

16. Fukui M, Suzuki K, Matsunaga T, Oh S, Takamochi K. Importance of smoking cessation on surgical outcome in primary lung cancer. Ann Thorac Surg. 2019;107(4):1005–9.

17. Parsons A, Daley A, Begh R, Aveyard P. Influence of smoking cessation after diagnosis of early stage lung cancer on prognosis: systematic review of observational studies with meta-analysis. BMJ. 2010;340:b5569.

18. Roach MC, Rehman S, DeWees TA, Abraham CD, Bradley JD, Robinson CG. It's never too late: smoking cessation after stereotactic body radiation therapy for non-small cell lung carcinoma improves overall survival. Pract Radiat Oncol. 2016;6(1):12–8.

19. Dresler CM. Is it more important to quit smoking than which chemotherapy is used? Lung Cancer. 2003;39(2):119–24.

20. Zhang J, Kamdar O, Le W, Rosen GD, Upadhyay D. Nicotine induces resistance to chemotherapy by modulating mitochondrial signaling in lung cancer. Am J Respir Cell Mol Biol. 2009;40(2):135–46.

21. Xu J, Huang H, Pan C, Zhang B, Liu X, Zhang L. Nicotine inhibits apoptosis induced by cisplatin in human oral cancer cells. Int J Oral Maxillofac Surg. 2007;36(8):739–44.

22. O'Malley M, King AN, Conte M, Ellingrod VL, Ramnath N. Effects of cigarette smoking on metabolism and effectiveness of systemic therapy for lung cancer. J Thorac Oncol. 2014;9(7):917–26.

23. Hughes AN, O'Brien ME, Petty WJ, Chick JB, Rankin E, Woll PJ, et al. Overcoming CYP1A1/1A2 mediated induction of metabolism by escalating erlotinib dose in current smokers. J Clin Oncol. 2009;27(8):1220–6.

24. Steuer CE, Jegede OA, Dahlberg SE, Wakelee HA, Keller SM, Tester WJ, et al. Smoking behavior in patients with early-stage NSCLC: a report from ECOG-ACRIN 1505 trial. J Thorac Oncol. 2021;16(6):960–7.

25. Garces YI, Yang P, Parkinson J, Zhao X, Wampfler JA, Ebbert JO, et al. The relationship between cigarette smoking and quality of life after lung cancer diagnosis. Chest. 2004;126(6):1733–41.

26. Daniel M, Keefe FJ, Lyna P, Peterson B, Garst J, Kelley M, et al. Persistent smoking after a diagnosis of lung cancer is associated with higher reported pain levels. J Pain. 2009;10(3):323–8.

27. Margolis ML, Christie JD, Silvestri GA, Kaiser L, Santiago S, Hansen-Flaschen J. Racial differences pertaining to a belief about lung cancer surgery: results of a multicenter survey. Ann Intern Med. 2003;139(7):558–63.
28. Dominguez DA, Ely S, Bach C, Lee T, Velotta JB. Impact of intercostal nerve blocks using liposomal versus standard bupivacaine on length of stay in minimally invasive thoracic surgery patients. J Thorac Dis. 2018;10(12):6873–9.
29. Hsu DS, Ely S, Alcasid NJ, Banks KC, Santos J, Wei J, et al. Reduced opioid utilization and post-operative pain in Asian vs. Caucasian populations after video-assisted thoracoscopic surgery lobectomy with liposomal bupivacaine-based intercostal nerve blockade. Ann Palliat Med. 2022;11:1635.
30. Louie BE, Farivar AS, Aye RW, Vallieres E. Early experience with robotic lung resection results in similar operative outcomes and morbidity when compared with matched video-assisted thoracoscopic surgery cases. Ann Thorac Surg. 2012;93(5):1598–604; discussion 604–5.
31. Cao C, Manganas C, Ang SC, Peeceeyen S, Yan TD. Video-assisted thoracic surgery versus open thoracotomy for non-small cell lung cancer: a meta-analysis of propensity score-matched patients. Interact Cardiovasc Thorac Surg. 2013;16(3):244–9.
32. Wei X, Yu H, Dai W, Mu Y, Wang Y, Liao J, et al. Patient-reported outcomes of video-assisted thoracoscopic surgery versus thoracotomy for locally advanced lung cancer: a longitudinal cohort study. Ann Surg Oncol. 2021;28(13):8358–71.
33. Bendixen M, Jorgensen OD, Kronborg C, Andersen C, Licht PB. Postoperative pain and quality of life after lobectomy via video-assisted thoracoscopic surgery or anterolateral thoracotomy for early stage lung cancer: a randomised controlled trial. Lancet Oncol. 2016;17(6):836–44.
34. Paci P, Madani A, Lee L, Mata J, Mulder DS, Spicer J, et al. Economic impact of an enhanced recovery pathway for lung resection. Ann Thorac Surg. 2017;104(3):950–7.
35. Dong Q, Zhang K, Cao S, Cui J. Fast-track surgery versus conventional perioperative management of lung cancer-associated pneumonectomy: a randomized controlled clinical trial. World J Surg Oncol. 2017;15(1):20.
36. Martin LW, Sarosiek BM, Harrison MA, Hedrick T, Isbell JM, Krupnick AS, et al. Implementing a thoracic enhanced recovery program: lessons learned in the first year. Ann Thorac Surg. 2018;105(6):1597–604.
37. Madani A, Fiore JF Jr, Wang Y, Bejjani J, Sivakumaran L, Mata J, et al. An enhanced recovery pathway reduces duration of stay and complications after open pulmonary lobectomy. Surgery. 2015;158(4):899–908; discussion −10.
38. Numan RC, Klomp HM, Li W, Buitelaar DR, Burgers JA, Van Sandick JW, et al. A clinical audit in a multidisciplinary care path for thoracic surgery: an instrument for continuous quality improvement. Lung Cancer. 2012;78(3):270–5.
39. Miller ED, Fisher JL, Haglund KE, Grecula JC, Xu-Welliver M, Bertino EM, et al. The addition of chemotherapy to radiation therapy improves survival in elderly patients with stage III non-small cell lung cancer. J Thorac Oncol. 2018;13(3):426–35.
40. Venuta F, Diso D, Onorati I, Anile M, Mantovani S, Rendina EA. Lung cancer in elderly patients. J Thorac Dis. 2016;8(Suppl 11):S908–S14.
41. Rivera C, Falcoz PE, Bernard A, Thomas PA, Dahan M. Surgical management and outcomes of elderly patients with early stage non-small cell lung cancer: a nested case-control study. Chest. 2011;140(4):874–80.
42. Detillon D, Aarts MJ, De Jaeger K, Van Eijck CHJ, Veen EJ. Video-assisted thoracic lobectomy versus stereotactic body radiotherapy for stage I nonsmall cell lung cancer in elderly patients: a propensity matched comparative analysis. Eur Respir J. 2019;53(6):1801561.
43. Watanabe K, Katsui K, Sugiyama S, Yoshio K, Kuroda M, Hiraki T, et al. Lung stereotactic body radiation therapy for elderly patients aged >/= 80 years with pathologically proven early-stage non-small cell lung cancer: a retrospective cohort study. Radiat Oncol. 2021;16(1):39.
44. Takeda A, Sanuki N, Eriguchi T, Kaneko T, Morita S, Handa H, et al. Stereotactic ablative body radiation therapy for octogenarians with non-small cell lung cancer. Int J Radiat Oncol Biol Phys. 2013;86(2):257–63.

45. Gajra A, Jatoi A. Non-small-cell lung cancer in elderly patients: a discussion of treatment options. J Clin Oncol. 2014;32(24):2562–9.
46. Driessen EJ, Bootsma GP, Hendriks LE, van den Berkmortel FW, Bogaarts BA, van Loon JG, et al. Stage III non-small cell lung cancer in the elderly: patient characteristics predictive for tolerance and survival of chemoradiation in daily clinical practice. Radiother Oncol. 2016;121(1):26–31.
47. Casaluce F, Sgambato A, Maione P, Spagnuolo A, Gridelli C. Lung cancer, elderly and immune checkpoint inhibitors. J Thorac Dis. 2018;10(Suppl 13):S1474–S81.
48. Chambers A, Routledge T, Pilling J, Scarci M. In elderly patients with lung cancer is resection justified in terms of morbidity, mortality and residual quality of life? Interact Cardiovasc Thorac Surg. 2010;10(6):1015–21.
49. Casiraghi M, Galetta D, Borri A, Tessitore A, Romano R, Diotti C, et al. Ten years' experience in robotic-assisted thoracic surgery for early stage lung cancer. Thorac Cardiovasc Surg. 2019;67(7):564–72.
50. Park BJ, Melfi F, Mussi A, Maisonneuve P, Spaggiari L, Da Silva RK, et al. Robotic lobectomy for non-small cell lung cancer (NSCLC): long-term oncologic results. J Thorac Cardiovasc Surg. 2012;143(2):383–9.
51. International Early Lung Cancer Action Program I, Henschke CI, Yankelevitz DF, Libby DM, Pasmantier MW, Smith JP, et al. Survival of patients with stage I lung cancer detected on CT screening. N Engl J Med. 2006;355(17):1763–71.
52. Onishi H, Shirato H, Nagata Y, Hiraoka M, Fujino M, Gomi K, et al. Stereotactic body radiotherapy (SBRT) for operable stage I non-small-cell lung cancer: can SBRT be comparable to surgery? Int J Radiat Oncol Biol Phys. 2011;81(5):1352–8.
53. Karliner LS, Patricia Kaplan C, Juarbe T, Pasick R, Perez-Stable EJ. Poor patient comprehension of abnormal mammography results. J Gen Intern Med. 2005;20(5):432–7.
54. Pietrzykowski T, Smilowska K. The reality of informed consent: empirical studies on patient comprehension-systematic review. Trials. 2021;22(1):57.
55. Ruske J, Sharma G, Makie K, He K, Ozaki CK, Menard MT, et al. Patient comprehension necessary for informed consent for vascular procedures is poor and related to frailty. J Vasc Surg. 2021;73(4):1422–8.
56. Engel KG, Heisler M, Smith DM, Robinson CH, Forman JH, Ubel PA. Patient comprehension of emergency department care and instructions: are patients aware of when they do not understand? Ann Emerg Med. 2009;53(4):454–61 e15.
57. Hasanpour Dehkordi A, Ebrahimi-Dehkordi S, Banitalebi-Dehkordi F, Salehi Tali S, Kheiri S, Soleimani BA. The effect of teach-back training intervention of breathing exercise on the level of dyspnea, six-minutes walking test and FEV1/FVC ratio in patients with chronic obstructive pulmonary disease; a randomized controlled trial. Expert Rev Respir Med. 2021;15(1):161–9.
58. Talevski J, Wong Shee A, Rasmussen B, Kemp G, Beauchamp A. Teach-back: a systematic review of implementation and impacts. PLoS One. 2020;15(4):e0231350.
59. Powers B. Reading level of lung cancer patient education materials. J Hosp Librariansh. 2007;6(4):69–74.
60. Shen Z, Herzfeld J. Floating orbitals reconsidered: the difference an imaginary part can make. ACS Omega. 2018;3(9):10992–8.
61. Zhao C, Dowzicky P, Colbert L, Roberts S, Kelz RR. Race, gender, and language concordance in the care of surgical patients: a systematic review. Surgery. 2019;166(5):785–92.
62. Diamond L, Izquierdo K, Canfield D, Matsoukas K, Gany F. A systematic review of the impact of patient-physician non-English language concordance on quality of care and outcomes. J Gen Intern Med. 2019;34(8):1591–606.
63. Ridgeway JL, Njeru JW, Breitkopf CR, Mohamed AA, Quirindongo-Cedeno O, Sia IG, et al. Closing the gap: participatory formative evaluation to reduce cancer screening disparities among patients with limited English proficiency. J Cancer Educ. 2021;36(4):795–803.
64. Pope JE, Tingey DP, Arnold JM, Hong P, Ouimet JM, Krizova A. Are subjects satisfied with the informed consent process? A survey of research participants. J Rheumatol. 2003;30(4):815–24.

Chapter 27
Achieving Health Equity in Lung Cancer Screening: Incorporation of Community Perspectives for Maximum Impact

Sydney C. Beache and Sandra E. Brooks

Background

There is accelerating interest and system level support for the advancement of health equity from a healthcare system perspective. A key element includes increasing the pace of adoption of evidence-based practices. It is estimated that 14% of scientific best practices for prevention and treatment disseminate into standard practice after an average of 17 years [1]. Given the magnitude of disparities in lung cancer outcomes, this time frame of wide adoption is not acceptable. Implementation of a successful lung cancer screening (LCS) program requires intentional engagement of key stakeholders to allow for sustainable translation of gold standards in clinical and public health practice into diverse community contexts. We provide a thematic overview of (1) inequities in lung cancer screening utilization and cancer outcomes; (2) barriers to LCS from the perspectives of clinicians and patients; (3) evidence-based strategies to reducing barriers; and (3) an introduction to the role of dissemination and implementation science in measuring the efficacy of community-based interventions designed to promote health equity.

S. C. Beache
Department of Surgery, Washington University in St. Louis, St. Louis, MO, USA
e-mail: beachesc@wustl.edu

S. E. Brooks (✉)
Independent Consultant and Faculty, Institute for Healthcare Improvement,
Philadelphia, PA, USA

Underutilization of Lung Cancer Screening as a Critical Quality Gap

Lung cancer is a leading cause of cancer death in the United States. The National Lung Screening Trial (NLST), a multi-center randomized control trial recruiting over 50,000 patients, demonstrated a clear reduction in mortality of up to 20% with early detection of lung nodules with low dose computed tomography (LDCT) in high-risk smoking populations [2]. The importance of early detection LDCT was validated in subsequent studies such as the NELSON trial, a Dutch-Belgian randomized control trial evaluating long-term mortality benefit of LCS [3]. Disparities in screening persist despite the United States Preventive Services Task Force (USPSTF) expansion of screening eligibility in 2021, with incidence rates and mortality for lung cancer disproportionately affecting non-Hispanic African American males and non-Hispanic White women [4]. Black males have the highest rates of age-adjusted lung cancer incidence among all US racial and ethnic groups, specifically 73.5 per 100,000 versus 63.5 per 100,000 for White males [4]. This racial disparity in incidence persists in both smokers and never-smokers [5]. Black males also have the highest lung cancer mortality compared with other racial/ethnic groups (62.1 vs 51.7 age-adjusted overall mortality) [4]. Black individuals develop lung cancer at an earlier age than White individuals (median age 67 vs 70 years) [6] and are more likely to present with advanced-stage disease (53% vs 49%) [7].

Disparities in mortality narrow when adjusting for stage at diagnosis and equal access to care, but little progress has been made in diagnosing lung cancer at an earlier stage over past decades [8]. Underutilization of LCS remains a barrier to improving these metrics, with only 12.7% of eligible individuals accessing screening per USPSTF guidelines according to recent data [9]. Population-based studies examining factors associated with increased utilization of screening services include diagnosis of a comorbid respiratory condition, previous cancer diagnoses, and age 65–74 years. Explanations for such trends may include healthcare utilization patterns in these populations, and reduced insurance coverage barriers for screening in the Medicare-eligible population. In this vein, uninsured individuals have lower odds of LCS uptake [10]. Prior studies demonstrate an association between access to healthcare and lung cancer survival [11].

Barriers to completion of screening are both primary care clinician and patient-facing: studies of clinicians describe low awareness of LCS guidelines, competing time and administrative burdens, and concerns about the sensitivity and specificity of screening with LDCT. At the same time patients report low knowledge of the role of LDCT in screening, and misperceptions about lung cancer diagnosis and treatment [6, 12–14]. The underutilization of lung cancer screening and the ensuing disparities in cancer morbidity and mortality are complex issues that require multi-modal solutions centered on understanding the barriers to implementation facing these key stakeholders.

Provider-Specific Considerations

Clinicians play a critical role in the landscape of healthcare and in building a high-quality LCS program. Since 2015, the Centers for Medicare and Medicaid Services (CMS) stipulated a counseling and shared decision-making (SDM) visit as a reimbursable prerequisite for LCS. Shared decision-making is rooted in patient-centered care principles of providing high quality, accessible knowledge to empower patients to make informed decisions about their medical care that align with their values. The CMS-required components of counseling and SDM for LCS includes: (1) assessment of screening eligibility; (2) SDM with the use of at least one decision aid; (3) counseling on the importance of annual screening; (4) review of the impact of comorbidities; (5) demonstrating willingness or ability to undergo diagnostic evaluation and treatment; and (6) smoking cessation counseling [2]. As such, LCS is the first cancer screening service with financial implications if SDM is not delivered before a patient is screened. Although CMS provides general guidance regarding expected activities, most of the decisions regarding SDM are left to providers and their organizations, making this requirement challenging to implement in practice. Further complicating the SDM conversation are lingering provider concerns about patient harms associated with annual LCS, including cumulative radiation exposure and detection of false-positive results and incidental findings. The challenge facing these organizations, and those wanting to help patients and clinicians balance the tradeoffs inherent with LCS, is how to move beyond a check-box documentation to a balanced discussion on the risks associated with tobacco exposure and screening with LDCT, as well as benefits associated with smoking cessation and LCS.

In the earliest stages of national LCS implementation, there was concern among primary care clinicians regarding the feasibility of LCS in community settings given logistical concerns and resource limitations, culminating in a 2013 statement by the American Academy of Family Physicians (AAFP) citing insufficient evidence for LCS in the setting of implementation concerns particularly in rural and urban underserved populations, as well as in communities of color. A subsequent retrospective review by Handy et al. of an integrated community health system based in Oregon reviewed approximately 6,000 LCS referrals over a 5-year period evaluated screening outcomes in the community health setting. They discovered similar rates of lung cancer diagnoses, interventions, and adverse events compared to larger tertiary care center data as in the NLST, suggesting that high quality LCS programs could be safely implemented in community health settings [15]. In 2021, the AAFP updated their position to endorse USPSTF guidelines of LCS [15].

Several studies have evaluated the role of implementing educational interventions aimed at increasing provider acceptance and adoption of LCS-unifying components including review of eligibility criteria, review of the evidence basis behind LCS, the risks and benefits to screening with LDCT, and concise models for implementing SDM that facilitate discussion informed decision-making [5, 7, 8]. There is a growing basis of community-based participatory research in the oncology prevention literature describing the role of non-clinician extenders such as nurses, medical assistants, and lay health navigators (community health workers) in reducing barriers to enrolling patients in screening services [5, 8]. Emerging research has also explored the role of checklists in implementing quality LCS programs, including structured mechanisms for reporting screening outcomes to facilitate communication among clinicians, radiologists, pulmonologists, and thoracic surgeons as they navigate lung nodule management [16]. Checklists widely used in the arena of perioperative care after a landmark World Health Organization international trial in 2009 are efficacious in reducing perioperative mortality and morbidity, and facilitating interdisciplinary communication [17].

Patient-Facing Concerns

Challenges to patient acceptance of LCS are multifactorial. Unequal healthcare access and insurance reimbursement structures may inadvertently widen LCS disparities: USPSTF guidelines for LCS ensure coverage of LDCTs for eligible Medicare recipients, but not Medicaid beneficiaries as Medicaid coverage is defined at the state level. Limitations in the reimbursement structure for LCS may represent a barrier to access for high-risk groups such as Black smokers, who are at risk of developing lung cancer at an earlier age compared to White smokers most notably in the 50–54-year-old age range. In addition, rural populations, who demonstrate earlier age of smoking initiation and greater smoking prevalence compared to metropolitan populations, may also face barriers to coverage for LCS [18]. Low community awareness of LCS and eligibility also limits LCS utilization, with multiple studies finding rates of LCS unawareness as high as 38–59% [19]. Furthermore, misperceptions about the role of LCS in prevention and early detection, personal risk for developing cancer, as well as fatalistic perceptions about lung cancer treatment options also serve to limit LCS uptake according to a qualitative study of clinicians and patients in an academic primary care setting in San Francisco, California [12].

While barriers to access are challenging to address given their systemic nature, experience from the breast, colorectal, and cervical cancer literature supports the use of community-based interventions in the form of partnerships with underserved communities to provide subsidized screening services [13]. There is an emerging evidence base for community-based interventions in the LCS literature: in 2018, a Los Angeles, California-based health system published their experience with securing a private grant to provide free LCS services, including transportation vouchers and personalized post-screening navigation services to underserved individuals in the region. In addition, a large body of evidence supports the effectiveness of engaging with lay people as community health workers (CHWs) to reach disparate populations to improve health knowledge and outcomes [20]. CHWs are credible and trusted sources of information; therefore, training them to present LCS information within the context of other cancer screenings may normalize the information, decrease stigma, raise awareness, and increase consideration of screening initiation. Community health workers are unique in that they share cultural or experiential backgrounds with the patients with whom they serve, which has shown to lend itself to successful community-based interventions [21]. Randomized control trials in the colorectal and breast cancer literature demonstrate greater utilization of preventive screening services and improved screening outcomes [22–24]. Despite the effectiveness of CHWs, there are notable implementation gaps in some regions of the United States that impede dissemination of evidenced-based interventions; more data is warranted on effective methods to establish CHW models in new areas.

Shared decision-making also represents an opportunity to address knowledge concerns regarding LCS. Nishi et al. examined the perception of SDM with recently screened patients. They determined that recently screened patients possessed varied LCS knowledge, answering an average of 41.4% of questions correctly. Patients valued finding cancer early over concerns about harms. Patients indicated that LCS benefits were presented to them by a health care provider far more often than harms (68.3% vs 20.8%, respectively), and 30.7% reported they received educational materials about LCS during the screening process. One-third of patients had some decisional conflict (33.6%) related to their screening decisions, whereas most patients (86.6%) noted that they were involved in the screening decision as much as they wanted. In multivariate models, non-White race and having less education were related to lower knowledge scores. Non-White patients and former smokers were also more likely to be conflicted about the screening decision. Most patients ($n = 227$ [85.3%]) indicated that a health care provider had discussed smoking cessation or abstinence with them.

Finally, efforts to increase screening engagement should address knowledge gaps and misperceptions regarding LCS among patients. A 2017 study of screening-eligible patients in the Appalachia region of Kentucky revealed a preference for personal testimonies on the LCS experience, life-saving benefits of early detection, and receiving messaging from trusted sources [21]. A systematic review by the Agency for Healthcare Research and Quality also highlighted the use of faith-based organizations to fulfill the role of a trusted source through community engagement efforts aimed at increasing preventive healthcare utilization [22].

Using Dissemination and Implementation Science to Measure the Process and Impact of Efforts to Increase Lung Cancer Screening

A recent World Health Organization report indicated that global healthcare expenditures have doubled over the past two decades, with spending in the United States accounting for over 40% of these costs [22]. Spending, however, does not equate to linear improvement in health outcome metrics like life expectancy, and as such there is growing interest in re-evaluating practices to improve the efficiency of healthcare systems. Dissemination and implementation science involves rigorous study of methods for translating evidence-based interventions into clinical practice with attention to principles of feasibility and sustainability across multiple socio-ecological levels [23]. While related to quality improvement initiatives in the goal of improving healthcare delivery, implementation science studies the process of improving uptake of an underutilized evidence-based intervention, and dissemination emphasizes the spread of such efforts across different practice settings. Outcomes of interest in dissemination and implementation science include rates of uptake of an evidence-based intervention, as well as an assessment of the quality of its use within a practice environment. Frameworks are a hallmark of dissemination and implementation science: frameworks provide a roadmap for data collection and analysis as the adoption of evidence-based practices are systematically evaluated. In 1999, Glasgow et al. introduced the eponymous RE-AIM model to guide evaluation of evidence-based intervention in terms of their reach, efficacy, adoption, implementation, and maintenance [24]. Damschroeder et al. developed the Consolidated Framework for Implementation Research (CFIR) in 2009 in a collaboration with the Veterans Affairs Diabetes Quality Enhancement Research Initiative (QUERI), offering constructs across five domains – intervention characteristics, outer setting, inner setting, individual characteristics, and implementation process – to guide the systematic assessment of barriers and facilitators associated with implementation [25]. Implementation studies can be combined with health services and health outcome–related research in hybrid study designs, whereby the process of implementing an evidence-based intervention can be studied alongside its effects on health metrics at the patient level.

We can apply dissemination and implementation science principles to rigorously evaluate efforts to engage patients in LCS. A study by Williams et al. used the RE-AIM framework to study implementation of a validated LCS educational program, which involved training CHWs to apply this intervention to medically under-served populations in Kentucky. Developed for readability at the sixth grade reading level, this intervention addressed LCS risk, benefits, and stigma. Researchers were successful in reaching CHWs to train them in educational intervention use, and in encouraging uptake of the intervention within their communities [26].

Final Thoughts

While this chapter identifies inequalities in outcomes related to lung cancer and LCS, we must recognize the limitations in drawing inferences on causality between these variables and our outcomes of interest as we think about designing interventions to address disparities. For example, while race is often reported as a variable of interest in health outcomes research, it is not race itself but the experience that one from a particular background experiences that serves as a critical determinant of health. To further extend this example, one's race may actually be considered a proxy for a multitude of social determinants, including income, wealth, quality of education, and cultural context that may be quite heterogeneous among people within one category [27]. In considering the various interventions designed to address healthcare inequity, we must also be mindful of an "inverse prevention law," a concept describing how those who would benefit from interventions may be the least likely to receive it, thereby propagating inequalities. It is of critical importance to keep in mind the complexity enmeshed within target predictor variables when interpreting health disparities research and designing and implementing interventions. Brownson et al. offer implementation science as a mechanism for achieving health equity with recommendations that include defining equity-relevant metrics, thoughtful stakeholder engagement, and tailoring of strategies for dissemination and implementation to meet contextual needs [28]. Community-based interventions represent an important path forward in this regard, by building upon existing community strengths and systems to enhance adoption and sustainability of interventions [29–33]. Focusing on health equity moves us away from a deficit conceptual model that focuses shortcomings on our healthcare system, to a solutions-based mindset wherein we are empowered to take action to address determinants of health.

References

1. Morris ZS, Wooding S, Grant J. The answer is 17 years, what is the question: understanding time lags in translational research. J R Soc Med. 2011;104:510. (sagepub.com).
2. National Lung Screening Trial Research Team, Aberle DR, Berg CD, et al. The National lung screening trial: overview and study design. Radiology. 2011;258(1):243–53. https://doi.org/10.1148/radiol.10091808.
3. Ru Zhao Y, Xie X, de Koning HJ, Mali WP, Vliegenthart R, Oudkerk M. NELSON lung cancer screening study. Cancer Imaging. 2011;11:S79–84. https://doi.org/10.1102/1470-7330.2011.9020. PMID: 22185865; PMCID: PMC3266562.
4. Cancer Facts & Figures 2019—Table 9. https://www.cancer.org/content/dam/cancer-org/research/cancer-facts-and-statistics/annual-cancer-facts-and-figures/2019/incidence-and-mortality-rates-for-selected-cancers-by-race-and-ethnicity-us-2011-2016.pdf. Accessed 8 Mar 2022
5. Akhtar A, Sosa E, Castro S, Sur M, Lozano V, D'Souza G, Yeung S, Macalintal J, Patel M, Zou X, Wu PC, Silver E, Sandoval J, Gray SW, Reckamp KL, Kim JY, Sun V, Raz DJ, Erhunmwunsee L. A lung cancer screening education program impacts both referral rates and provider and medical assistant knowledge at two federally qualified health centers. Clin Lung Cancer. 2021;23:356. https://doi.org/10.1016/j.cllc.2021.12.002. (clinical-lung-cancer.com). Accessed 12 Dec 2021.
6. Volk RJ, Foxhall LE. Readiness of primary care clinicians to implement lung cancer screening programs. Prev Med Rep. 2015;2:717–9. https://doi.org/10.1016/j.pmedr.2015.08.014. Published 2015 Aug 24.
7. Lowenstein LM, Deyter GMR, Nishi S, Wang T, Volk RJ. Shared decision-making conversations and smoking cessation interventions: critical components of low-dose CT lung cancer screening programs. Transl Lung Cancer Res. 2018;7(3):254–71. https://doi.org/10.21037/tlcr.2018.05.10.
8. Salazar AS, Sekhon S, Rohatgi KW, Nuako A, Liu J, Harriss C, et al. A stepped-wedge randomized trial protocol of a community intervention for increasing lung screening through

engaging primary care providers (I-STEP). Contemp Clin Trials. 2020;91:105991. https://doi. org/10.1016/j.cct.2020.105991. Accessed 10 Mar 2022.

 9. Richards TB, Soman A, Thomas CC, et al. Screening for lung cancer—10 states, 2017. MMWR Morb Mortal Wkly Rep. 2020;69:201–6. https://doi.org/10.15585/mmwr.mm6908a1.

10. Zgodic A, Zahnd WE, Miller DP Jr, Studts JL, Eberth JM. Predictors of lung cancer screening utilization in a population-based survey. J Am Coll Radiol. 2020;17(12):1591–601. https://doi. org/10.1016/j.jacr.2020.06.015. Epub 2020 Jul 16.

11. Ganti AK, Subbiah SP, Kessinger A, Gonsalves WI, Silberstein PT, Loberiza FR Jr. Association between race and survival of patients with non–small-cell lung cancer in the United States veterans affairs population. Clin Lung Cancer. 2014;15:152–8.

12. Lowenstein M, Vijayaraghavan M, Burke NJ, Karliner L, Wang S, Peters M, Lozano A, Kaplan CP. Real-world lung cancer screening decision-making: barriers and facilitators. Lung Cancer. 2019;133:32–7.

13. Love MB, Gardner K, Legion V. Community health workers: who they are and what they do. Health Educ Behav. 1997;24:510–22.

14. Lewis JA, Chen H, Weaver KE, Spalluto LB, Sandler KL, Horn L, Dittus RS, Massion PP, Roumie CL, Tindle HA. Low provider knowledge is associated with less evidence-based lung cancer screening. J Natl Compr Cancer Netw. 2019;17(4):339–46. Accessed 28 Feb 2022. https://jnccn.org/view/journals/jnccn/17/4/article-p339.xml

15. Handy JR, Skokan M, Rauch E, Zinck S, Sanborn RE, Kotova S, Wang M. Results of lung cancer screening in the community. Ann Fam Med. 2020;18(3):243–9. (annfammed.org).

16. Mulshine JA. Implementing lung cancer screening: a checklist. Lung Cancer Manag. 2014;3(1):1. (futuremedicine.com).

17. Haynes AB, Weiser TG, Berry WR, Lipsitz SR, Breizat AH, Dellinger EP, Herbosa T, Joseph S, Kibatala PL, Lapitan MC, Merry AF, Moorthy K, Reznick RK, Taylor B, Gawande AA, Safe Surgery Saves lives Study Group. A surgical safety checklist to reduce morbidity and mortality in a global population. N Engl J Med. 2009;360(5):491–9. https://doi.org/10.1056/ NEJMsa0810119. Epub 2009 Jan 14. PM.

18. Wang GX, Baggett TP, Pandharipande PV, Park ER, Percac-Lima S, Shepard J, Fintelmann FJ, Fllores EF. Barriers to lung cancer screening engagement from the patient and provider perspective. Radiology. 2019;290(2):278. https://doi.org/10.1148/radiol.2018180212.

19. Lee C. Screening for lung cancer: effective recruitment methods. Am J Roentgenol. 2018;210(3):514–7. (ajronline.org).

20. Raphael JL, Rueda A, Lion KC, et al. The role of lay health workers in pediatric chronic disease: a systematic review. Acad Pediatr. 2013;13:408–20.

21. Roland KB, Milliken EL, Rohan EA, et al. Use of community health workers and patient navigators to improve cancer outcomes among patients served by federally qualified health centers: a systematic literature review. Health Equity. 2017;1:61–76.

22. Russell KM, Champion VL, Monahan PO, et al. Randomized trial of a lay health advisor and computer intervention to increase mammography screening in African American women. Cancer Epidemiol Biomark Prev. 2010;19:201–10.

23. Cardarelli R, Roper KL, Cardarelli K, et al. Identifying community perspectives for a lung cancer screening awareness campaign in Appalachia Kentucky: the terminate lung cancer (TLC) study. J Cancer Educ. 2017;32(1):125–34. https://doi.org/10.1007/s13187-015-0914-0. PMID: 26411308; PMCID: PMC5569580.

24. Berkman ND, Sheridan SL, Donahue KE, Halpern DJ, Viera A, Crotty K, Holland A, Brasure M, Lohr KN, Harden E, Tant E, Wallace I, Viswanathan M. Health literacy interventions and outcomes: an updated systematic review. Evidence report/technology assessment No. 199. Rockville, MD: Agency for Healthcare Research and Quality; 2011. Prepared by RTI International–University of North Carolina Evidence-based Practice Center under contract No. 290–2007-10056-I. AHRQ publication number 11-E006.

25. WHO. Global expenditure on health: public spending on the rise? Geneva: World Health Organization; 2021. 9789240041219-eng.pdf (who.int).
26. Bauer MS, Damschroder L, Hagedorn H, Smith J, Kilbourne AM. An introduction to implementation science for the non-specialist. BMC Psychol. 2015;3(1):32. https://doi.org/10.1186/s40359-015-0089-9. PMID: 26376626; PMCID: PMC4573926.
27. Glasgow RE, Vogt TM, Boles SM. Evaluating the public health impact of health promotion interventions: the RE-AIM framework. Am J Public Health. 1999;89(9):1322–7. (aphapublications.org).
28. Damschroder LJ, Aron DC, Keith RE, Kirsh SR, Alexander JA, Lowery JC. Fostering implementation of health services research findings into practice: a consolidated framework for advancing implementation science. Implement Sci. 2009;4:50. https://doi.org/10.1186/1748-5908-4-50. PMID: 19664226; PMCID: PMC2736161.
29. Williams LB, Shelton BJ, Gomez ML, et al. Using implementation science to disseminate a lung cancer screening education intervention through community health workers. J Community Health. 2021;46:165–73. https://doi.org/10.1007/s10900-020-00864-2.
30. Haddad DN, Sandler KL, Henderson LM, Rivera MP, Aldrich MC. Disparities in lung cancer screening: a review. Ann Am Thorac Soc. 2020;17(4):399–405. https://doi.org/10.1513/AnnalsATS.201907-556CME.
31. VanderWeele TJ, Robinson WR. On the causal interpretation of race in regressions adjusting for confounding and mediating variables. Epidemiology. 2014;25(4):473–84. https://doi.org/10.1097/EDE.0000000000000105.
32. Brownson, et al. Implementation science should give higher priority to health equity. Implement Sci. 2021;16:28. https://doi.org/10.1186/s13012-021-01097-0.
33. Ward M, Schulz AJ, Israel BA, Rice K, Martenies SE, Markarian E. A conceptual framework for evaluating health equity promotion within community-based participatory research partnerships. Eval Program Plann. 2018;70:25–34. https://doi.org/10.1016/j.evalprogplan.2018.04.014.

Part VI
Determining Impact at the Population Level

Chapter 28
Lung Cancer Screening: Addressing Disparities

Christine S. Shusted and Gregory C. Kane

Background

When a new preventive health measure is first introduced, racial and socioeconomic disparities emerge in uptake. These gaps in care tend to decline with time, but inequities at some level endure [1–3]. As a screening test endorsed nationally within the last decade, lung cancer screening with low-dose computed tomography (LDCT) follows this pattern. In addition to disparate test use, newer screening mechanisms are associated with disparities in stage at diagnosis, treatment, and mortality [1–5].

Disparities, driven in large part by a lack of equity and equality, occur across several facets, including race, ethnicity, sex assigned at birth, gender identity, sexual orientation, age, geography, socioeconomic status, disability, veteran status, educational attainment, insurance status, foreign-born nativity, as well as other demographic and social factors [6, 7]. Disparities are often exacerbated by intersectionality and the complex interplay of individual, interpersonal, organization, community, environmental, and policy factors. Fully understanding that lung cancer disparities are not based solely on one factor but rather at the intersection of individual characteristics, social identities, outside influences, and predetermined factors is essential to working toward a more equitable lung cancer screening landscape.

C. S. Shusted (✉)
Division of Pulmonary and Critical Care Medicine, Department of Medicine, Sidney Kimmel Medical College at Thomas Jefferson University, Philadelphia, PA, USA
e-mail: Christine.Shusted@Jefferson.edu

G. C. Kane
Department of Medicine, Thomas Jefferson University, Philadelphia, PA, USA
e-mail: Gregory.Kane@Jefferson.edu

G. C. Kane et al. (eds.), *Lung Cancer Screening*,
https://doi.org/10.1007/978-3-031-33596-9_28

Familiarizing oneself with how to view a known disparity through a multifaceted lens is imperative to successfully reduce disparate care and improve patient outcomes; however, it can be intimidating to those unaccustomed to the practice. To illustrate, compared to whites, blacks are more likely to be unaware of lung cancer screening; compounding this issue, they are also more likely to be underinsured, have low levels of trust in clinicians, experience provider bias, have limited health literacy, and to live in poverty – all factors that contribute to decreased screening rates [1, 3, 8–10]. Further, blacks are more likely to present with advanced disease, experience infrequent guideline-concordant treatment, have less favorable lung cancer outcomes, and have lower rates of long-term survival [1, 3, 4]. Blacks are less likely to meet screening eligibility criteria, despite recent revisions expanding eligibility; among those eligible, they are also less likely to undergo screening; paradoxically, blacks experience a greater reduction in mortality from screening with LDCT compared to whites [3, 11–15]. Despite these differences, black men experience a mortality rate for lung cancer per 100,000 persons that is 15% greater than that of white men and black women experience a 17% greater mortality than white women [16].

Lung Cancer Screening Eligibility

There has been increased momentum surrounding health equity and equality – both in a healthcare setting and in society as a whole. This may have been catalyzed by the COVID-19 pandemic. Driven in part by this momentum, the United States Preventive Services Taskforce (USPSTF) broadened lung cancer screening eligibility in March 2021. These newly implemented guidelines lowered the minimum age to 50 years and lessened the smoking intensity threshold to 20 pack-years [17]. The expanded criteria encompasses an additional 6.5 million individuals eligible for lung cancer screening [13, 18]. While the hope of the expanded guidelines is to improve screening eligibility among individuals who have previously experienced under-screening through the USPSTF 2013 guidelines – particularly for black, Hispanic, and female patients, in part due to the fact the criteria was based upon the National Lung Screening Trial (NLST), which was comprised of less than 10% non-white participants [19, 20]. However, the updated criteria likely will not be as efficacious at closing gaps in uptake as initially imagined. Recent data indicated that USPSTF 2020 guidelines increased eligibility across all races; however, that increase was not uniform in nature. Eligibility increased by 16%, 14%, 8%, and 10% for whites, blacks, Asians, and Hispanic populations, respectively. Based on the 2013 guidelines, an estimated 55% of lung cancer deaths would be averted among whites compared to 30–40% of other races and ethnicities. While the updated criteria provided an increased mortality benefit across races, an estimated 41–54% of lung cancer deaths will be prevented for non-white races – less than the averted deaths for whites from the original USPSTF 2013 guidelines [13, 21].

Despite the improvement in guideline inclusivity, some experts believe race-specific adjustment of screening guidelines or individualized risk calculations would improve eligibility equity [15, 22, 23]. Racial minorities are more likely to be light smokers than white adults and, therefore, may not meet the pack-year guidelines; regardless of lesser smoking duration and intensity, blacks are at higher risk for lung cancer than whites [15, 24]. Additionally, black individuals are twice as likely as whites to be diagnosed with lung cancer under 50 – rendering the guidelines useless as individuals under 50 years are not eligible [25]. Moreover, a recent examination of the USPSTF 2021 guidelines found women more likely to be ineligible than men due to a shorter smoking duration, despite an increased lung cancer risk [8, 22]. However, 27% of women ineligible based on the screening guidelines were eligible based on the PLCOm2012 6-year lung cancer risk score $\geq$ 1.0% [22, 26].

The USPSTF 2020 guidelines move screening eligibility in the right direction, yet, regardless of how wide the criteria become, disparities across the lung cancer screening and care continuum will persist until society moves to address the complex roots of disparate care and works to eradicate barriers to screening.

Lung Cancer Screening Uptake

Lung cancer is the leading cause of cancer-related mortality in the United States; cigarette smoking is linked to the majority of lung cancer cases, making it one of the most preventable cancer deaths [27]. Aside from smoking cessation, annual lung cancer screening with LDCT is one of the most effective mechanisms for reducing lung cancer mortality [20]. Even with a relative reduction in lung cancer mortality of 20%, lung cancer screening with LDCT rates remain in the single digits [20, 21, 28, 29]. Despite strong evidence in favor of lung cancer screening, uptake among eligible individuals in the United States ranges from 1.9% to 13%, with variations based on geographic location [21, 28–31]. While the USPSTF broadened eligibility criteria for screening, reducing screening uptake requires dismantling extensive barriers and working through multifarious implementation issues.

The underutilization of lung cancer screening is driven by complex factors and barriers across all levels of the social-ecological model, which in turn widen gaps in care. Racial and ethnic disparities in LDCT uptake are the perfect example of why viewing disparities through a lens of intersectionality is critical. Black individuals are less likely to undergo lung cancer screening, even after a LDCT referral order is placed compared to other races [12, 32]. A contributing factor to this disparity is likely the increased level of mistrust in healthcare providers and the healthcare system among black and Hispanic populations [33]. Racial and ethnic minorities are more likely to express fatalism, nihilism, and be skeptical of medical intervention; these beliefs fuel hesitancy in seeking preventive care [34, 35]. Further, the stigma surrounding lung cancer and tobacco use discourages eligible individuals from undergoing screening. Black and Hispanic individuals are more likely than other races to fear adverse outcomes from screening, including harm from radiation exposure [36]. Racial and ethnic minorities are more likely than whites to live in poverty, have lower levels of educational attainment, and be uninsured – all of which are linked to a reduced level of lung cancer screening.

Insurance status is a key factor in the decision to undergo preventive health measures; in fact, among all individuals eligible for lung cancer screening; those without insurance had rates three times lower than those with insurance [37, 38]. Highlighting the interplay of factors, black individuals are almost twice as likely to be uninsured and more than twice as likely to have Medicaid compared to individuals of other races [39, 40]. Racial and ethnic minorities as a whole are more likely to be uninsured [41]. Regardless of race, over half of the screening eligible individuals not yet qualified for Medicare (age 50–64 years) have Medicaid or are uninsured [27, 40]. While many private insurers and Medicare plans cover lung cancer screening with LDCT, Medicaid coverage is determined on a state-by-state basis [8]. The lack of universal coverage for individuals with Medicaid leaves many high-risk persons without the opportunity to screen. Medicaid covers low socioeconomic status individuals, who also have an increased propensity for smoking cigarettes, therefore, placing them at an increased risk for lung cancer, underlining the importance of screening [42].

Further highlighting the significance of socioeconomic factors, lung cancer screening rates vary drastically based on median household income. Eligible persons with lower household incomes are more likely not to undergo LDCT [3, 43, 44]. Many individuals of low socioeconomic status work jobs with inflexible hours, thus making it impossible to undergo an LDCT scan during typical screening center hours. Creating a choice between taking time off and being screened for lung cancer widens already existing socioeconomic disparities in LDCT uptake.

The southeastern United States is the poorest region of the nation, boasts the highest smoking prevalence, and has the highest lung cancer incidence rate – yet has the lowest number of accredited lung cancer screening sites [8, 45]. Amplifying this disparity is that the southeast has the most significant proportion of black individuals, who are at disproportionately high risk for lung cancer incidence [45]. This incongruity is concerning as those at the highest risk for lung cancer have the least access to preventive care. Geographic disparities are not limited to the region; urbanization also leads to inequalities in access to LDCT and knowledge of lung cancer screening. An estimated 22% of Americans eligible for screening living in a rural area reside within a 30-min drive of a screening center compared to 83% of those who live in urban areas [46]. Once again, there is a discrepancy between the distributions of at-risk individuals and access to lung cancer screening. In this case, rural residents who are at an increased risk for lung cancer mortality compared to those who live in urban areas are unable to access an LDCT scan as easily as those at lower risk [46, 47]. Interestingly, screening sites are more readily available in urban areas; knowledge of lung cancer screened skews toward those living in rural areas [8, 48]. Urbanites are the least likely to be aware of lung cancer screening and the most likely to be undecided about undergoing LDCT compared to those living in suburban and rural areas [3].

Adherence to Follow-Up

Adherence to follow-up in lung cancer screening tends to be more complex than other cancer screening tests; depending on LDCT results, recommendations may include an annual follow-up LDCT, 6-month follow-up scan, 3-month follow-up, referral to advanced imaging or surgery, as well referral for workup for incidental findings. Because of the variation and complex follow-up, patients have many opportunities to fall through the cracks. Timely follow-up is critical for the full benefits of lung cancer screening to be realized. Despite the increased mortality benefit experienced by black individuals, blacks have 33% lower odds of adhering to recommended follow-up than whites [49]. Regardless of the finding of the LDCT scan, blacks have disparate follow-up compared to whites. Of patients with the highest risk of malignancy, blacks have 44% lower odds of completing follow-up [49]. Blacks are more likely than white individuals to be diagnosed with late-stage lung cancer, which may partly be due to lack of adherence to follow-up. Further, black individuals undergoing screening through a decentralized program experience a 27% reduction in annual lung cancer screening adherence [50]. Despite known racial disparities in adherence, there is minimal additional investigation into potential confounders such as socioeconomic status, educational attainment, income, and insurance status.

Treatment

Treatment for lung cancer has improved over the last decade; targeted immunotherapy and molecular testing have allowed for customized treatment regimens and decreased mortality. However, not all individuals with lung cancer receive the same treatment options, even if their cancers are identical. Black lung cancer patients are less likely to receive stage-appropriate treatment than other races [35, 51]. Racial disparities, in part, might be due to attitudes and cultural beliefs. Black and Hispanic individuals are more likely to report high levels of fatalism and distrust in clinicians [34, 35]. Consequences of these feelings include lower follow-up rates for diagnostic workup and treatment refusal [35]. A fatalistic perspective regarding treatment is likely why black and Hispanic lung cancer patients are less likely to receive guideline-concordant treatment. A common belief among black communities is that surgical intervention will cause lung cancer to spread throughout the body; this belief, along with other views, likely contribute to the incongruent treatment across races and the fact blacks are less likely to undergo surgery with curative intent [35]. It is of particular concern that black individuals are not receiving appropriate treatment as they present, more often, with late-stage disease and have the most significant lung cancer mortality burden of all races [1, 3, 4, 16].

Individuals with public insurance are more likely to delay or decline guideline-concordant treatment for lung cancer [51, 52]. Other socioeconomic factors increase the risk of receiving guideline discordant care, such as low educational attainment, living in a rural area, having Medicaid or being uninsured, low-income level, and being non-white; as the number of factors increases, the odds of the patient declining therapy rises dramatically [53].

Individuals living in poverty are more likely to present with late-stage lung cancer and less likely to undergo surgical resection or receive guideline-concordant therapy[25, 51, 54]. Conversely, individuals from higher socioeconomic status are more likely to undergo a brain MRI, surgical resection, palliative radiation, and adjuvant chemotherapy [51, 54]. Black and Hispanic individuals are over two times as likely to live in poverty compared to whites [55]. Socioeconomic status and minority status are inescapably linked, each associated with reduced screening uptake, subpar treatment, and poor lung-cancer-related outcomes.

Lung Cancer Outcomes and Mortality

The 5-year survival rate for lung cancer is 22%, which increases to 60% if diagnosed at a localized stage, making early diagnosis key to favorable outcomes, making lung cancer the leading cause of cancer-related mortality [16]. Out of all groups, black men have the highest lung cancer mortality, though disparate racial mortality tightens when adjusting for stage and access to care [56]. In line with fatalistic views held by certain racial minorities, individuals may refuse treatment or avoid seeking care, thus leading to poor long-term outcomes.

Racial and ethnic minorities are more likely to have Medicaid or lack insurance [39, 40]. Patients with Medicaid are more likely to die the same month of their diagnosis, and uninsured patients have an increased hazard of death [57].

Over the last half-decade, lung cancer mortality has steadily increased among those in lower socioeconomic brackets and declined for those in upper-income brackets. This trend follows the rise and fall of cigarette smoking in socioeconomically advantaged groups [8, 58]. Individuals that live in low-income areas are more likely to have environmental and workplace exposures that lead to lung cancer [8]. Compounding the burden of living in poverty, individuals are more likely to be a racial or ethnic minority, thus increasing their lung cancer mortality risk. Low-income neighborhoods are more likely to be segregated, another factor influencing lung cancer mortality [59]. As neighborhoods become more segregated, there is an increase in lung cancer mortality among blacks; conversely, as segregation increases, mortality decreases among whites [59]. Neighborhoods are not the only type of geography that impacts mortality; those who live in rural areas experience increased economic deprivation and thus an increase in mortality [33, 60].

Disparities in lung cancer mortality are a complex web, with many factors, directly and indirectly, influencing one another. Only by understanding these interrelated socio-ecological forces can we hope to address these disparities directly.

Working Toward Equity

Throughout the United States, racial and socioeconomic disparities account for 37% of premature cancer deaths. The most significant socioeconomic disparity across disease types is observed in lung cancer; lung cancer mortality is five times greater among the least educated men ($\leq$ 12 years of education) compared to the most educated ($\geq$16 years of education) [8, 61]. Disparities are initiated by a lack of equity and equality in the multifaceted interaction of individual, interpersonal, organization, community, environmental, and policy factors.

The intersectional nature of disparities requires working toward equity utilizing a multi-pronged approach. Thoughtful and steadfast efforts are needed to dismantle barriers to lung cancer screening and prevent already pervasive gaps in care from widening. The first step is to consider the implementation of broadening eligibility criteria to include race-specific or individualized lung cancer risk score calculations in an effort to provide eligibility that is more equitable. Utilizing the USPSTF 2020 guidelines and the Life-Years From Screening With Computed Tomography (LYFS-CT) model eliminated disparities for black individuals, marginally reduced disparities among Hispanic individuals, and had no impact on Asians [13]. Additional resources should focus on unraveling the complex, intertwining web of lung cancer disparities while simultaneously narrowing gaps in care. However, risk-based eligibility criteria would be time-consuming for providers to roll out and could further widen disparities as community clinics where underserved patients often seek care may be overburdened with new sets of calculations [28].

After considering a roll-out of more equitable lung cancer screening criteria, additional work is still needed to minimize disparity gaps. Implementation scientists, community stakeholders, lung cancer screening experts, and patient advocates should consider joining forces to strategize how to tackle disparities across the lung cancer screening and care continuum. These strategies might include free screening to those without insurance, mobile LDCT units to reach rural areas, and culturally competent patient navigation to ensure timely follow-up of clinically significant findings.

As we collectively move toward health equity, it is worth remembering that disparities exist across the lung cancer care continuum. If we are to realize the full benefit of lung cancer screening, it must be deployed so that all persons at risk for lung cancer are able to undergo an LDCT without an added burden on the patient. Examining the intersection of individual characteristics, social identities, outside influences, and predetermined factors is a critical step in achieving health equity and ultimately saving lives.

References

1. Shusted CS, Barta JA, Lake M, Brawer R, Ruane B, Giamboy TE, et al. The case for patient navigation in lung cancer screening in vulnerable populations: a systematic review. Popul Health Manag. 2019;22(4):347–61.

2. Phelan JC, Link BG, Diez-Roux A, Kawachi I, Levin B. "Fundamental causes" of social inequalities in mortality: a test of the theory. J Health Soc Behav. 2004;45(3):265–85.
3. Carter-Harris L, Slaven JE Jr, Monahan PO, Shedd-Steele R, Hanna N, Rawl SM. Understanding lung cancer screening behavior: racial, gender, and geographic differences among Indiana long-term smokers. Prev Med Rep. 2018;10:49–54.
4. Blom EF, Kt H, Arenberg DA, Koning HJ. Disparities in receiving guideline-concordant treatment for lung cancer in the United States. Ann Am Thorac Soc. 2020;17(2):186–94.
5. Lutfi W, Martinez-Meehan D, Sultan I, Evans N 3rd, Dhupar R, Luketich JD, et al. Racial disparities in local therapy for early stage non-small-cell lung cancer. J Surg Oncol. 2020;122(8):1815–20.
6. Meyer PA, Yoon PW, Kaufmann RB. Introduction: CDC health disparities and inequalities report-United States, 2013. MMWR Suppl. 2013;62(3):3–5.
7. Braveman P. Health disparities and health equity: concepts and measurement. Annu Rev Public Health. 2006;27:167–94.
8. Rivera MP, Katki HA, Tanner NT, Triplette M, Sakoda LC, Wiener RS, et al. Addressing disparities in lung cancer screening eligibility and healthcare access. Am J Respir Crit Care Med. 2020;202(7):e95–e112.
9. Gordon HS, Street RL Jr, Sharf BF, Kelly PA, Souchek J. Racial differences in trust and lung cancer patients perceptions of physician communication. J Clin Oncol. 2006;24(6):904–9.
10. Muvuka B, Combs RM, Ayangeakaa SD, Ali NM, Wendel ML, Jackson T. Health literacy in African-American communities: barriers and strategies. Health Lit Res Pract. 2020;4(3):e138–e43.
11. Tanner NT, Gebregziabher M, Hughes Halbert C, Payne E, Egede LE, Silvestri GA. Racial differences in outcomes within the National lung screening trial. Implications for widespread implementation. Am J Respir Crit Care Med. 2015;192(2):200–8.
12. Lake M, Shusted CS, Juon H-S, McIntire RK, Zeigler-Johnson C, Evans NR, et al. Black patients referred to a lung cancer screening program experience lower rates of screening and longer time to follow-up. BMC Cancer. 2020;20(1):561.
13. Landy R, Young CD, Skarzynski M, Cheung LC, Berg CD, Rivera MP, et al. Using prediction models to reduce persistent racial and ethnic disparities in the draft 2020 USPSTF lung cancer screening guidelines. J Natl Cancer Inst. 2021;113(11):1590–4.
14. Narayan AK, Chowdhry DN, Fintelmann FJ, Little BP, Shepard J-AO, Flores EJ. Racial and ethnic disparities in lung cancer screening eligibility. Radiology. 2021;301(3):712–20.
15. Aldrich MC, Mercaldo SF, Sandler KL, Blot WJ, Grogan EL, Blume JD. Evaluation of USPSTF lung cancer screening guidelines among African American adult smokers. JAMA Oncol. 2019;5(9):1318–24.
16. Siegel RL, Miller KD, Fuchs HE, Jemal A. Cancer statistics, 2022. CA Cancer J Clin. 2022;72(1):7–33.
17. United States Preventive Services Task Force. 2021; Pages. Accessed at United States Preventive Services Task Force at https://www.uspreventiveservicestaskforce.org/uspstf/recommendation/lung-cancer-screening on 10 Aug 2021.
18. Meza R, Jeon J, Toumazis I, ten Haaf K, Cao P, Bastani M, et al. Evaluation of the benefits and harms of lung cancer screening with low-dose computed tomography: modeling study for the US preventive services task force. JAMA. 2021;325(10):988–97.
19. Reese TJ, Schlechter CR, Potter LN, Kawamoto K, Del Fiol G, Lam CY, et al. Evaluation of revised US preventive services task force lung cancer screening guideline among women and racial/ethnic minority populations. JAMA Netw Open. 2021;4(1):e2033769-e.
20. National Lung Screening Trial Research Team, Aberle DR, Adams AM, Berg CD, Black WC, Clapp JD, et al. Reduced lung-cancer mortality with low-dose computed tomographic screening. N Engl J Med. 2011;365(5):395–409.
21. Fedewa SA, Silvestri GA. Reducing disparities in lung cancer screening: It's not so Black and white. J Natl Cancer Inst. 2021;113(11):1447–8.

22. Pasquinelli MM, Tammemägi MC, Kovitz KL, Durham ML, Deliu Z, Guzman A, et al. Addressing sex disparities in lung cancer screening eligibility: USPSTF vs PLCOm2012 criteria. Chest. 2022;161(1):248–56.
23. Pasquinelli MM, Tammemägi MC, Kovitz KL, Durham ML, Deliu Z, Rygalski K, et al. Risk prediction model versus United States preventive services task force lung cancer screening eligibility criteria: reducing race disparities. J Thorac Oncol. 2020;15:1738.
24. U.S. National Cancer Institute. A socioecological approach to addressing tobacco-related health disparities. Bethesda, MD: Department of Health and Human Services, National Institutes of Health, National Cancer Institute; 2017.
25. Ryan BM. Lung cancer health disparities. Carcinogenesis. 2018;39(6):741–51.
26. Tammemagi MC, Katki HA, Hocking WG, Church TR, Caporaso N, Kvale PA, et al. Selection criteria for lung-cancer screening. N Engl J Med. 2013;368(8):728–36.
27. Jemal A, Fedewa SA. Lung cancer screening with low-dose computed tomography in the United States—2010 to 2015. JAMA Oncol. 2017;3(9):1278–81.
28. Fedewa SA, Kazerooni EA, Studts JL, Smith RA, Bandi P, Sauer AG, et al. State variation in low-dose computed tomography scanning for lung cancer screening in the United States. J Natl Cancer Inst. 2021;113(8):1044–52.
29. Carter-Harris L, Gould MK. Multilevel barriers to the successful implementation of lung cancer screening: why does it have to be so hard? Ann Am Thorac Soc. 2017;14(8):1261–5.
30. Pham D, Bhandari S, Oechsli M, Pinkston CM, Kloecker GH. Lung cancer screening rates: data from the lung cancer screening registry. J Clin Oncol. 2018;36(15_suppl):6504.
31. Yong PC, Sigel K, Rehmani S, Wisnivesky J, Kale MS. Lung cancer screening uptake in the United States. Chest. 2020;157(1):236–8.
32. Japuntich SJ, Krieger NH, Salvas AL, Carey MP. Racial disparities in lung cancer screening: an exploratory investigation. J Natl Med Assoc. 2018;110(5):424–7.
33. Haddad DN, Sandler KL, Henderson LM, Rivera MP, Aldrich MC. Disparities in lung cancer screening: a review. Ann Am Thorac Soc. 2020;17(4):399–405.
34. Niederdeppe J, Levy AG. Fatalistic beliefs about cancer prevention and three prevention behaviors. Cancer Epidemiol Biomark Prev. 2007;16(5):998–1003.
35. Lin JJ, Mhango G, Wall MM, Lurslurchachai L, Bond KT, Nelson JE, et al. Cultural factors associated with racial disparities in lung cancer care. Ann Am Thorac Soc. 2014;11(4):489–95.
36. Jonnalagadda S, Bergamo C, Lin JJ, Lurslurchachai L, Diefenbach M, Smith C, et al. Beliefs and attitudes about lung cancer screening among smokers. Lung Cancer. 2012;77(3):526–31.
37. Zahnd WE, Eberth JM. Lung cancer screening utilization: a behavioral risk factor surveillance system analysis. Am J Prev Med. 2019;57(2):250–5.
38. Sun J, Perraillon MC, Myerson R. The impact of Medicare health insurance coverage on lung cancer screening. Med Care. 2022;60(1):29–36.
39. Cohen RA, Terlizzi EP, Martinez ME. Health insurance coverage: early release of estimates from the National Health Interview Survey 2018. Hyattsville, MD: National Center for Health Statistics; 2018.
40. Lozier JW, Fedewa SA, Smith RA, Silvestri GA. Lung cancer screening eligibility and screening patterns among Black and white adults in the United States. JAMA Netw Open. 2021;4:10–e2130350-e.
41. Barnett JC, Vornovitsky MS. Health insurance coverage in the United States: 2015. Washington, DC: US Government Printing Office; 2016.
42. Jamal A, Phillips E, Gentzke AS, Homa DM, Babb SD, King BA, et al. Current cigarette smoking among adults—United States, 2016. MMWR Morb Mortal Wkly Rep. 2018;67(2):53–9.
43. Steiling K, Loui T, Asokan S, Nims S, Moreira P, Rebello A, et al. Age, race, and income are associated with lower screening rates at a safety net hospital. Ann Thorac Surg. 2020;109(5):1544–50.
44. Castro S, Sosa E, Lozano V, Akhtar A, Love K, Duffels J, et al. The impact of income and education on lung cancer screening utilization, eligibility, and outcomes: a narrative review of socioeconomic disparities in lung cancer screening. J Thorac Dis. 2021;13(6):3745–57.

45. Wiener RS, Rivera MP. Access to lung cancer screening programs in the United States: perpetuating the inverse care law. Chest. 2019;155(5):883–5.
46. Eberth JM, Bozorgi P, Lebrón LM, Bills SE, Hazlett LJ, Carlos RC, et al. Geographic availability of low-dose computed tomography for lung cancer screening in the United States, 2017. Prev Chronic Dis. 2018;15:E119.
47. Jenkins WD, Matthews AK, Bailey A, Zahnd WE, Watson KS, Mueller-Luckey G, et al. Rural areas are disproportionately impacted by smoking and lung cancer. Prev Med Rep. 2018;10:200–3.
48. Rohatgi KW, Marx CM, Lewis-Thames MW, Liu J, Colditz GA, James AS. Urban-rural disparities in access to low-dose computed tomography lung cancer screening in Missouri and Illinois. Prev Chronic Dis. 2020;17:E140-E.
49. Kunitomo Y, Bade B, Gunderson CG, Akgün KM, Brackett A, Cain H, et al. Racial differences in adherence to lung cancer screening follow-up: a systematic review and meta-analysis. Chest. 2022;161(1):266–75.
50. Kim RY, Rendle KA, Mitra N, Saia CA, Neslund-Dudas C, Greenlee RT, et al. Racial disparities in adherence to annual lung cancer screening and recommended follow-up care: a multicenter cohort study. Ann Am Thorac Soc. 2022;19:1561.
51. Evans N III, Grenda T, Alvarez NH, Okusanya OT. Narrative review of socioeconomic and racial disparities in the treatment of early stage lung cancer. J Thorac Dis. 2021;13(6):3758–63.
52. Obrochta CA, Murphy JD, Nara A, Thompson CA. Disparities in receipt of guideline concordant treatment for early-stage non-small cell lung cancer (NSCLC) patients in California. J Clin Oncol. 2019;37(27_suppl):160.
53. Ebner PJ, Ding L, Kim AW, Atay SM, Yao MJ, Toubat O, et al. The effect of socioeconomic status on treatment and mortality in non-small cell lung cancer patients. Ann Thorac Surg. 2020;109(1):225–32.
54. Shah M, Parmar A, Chan KKW. Socioeconomic disparity trends in diagnostic imaging, treatments, and survival for non-small cell lung cancer 2007-2016. Cancer Med. 2020;9(10):3407–16.
55. Gradín C. Poverty among minorities in the United States: explaining the racial poverty gap for blacks and Latinos. Appl Econ. 2012;44(29):3793–804.
56. Howlader N NA, Krapcho M, Miller D, Bresi A, Yu M, Ruhl J, Tatalovich Z, Mariotto A, Lewis DR, Chen HS, Feuer EJ, Cronin KA. 2020; Pages. Accessed at National Cancer Institute at https://seer.cancer.gov/csr/1975_2017/on. 18 Jan 2021.
57. Slatore CG, Au DH, Gould MK. An official American Thoracic Society systematic review: insurance status and disparities in lung cancer practices and outcomes. Am J Respir Crit Care Med. 2010;182(9):1195–205.
58. Heidary F, Rahimi A, Gharebaghi R. Poverty as a risk factor in human cancers. Iran J Public Health. 2013;42(3):341–3.
59. Hayanga AJ, Zeliadt SB, Backhus LM. Residential segregation and lung cancer mortality in the United States. JAMA Surg. 2013;148(1):37–42.
60. Yang R, Cheung MC, Byrne MM, Huang Y, Nguyen D, Lally BE, et al. Do racial or socioeconomic disparities exist in lung cancer treatment? Cancer. 2010;116(10):2437–47.
61. Siegel R, Ward E, Brawley O, Jemal A. Cancer statistics, 2011: the impact of eliminating socioeconomic and racial disparities on premature cancer deaths. CA Cancer J Clin. 2011;61(4):212–36.

Chapter 29
Connecting the Dots: Geocoding and Assessing a Program's Impact

Christine S. Shusted, Russell K. Mcintire, and Charnita Zeigler-Johnson

Background

Lung cancer is the leading cause of cancer-related mortality in the United States, causing 1 in 5 cancer deaths [1]. Lung cancer is among the deadliest of cancers, with over half of individuals diagnosed dying within a year [2]. Lung cancer carries a 5-year survival rate of just over 18%, however, survival increases dramatically (56%) if it is caught at a localized stage. However, just 16% of lung cancer diagnoses are made early [2]. Therefore, early detection of lung cancer is critical. Aside from smoking cessation, annual lung cancer screening with low-dose computed tomography (LDCT) is one of the most effective mechanisms for reducing lung cancer mortality. Despite providing a 20% relative reduction in lung cancer mortality, screening uptake remains in the single digits nationally [3, 4].

Lung cancer incidence and mortality have a disparate impact nationally, with disparities existing across the cancer care continuum. Disparities exist in lung cancer by race, ethnicity, sex assigned at birth, gender identity, sexual orientation, age, socioeconomic status, disability, veteran status, educational attainment, insurance

C. S. Shusted (✉)
Division of Pulmonary and Critical Care Medicine, Department of Medicine, Sidney Kimmel Medical College at Thomas Jefferson University, Philadelphia, PA, USA
e-mail: Christine.Shusted@Jefferson.edu

R. K. Mcintire
Department of Population Health, Thomas Jefferson University, Philadelphia, PA, USA
e-mail: Russell.McIntire@Jeffeson.edu

C. Zeigler-Johnson
Cancer Prevention and Control, Communicyt Outreach and Engagement, Fox Chase Cancer Center, Philadelphia, PA, USA
e-mail: Charnita.Zeigler-Johnson@Jefferson.edu

G. C. Kane et al. (eds.), *Lung Cancer Screening*,
https://doi.org/10.1007/978-3-031-33596-9_29

status, foreign-born nativity, geography, as well as other demographic and social factors. An often underappreciated influence is geography, whether that be rural vs. urban, region of the country, or zip code. Life expectancy, health-related outcomes, and income can be drastically impacted by neighborhood. In Philadelphia, the average life expectancy in the Spring Garden neighborhood is 87 years, 10 min down the road, the Mantua neighborhood has an average life expectancy of just 66 years [5].

The impact of geography on lung cancer screening is immense, and screening programs should frequently evaluate geographic data to provide equitable care. In the United States, despite having a higher lung cancer burden, many Southern states screen less than 4% of eligible adults for lung cancer, whereas several Northeastern states that have lower incidence rates of lung cancer screen a significantly greater proportion of eligible adults (>12%) [6]. These geographic patterns have been previously observed in other preventive health measures, indicating geographic disparities cross all aspects of healthcare [6–9]. The root cause of these disparities is multifaceted and spans all levels of the social ecological model. Southern states have the greatest incidence of lung cancer, likely due to weak tobacco control policies, a higher proportion of the population living at a lower socioeconomic level, and minimal tobacco cessation efforts [6, 10]. Minimal government intervention is further driving lung cancer incidence, many southern states register tobacco tax at less than $1.00 per pack, whereas northeastern states charge upward of $4.00 a pack [11, 12]. Additionally, many southern states lack smoke-free air laws in 2022, meaning exposure to second-hand smoke is frequent and indiscriminate [11, 13].

Exacerbating existing disparities in the southern United States is the volume of rural areas. Rural areas have higher rates of poverty, uninsured people, low educational attainment, greater rates of elderly individuals, all factors that increase smoking and lung cancer risk. This is underscored in the deep south, where poverty rates, smoking rates, and lung cancer incidence are the highest nationally [7, 14, 15].

Smokers living in the South have an uphill battle when it comes to getting screened for lung cancer. There is drastic misalignment between lung cancer burden and access to screening centers, with the states with the fewest screening centers having the highest lung cancer incidence [6, 11, 16]. Further, screening centers are typically clustered in urban areas, making it difficult for those living in rural areas to make the trip, despite having greater incidence and mortality than their urban counterparts [7, 17, 18]. Further, individuals living in the Southern United States are more frequently diagnosed with late stage lung cancer and have access to fewer treatment options compared to their Northern counterparts [7, 17, 18].

More than 40% of the eligible screening population residents in the South, 26% of eligible persons live in the Midwest, and just 15% of eligible individuals live in the Northeast, yet the highest screening utilization is over twice that of the Southern United States [7]. The geographic disparities in lung cancer screening are staggering, and underscore the importance of analyzing geography when conducting cancer research.

Identifying Geographic Distribution of Disease

Describing the geographic distribution of disease is an important process, especially when considering provision of cancer screening services. Descriptive epidemiology is a branch of epidemiology that characterizes the "what, who, where, and when" of disease characteristics as they exist among populations. Descriptive epidemiology typically measures the burden of disease by generating incidence rates, which characterize new cases of disease, and mortality rates, which characterize disease-related deaths, during certain time-periods and among certain subgroups of people. Important considerations when conducting descriptive epidemiologic studies are the following: Which disease is under question? How is/was the disease measured? Self-reports by patients, diagnoses by practitioners, observations by researchers? Do you have data on the number of cases, percentage of cases, or rates (number of cases/total population, or per at-risk population)? All of these factors should be considered and reported in descriptive epidemiologic studies. In addition to the data that describes the disease, descriptive epidemiological studies include measurements of "person, place, and time."

Person: Determining disease characteristics related to person include asking questions such as: Is your descriptive study focused only on those who are at-risk of acquiring the disease, or all people in the population? Does it just focus on adults (vs those of any age)? Women (as opposed to women and men)?

Place: Characteristics related to place include determining where, geographically, the data describes. Do you have rates that describe counties in the United States? Countries in Africa?

Time: Characteristics related to time focus on the time-period in which the data was collected. Does the data describe the current state of disease within the population, in real-time? Does the data describe some historical time period? Was all of the data collected at one time point, or was it collected over a period of years at many time points?

Identifying geographic distribution requires the researcher to consider the geographic unit of analysis for which the data describes. For example, lung cancer mortality rates may be generated for the state of Pennsylvania by county for the time period 2008–2018. In this case, each county in Pennsylvania has a distinct mortality rate, which could be viewed in isolation or in comparison with other counties. The geographic unit of analysis is the county in this example. The data may also be expressed by a larger geographic unit (e.g., states) or a smaller geographic unit (e.g., US Postal Service zip codes (average population = 30,000) or census tracts (average population = 4000)). When the popular press describes a geographic unit of analysis, they often refer to zip codes. Yet, zip codes do not describe geographic boundaries; they describe delivery routes for the US Postal Service. Zip codes are not created by the US Census and therefore do not always align with data collected by the census.

Additionally, although zip codes are easily accessible, there is more variation among people who live in the same zip code, compared to smaller area units, especially those created by the U.S. Census Bureau. Within counties, researchers more often focus on census tracts, census blocks, or blocks, as depicted by

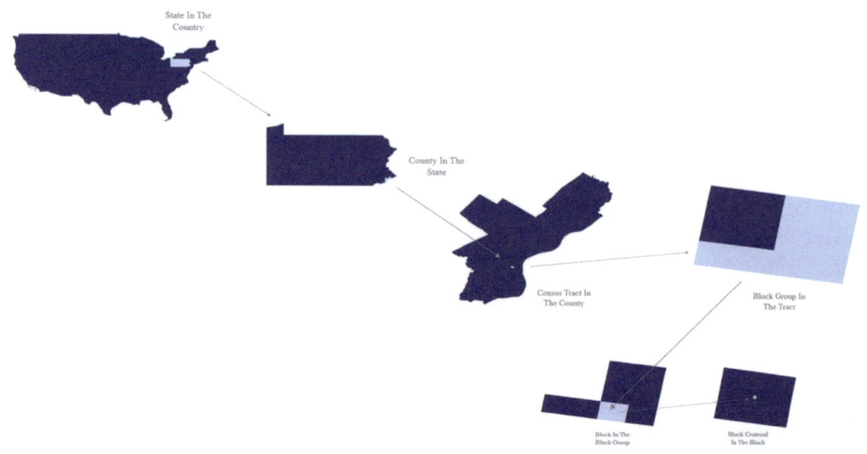

Fig. 29.1 Nested Geographic Units of Analysis

Fig. 29.1. Studies have shown that zip code–based cancer mortality analyses do not perform well compared to those utilizing smaller geographic units, such as census tracts [19].

The geographic units of analysis depicted in this Figure have common boundaries that are nested so that the higher level units are composed of the units in the level immediately adjacent. Zip codes do not always share borders with these geographies, and are bisected not just by census tracts, but by counties or even states! For the most accurate geographic analysis, the best practice is to use the smallest geographic unit of analysis available for your study. While zip codes are not ideal area units, they may be the best choice for your analysis, depending on the data available and the objectives of the study [20].

Geocoding for Cancer Control

The evolution and increasing ease-of-use of geographic information systems (GIS) during in the past 50 years have made describing and analyzing geographic relationships for cancer prevention much easier and more accurate. Identifying the geographic distribution of disease among patients includes linking disease characteristics to geographical areas.

An advantage to working on cancer studies within a hospital system is that patient information on geography is typically collected in electronic medical records (EMR). Hospital systems use EMRs to collect and organize data about their patients, characterize patient conditions, and identify services provided. Researchers can use geographic data contained in EMRs to identify where patients with certain conditions live through geocoding. Geocoding is "the process by which an entity on the earth's surface, a household, for example, is given a label identifying its location with respect to some common point or frame of reference" [21]. In practice, this is the process of linking geographic data contained in spreadsheets or databases to latitude and longitude data on a map [22]. The process of geocoding is complicated as it links spreadsheet data to data represented on a three-dimensional surface of the earth, and displays it on a two-dimensional map or computer screen. Ultimately, the output of geocoding patients through GIS is a series of points on a map representing the geographic location of patients. These locations might be at the residential level, neighborhood level, or a higher geographical level.

Process of Geocoding

While there are many comprehensive reports on the process of geocoding, and geocoding within cancer prevention [23, 24], this text will discuss some important considerations while geocoding cancer patient data.

When conducting lung cancer research, the geocoding system utilizes address data including: street, unit, city, state, and zip code. Typically, that information can be extracted through the EMR. However, it is worth noting that geocoding can be performed with other means of identifying locations including X, Y coordinates, mailing addresses, named places, relative locations, and even approximated through digitizing locations in GIS software [24]. Geocoding requires a reference file that contains a collection of street segments with associated address ranges, called an address locator. GIS software utilizes the reference file to locate each geographic location on a map automatically.

Geocoding Quality and Match Rate

Despite GIS software performing automated geocoding, the process still requires manual intervention. Immediately following the completion of geocoding, approximately 60–80% of the addresses will be identified on a map. Locations that successfully mapped to a candidate location are marked as "M" (matched), each matched address is given a score to gauge the sensitivity of how accurate the location entered was to the candidate location it was matched to. Addresses that were not able to be matched based on the address locator will be marked as "U" (unmatched) or T (tied; more than one candidate location). A review of the unmatched and tied candidates are required, and often can be rectified with minor spelling corrections. Three passes at correcting any errors in the address data is recommended. Geocoding accuracy is measured by the sensitivity and specificity of each match, and a match rate of at least 85% per location is essential to maintain spatial patterns and allow for advanced analyses [25].

Confidentiality and Privacy

Assessing lung cancer burden and other relevant data requires individual-level address and health data. Geocoding, spatial analyses, and associated mapping rely heavily on individual-level data, which is critical to identifying geographic patterns of disease [26, 27]. However, individual-level data requires special handling as to persevere confidentiality. Address, demographics, and relevant health information such as lung cancer diagnosis or smoking history are all protected health information (PHI) under the Health Insurance Portability and Accountability Act (HIPAA). Ensuring confidentiality and observance of HIPAA statues is compulsory when geocoding patient data.

There are several considerations when handling geographic data. Releasing individual-level address data breaches confidentiality laws and is prohibited. Efforts to protect confidentiality do not always meet the mark. For example, sharing the longitude and latitude of an individual's home allows for this location to be plotted on a map, and then be identified as a residential address [26]. Furthermore, distributing a map with geocoding addresses identified as dots allows for the potential of reverse geocoding; a process of determining the street address of a location from a published work [26, 28]. Reverse geocoding requires special consideration when mapping cancer incidence in small communities where individuals would be easily identifiable.

Rather than disseminating a map with individual points, circulating data in its spatially aggregated form is a common method to protect confidentiality (Fig. 29.2). However, even spatially aggregated maps require special care when dealing with highly sensitive health information, especially in insular communities.

Geographic masking is the gold standard to limit the re-identification of individual-level data as it makes reverse geocoding extremely challenging [26]. There is no consensus regarding masking methodology, but there are two overarching categories of geographic masking. The first, and more common, are affine transformations, which displace locations utilizing translations, changes in scale, and rotation. Affine transformations allow for spatial statistics to be performed and patterns maintained. Random perturbation which simply displaces points by adding indiscriminate noise to the coordinates is used less frequently as it can conceal valuable patterns [26].

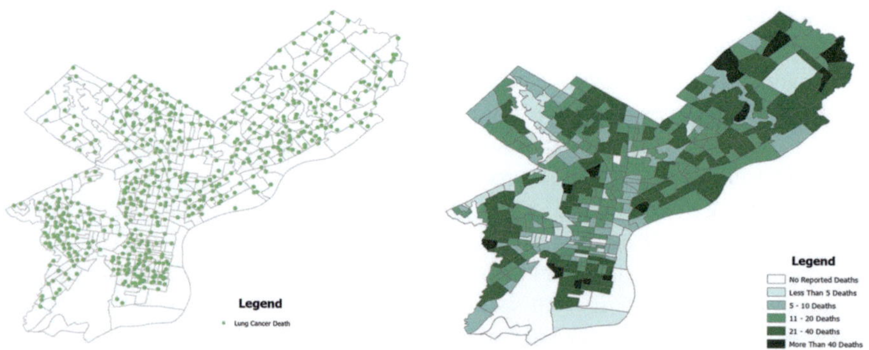

Fig. 29.2 Lung Cancer Mortality in Philadelphia; demonstrates how switching from individual-level point data to aggregated data helps protect identity by obscuring the true location

Random perturbation conceals PHI more so than affine transformations as it cannot be reverse engineered, thus allowing for the identification of individual-level data.

While there is no standardization of methodology protecting individual-level geographic data across the cancer research field, privacy concerns and adherence to HIPAA must be given the utmost deference when geocoding patient data.

Geographic Patterns and Mapping

Describing the distribution of cancer data rarely ends at geocoding. Are you interested in aggregating by some geographic unit of analysis? Are you interested in identifying clusters? Are you interested in analyzing the proximity of resources to patients, calculating travel times, or characterizing the neighborhood around patients? GIS plays a key role in lung cancer screening programs, and can be used to identify areas with high lung cancer burden, clusters of asbestoses exposure, pockets of high smoking prevalence, and more! Maps created highlighting these geographic patterns can then be used to target community outreach, identify where to send resources, and even detect emerging disease patterns.

While cartographers have carte blanche with map design, selecting the most appropriate mapping technique is critical to effectively use GIS software. Figure 29.3

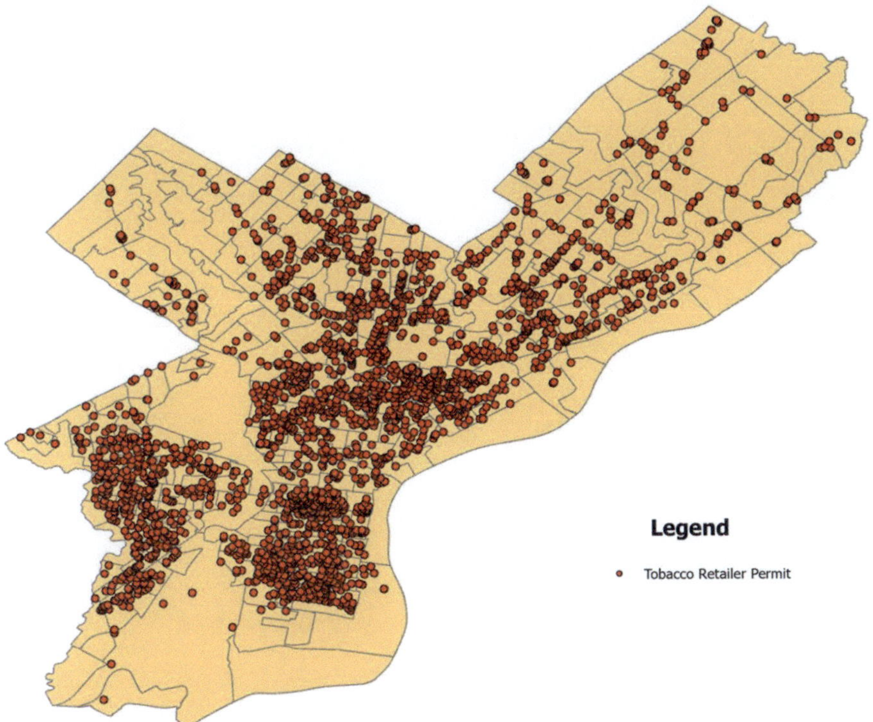

Fig. 29.3 Tobacco Retailer Permits in Philadelphia Dot Map

showcases the address of each approved tobacco retailer permit in Philadelphia. This dot map has an excess of overlapping points, and it is difficult to ascertain any helpful information. Therefore, a choropleth map may be better suited to map the number of retailers by census tract as shown in Fig. 29.4. The choropleth map makes clustering easier to visualize, allowing the viewer to point out the census tracts with the highest number of tobacco retailers. As demonstrated with the change in map formatting for tobacco retailers, it is vital to utilize the mapping methodology best-suited to display the data of interest.

In the following text are brief overviews of some of the most common types of maps.

Choropleth Maps

Choropleth maps utilize color-coded polygons to represent numeric attributes most commonly; however, qualitative data can also be displayed utilizing this mapping technique. Choropleth stems from the Greek *choro* meaning land or region [29]. Choropleth maps demonstrate the relative magnitude of the variable of interest. The

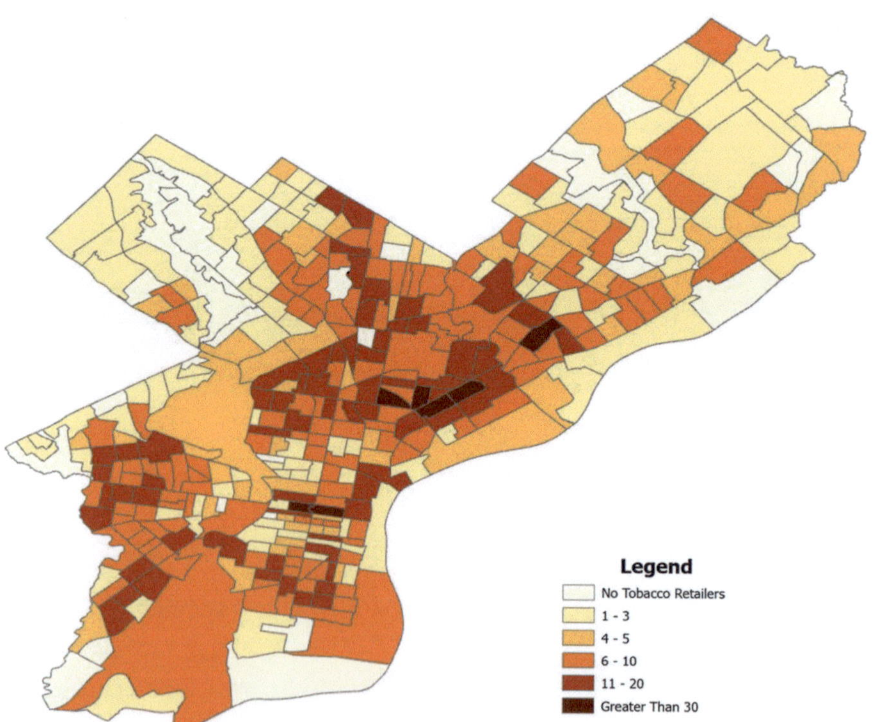

Fig. 29.4 Choropleth Map of Tobacco Retailer Permits in Philadelphia

maps are comprised of color-coded polygons that represent a numeric attribute or qualitative value.

Figure 29.5 displays a choropleth map of annual median household income in Philadelphia by census tract. The lightest of blue represents census tracts with an annual household income of less than $15,000, whereas the darkest blue represents tracts where the median income is greater than $100,000. This map shows the clustering of low income tracts in the center of the map, an area referred to as North Philadelphia by locals, an area full of poverty and underserved communities.

Depending on the variable of interest, choropleth maps can utilize graduated colors where values are transformed into a color scale, or unique colors where each value is given a specific color. Users are able to select the option that works best for their mapping interest. As shown in Figs. 29.6 and 29.7, poverty rates in Philadelphia by zip code is better suited for graduated colors than unique values. Typically, continuous variables are better represented by graduated colors whereas unique colors tend to better represent categorical variables.

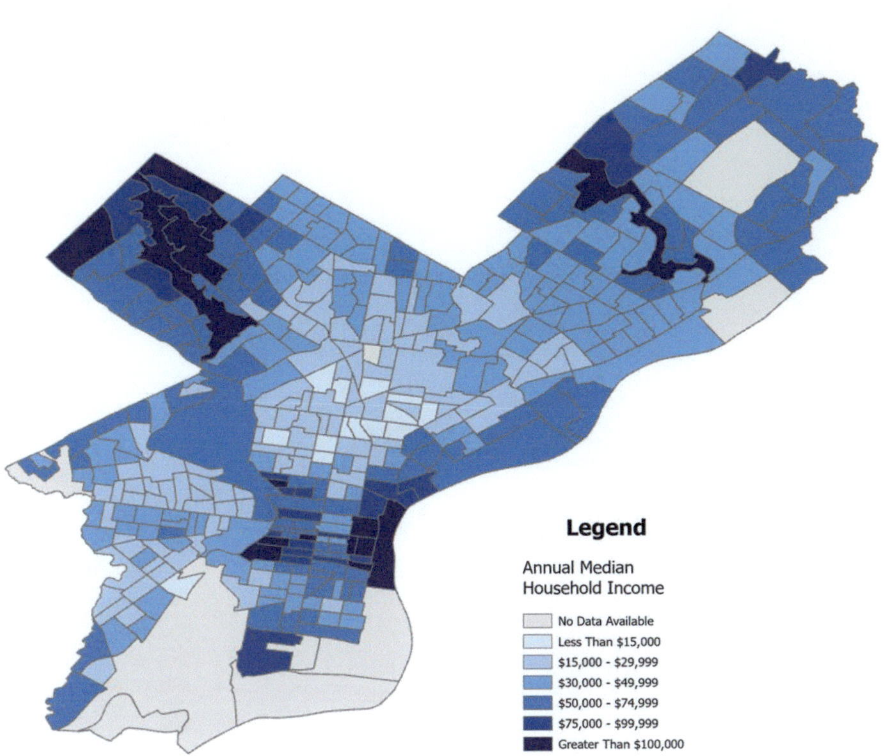

Fig. 29.5 Choropleth Map of Median Annual Household Income by Philadelphia Census Tract

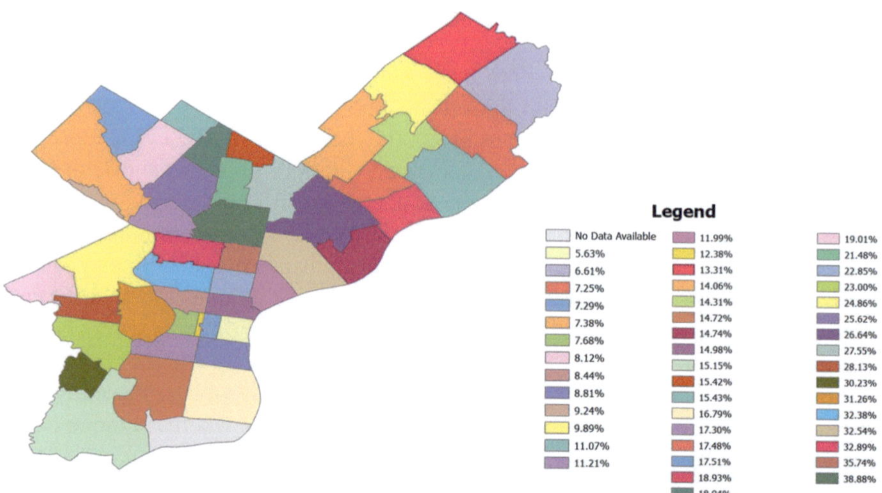

Fig. 29.6 Poverty Rate in Philadelphia by Zip Code; map made using unique values which makes it difficult to ascertain any meaningful information

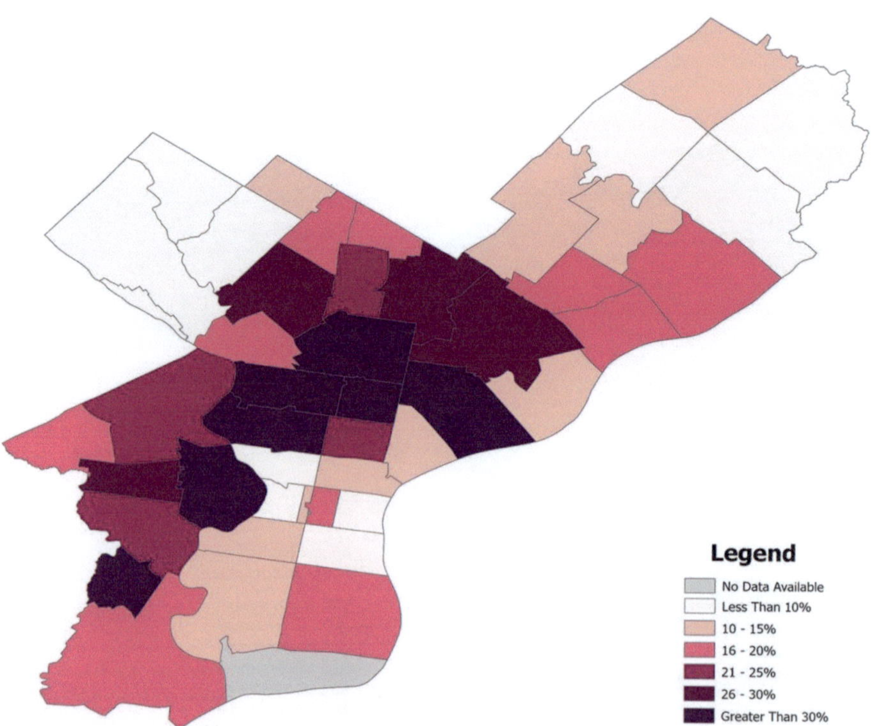

Fig. 29.7 Poverty Rate in Philadelphia by Zip Code; map made using graduated colors which allows for easy interpretation

Dot Density Maps

Dot density maps display a random pattern of dots placed within each unit of geography proportional to the attribute value associated with that geographic unit. Most frequently dot density maps are used to represent quantitative data. The map in Fig. 29.8 displays lung cancer incidence in Philadelphia, with each dot representing twenty cases of lung cancer.

Maps with Graduated Symbology Maps

Graduated symbols on a map are utilized to show the quantitative difference by symbol size [30]. The raw data is split into ranges, and each range is associated with a symbol size. The symbols do not vary in color or shape, the size simply changes based on range [30]. The map in Fig. 29.9 showcases adult smoking prevalence in Philadelphia by planning district with graduated symbology. Each size circle represents a classified range, with increasing size correlating to increase in smoking prevalence.

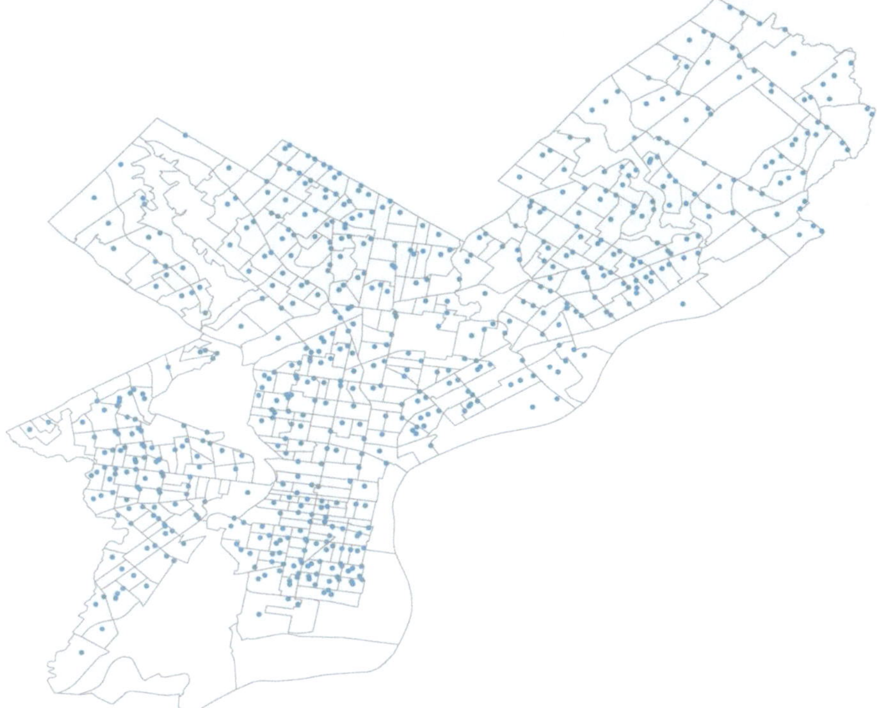

Fig. 29.8 Dot Density Map of Lung Cancer Cases in Philadelphia; one dot represents 20 cases

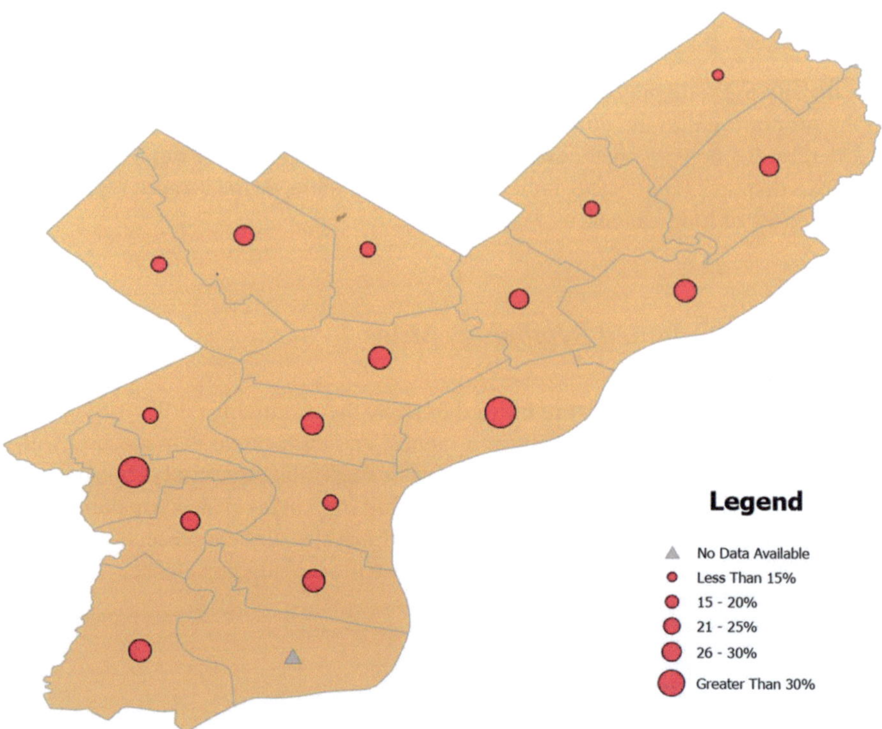

Fig. 29.9 Graduated Symbol Map of Adult Smoking Prevalence by Zip Code

Maps with Proportional Symbology

Proportional symbology displays relative differences, and is similar to graduated symbology, as both vary symbol size relative to the magnitude of the attribute [31]. Proportional symbology does not distribute raw data into ranges, rather each symbol represents quantitative values [31]. Figure 29.10 displays smoking attributable mortality in Philadelphia by planning district with proportional symbology.

Point and Kernel Density Maps for Clustering

Density mapping showcases where points are concentrated in a specific geographic unit. Point and Kernel Density maps are useful for analyzing clustering, such as a particular neighborhood with an abnormally high lung cancer incidence rate. Kernel density calculates the density of the feature of interest in a geographic area around those features [32]. Density can also be calculated for points, known as point

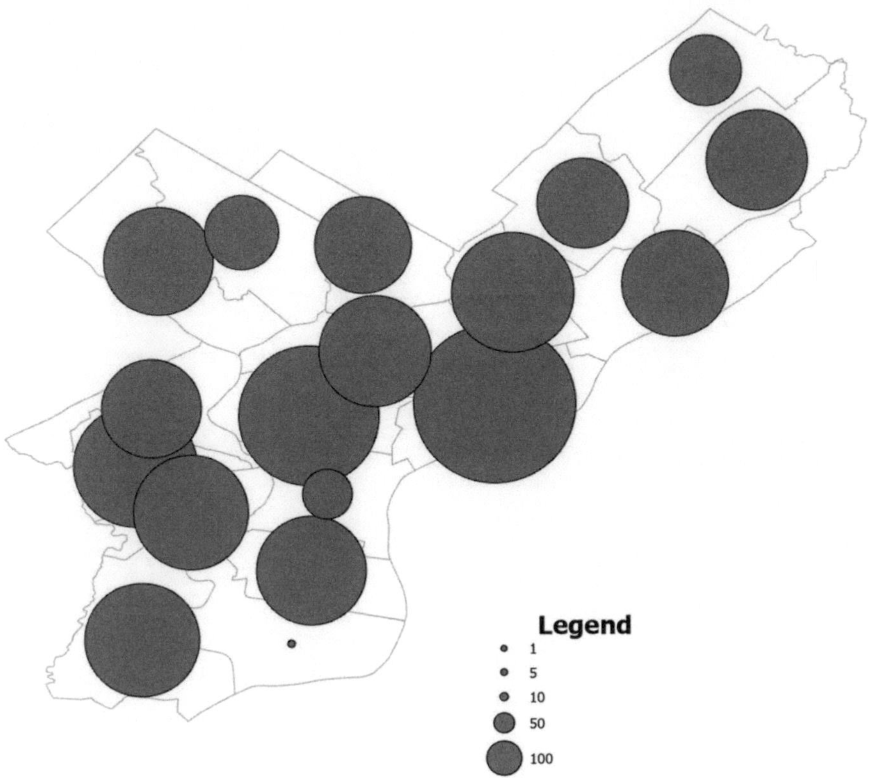

Fig. 29.10 Zip Code Map of Philadelphia Displaying Smoking Attributable Mortality with Proportional Symbology

density [33]. A kernel density map of lung cancer incidence can be found in Fig. 29.11, comparatively, a point density analysis for lung cancer incidence can be found in Fig. 29.12.

Hot Spot Analysis and Heat Maps to Express Continuous Variables

One way to identify geographic distribution of disease is through utilizing spatial and cluster analyses. These analyses can be used to visualize areas of high density or where a cluster of activity occurs. A common tool to display areas of concern is through hot spot analysis.

A common misconception surrounding hot spot analysis is that it can be used interchangeably with the phrase heat map, however, these two tools vary slightly. Heat maps are commonplace, proudly displaying their trademark bright red hues in high-density areas and cooler blues in low-density areas. Heat maps are simply the

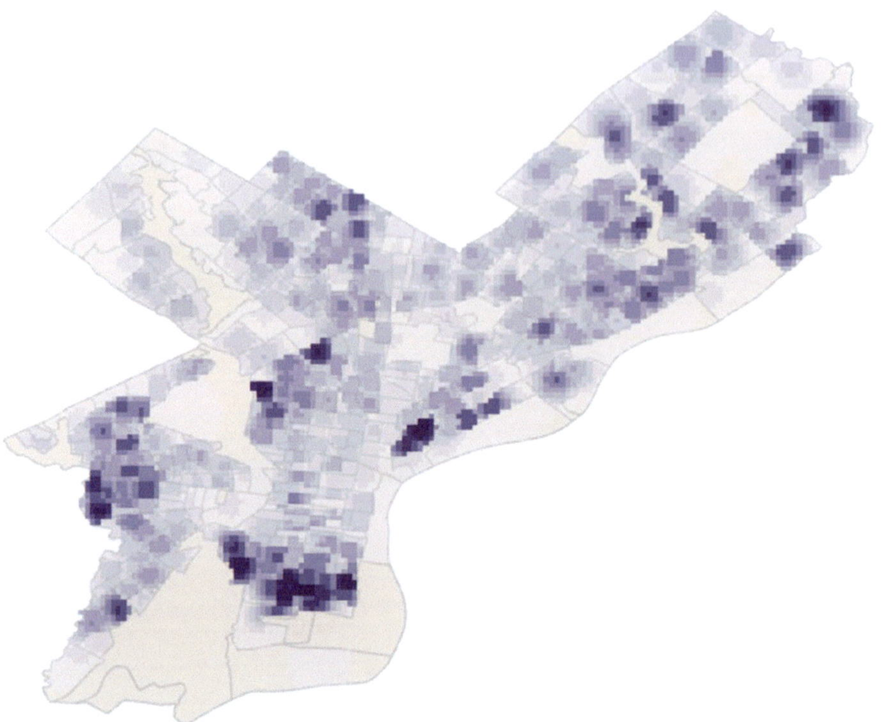

Fig. 29.11 Kernel Density Map of Philadelphia Showcasing Lung Cancer Incidence

result, the physical map, that displays the density of occurrence (Fig. 29.13). However, the visualization is subjective in a sense – the cutoff values for what appears in different colors is up to the cartographer. On one hand this is beneficial as the mapmaker is able to amplify areas of concern, thus influencing the way viewers of the map digest the data [34, 35]. On the other hand, if the visualization will be used to direct resources, drive decisions, or be presented as trustworthy then the validity of the data is paramount [34]. To combat the subjectivity of heat maps, cartographers often conduct a hot spot analysis [34].

A hot spot analysis is a mathematically driven analysis, with the end result presenting statistically significant clusters of increased incidence, displayed in red, and statistically significant clusters of markedly reduced incidence appear in blue [34] (Fig. 29.14). Instead of the mapper having discretion over which elements appear red and which appear blue, a hot spot analysis bases coloration on statistical significance. This allows any decisions based on the interpretation of the map to be rooted in fact, rather than subjective in nature.

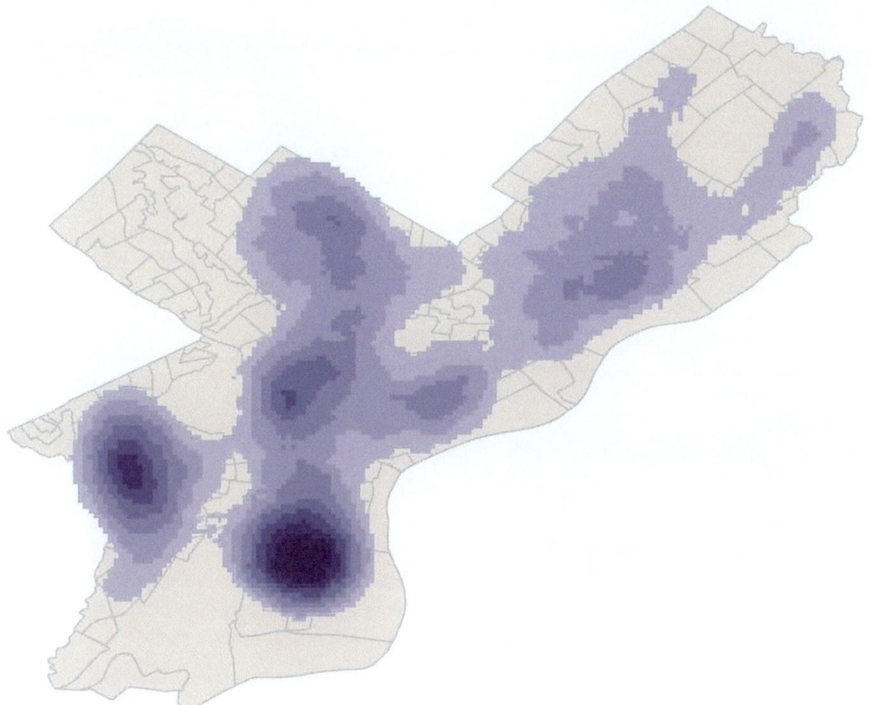

Fig. 29.12 Point Density Map Showing Lung Cancer Incidence In Philadelphia

Time-Series Maps

Time-series maps are useful to view trends over time. All types of maps referenced earlier can be turned into a time-series map by simply including many maps in a layout.

Geographic Targeting for Community-Based Interventions

Eligibility for lung cancer screening by geographic areas smaller than counties are not typically available, and recent studies have estimated lung cancer screening eligibility by neighborhoods [36]. A recent study produced estimates of the number of people eligible for lung cancer screening, the percentage of ever-smokers that were eligible for LCS, and the percentage of older adults eligible for LCS. These types of measures would be helpful in different scenarios where programs are doing outreach to different demographics for LCS services or education.

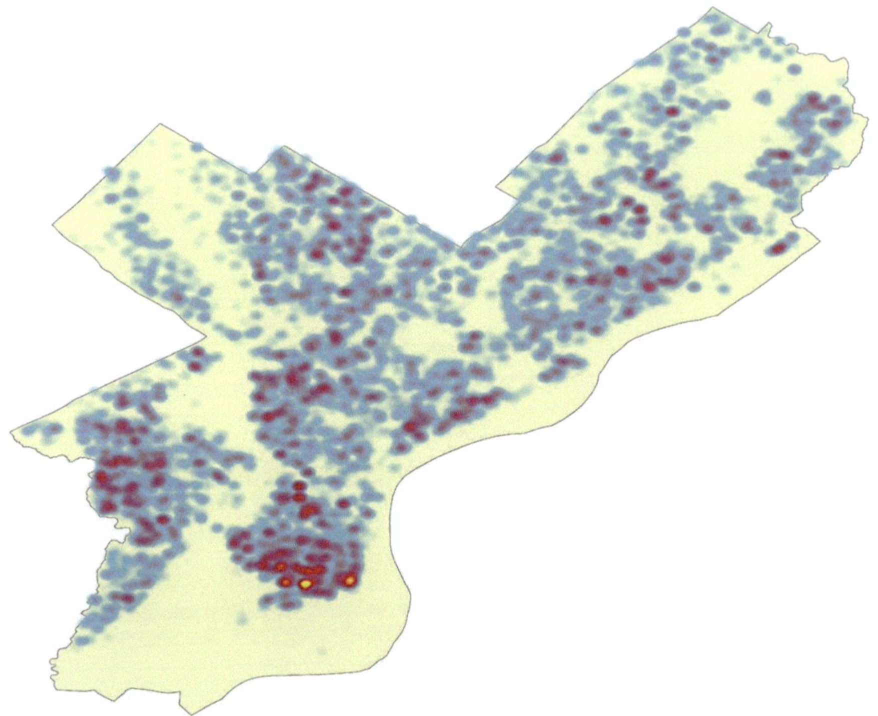

Fig. 29.13 Heat Map of Lung Cancer Incidence in Philadelphia

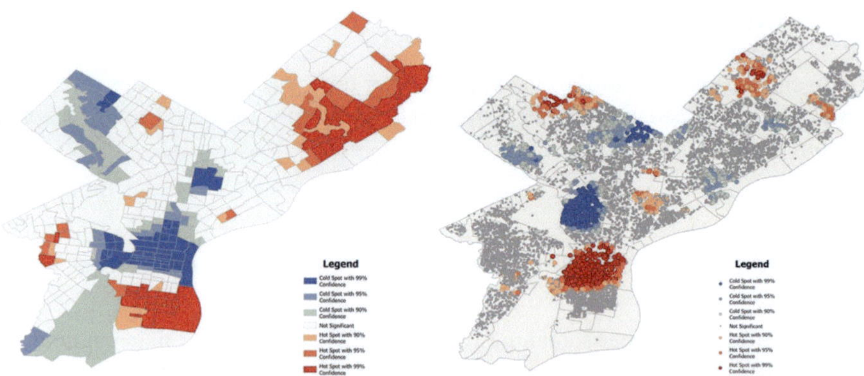

Fig. 29.14 Hot Spot Analysis of Lung Cancer Mortality by Philadelphia Census Tract; hot spot analyses can be choropleth or point in nature

Geocoding and Assessing a Program's Impact

Cancer incidence, mortality, and risk factors show strong geographic patterns. These patterns can inform the etiology of disease, and guide intervention and implementation strategies to reduce cancer risk and poor disease outcomes [37]. Our program has developed an example of using GIS to guide research protocols and identify the geographic areas where evidence-based lung cancer screening interventions can be most impactful. GIS-informed interventions have the potential to identify sub-groups of populations that are most vulnerable and to highlight environmental threats and community-based risk factors that need to be targeted to adequately address health risks. Studies suggest that interventions, such as community-based education and screening programs, have greater impact when they are targeted to at-risk populations that have been underserved and are most likely to benefit [38–40]. A growing number of programs and planning activities rely upon GIS methods to guide health resources to those areas that are most in need of equitable care [40–42].

A geographic approach was undertaken to identify geographic disparities in access to lung cancer screening facilities in the United States [43]. Geographic areas outside of a 40-mile radius of a screening facility were considered unserved. Areas with low access to screening, high smoking prevalence estimates, and high lung cancer mortality rates were identified as priority areas for lung cancer screening services [43]. The goal of our GIS-informed project is to determine areas of need that can be targeted for primary care-based interventions (to help navigate eligible patients to our health system's centralized lung cancer screening program) and community education/outreach to increase lung cancer screening rates of eligible residents in Philadelphia. We have developed a step-by-step process for determining areas of need and primary care providers within our health care system that serve patients in those high-risk areas (Fig. 29.15).

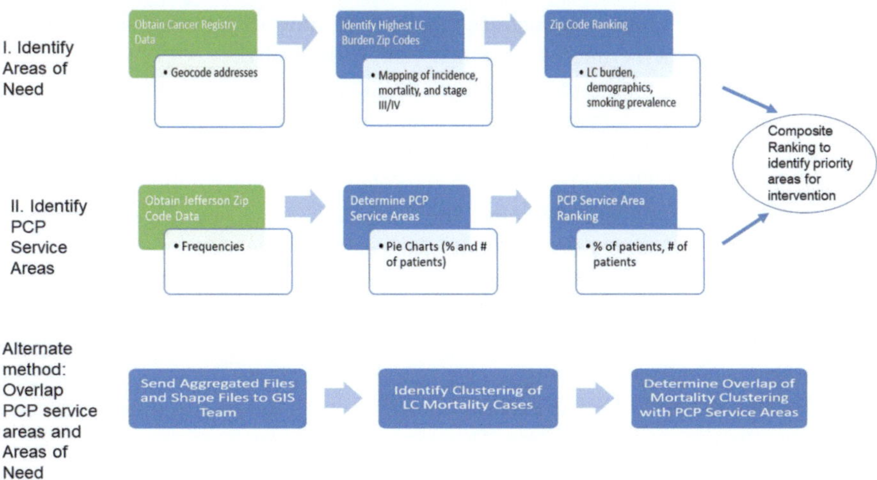

Fig. 29.15 Process for Determining Areas of Need for Clinic- and Community-Based Interventions

The first step in our process is to identify areas of need. We obtain lung cancer data and patient addresses at diagnosis from the state cancer registry. ArcGIS is used to geocode the addresses for mapping. Lung cancer burden is calculated for each zip code represented in the cancer registry. (Smaller geographic areas can be used if data are available.) Lung cancer burden is defined by summing age-standardized incidence rates (SIR), age-standardized mortality rates (SMR), and mean stage at diagnosis [39]. We rank the zip codes by characteristics (e.g., smoking prevalence and older age) that increase lung cancer risk. Zip codes with the highest combined rankings (highest lung cancer burden, oldest median population, and highest smoking prevalence) are designated areas of need for lung cancer screening and smoking cessation efforts. Additional factors that may help identify areas with high percentage of vulnerable populations (% low SES, % minority groups) may be used to further define and target priority areas for interventions.

The second step is to identify local primary care clinic partners within our healthcare system to provide preventive lung cancer care for areas of need. Primary care clinics will provide a linkage to smoking cessation resources for current smokers and determine the eligibility status for lung cancer screening based upon current United States Preventive Services Task Force recommendations. Eligible patients will be referred to local screening programs located in nearby cancer center facilities. Additional resources can be targeted to clinics that serve patients in previously identified areas of need to facilitate the referral process. The key to this step is to target the clinics that serve large numbers of patients residing in affected communities so that we can make impact where it is needed most. Rather than assume that the population served by the clinic are from the immediate surrounding area (zip codes), we will evaluate the residential zip code composition of the current patient population seeking care at each clinic. To accomplish this, we will obtain patient data (race/ethnicity, age, and residential zip code) from our electronic medical records. The patient data will reflect the primary care population within a defined area of our healthcare system's catchment area. We will sort the patient data by zip code and create pie charts to illustrate the absolute number and percentage of our patients served by each clinic over the last year. (Fig. 29.16).

After the creation of the pie charts, we will sort the clinics by the number and percent of patients they serve in each zip code of need. We will prioritize areas with clinics that serve the largest number of patients in the zip codes of greatest need (composite ranking). These clinics will be targeted as partners for clinical education and support for lung cancer referrals. The communities will be targeted for community outreach and education about lung cancer screening.

An alternate method for identifying areas of need is to use GIS techniques to map health system primary care clinics and zip code–level cases of lung cancer mortality (or burden, if preferred) using state cancer registry data (Fig. 29.1). A choropleth map can be created for each primary care practice that shows the % of patients (out of total in Philadelphia) per zip code. This will help us to identify practice service areas for each primary care practice. The service area for each primary care practice should be composed of zip codes that meet the criterion of a sizable percentage and number of patients in the area that are served by the clinic. The cut-point that is used

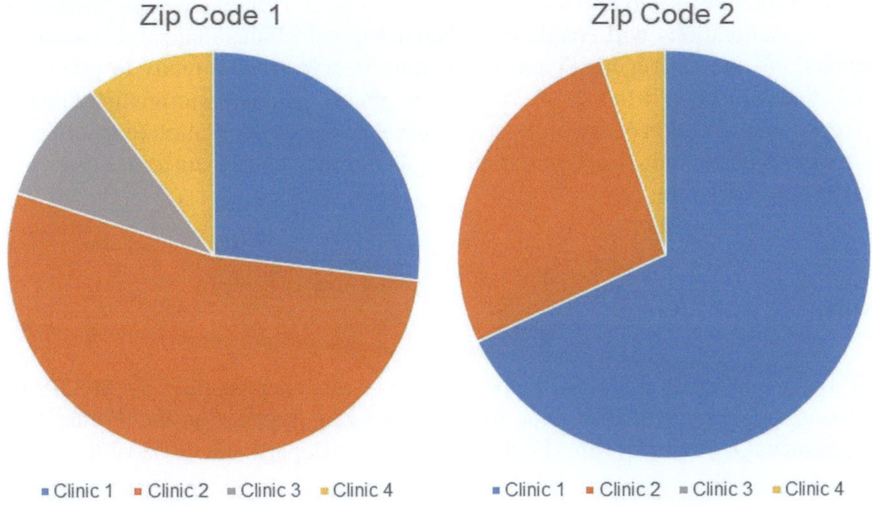

Fig. 29.16 Example of Pie Charts to Guide Prioritization of Primary Care Clinics

to fulfill the criterion may be somewhat arbitrary, depending on the distribution of zip codes served by each clinic. Based upon our preliminary analysis of Jefferson primary care clinics, we observed a range of 1–60% of patients served by our primary care clinics reside in specific zip codes. We found that we can account for more than 50% of our total patient population in each zip code by including clinics serving ≥10% of our patients. To determine each clinic's service area, we will use ≥10% as our cut point for percent of patients served in each zip code. A minimum number of patients from an area with high lung cancer burden may also be considered when defining a clinic's likelihood to engage with and impact a population of great need.

If it has been determined that clinics serve the majority of the populations in the immediate vicinity, then clinics can be chosen based on proximity to the area of greatest need (with the greatest lung cancer mortality). Additional mapping can be conducted to overlay other area-level characteristics describing lifestyle behaviors and sociodemographics (e.g., prevalence of smoking, older age-groups) for additional layers of prioritization. Another benefit of mapping is that a decision can be made to combine contiguous zip codes (rather than individual zip codes) in the assessment of the criterion for serving a specific percentage (and number) of the patient population in a geographic area. The resulting maps will indicate geographic areas with greatest need and the nearby clinics that are most likely to serve the greatest number of patients in those areas.

Ultimately, our plan is to use these techniques to identify and engage primary care practices in the delivery of evidence-based interventions. We plan to develop a health-system wide primary care–based lung cancer screening initiative involving clinical practices that serve areas of need. Carefully placed screening access can help minimize costs and provide timely medical care to vulnerable populations [44]. These collaborations will enable us to better support clinics that serve vulnerable populations and deliver lung cancer screening interventions directly to patients in areas that will benefit the most. We will be able to evaluate various methods for effective identification of areas of need, intervention implementation (e.g., intervention reach, barrier reduction), and improvement of lung cancer outcomes (e.g., lung cancer screening rates).

Note

All maps were created solely for the purpose of this chapter utilizing ArcGIS Pro utilizing publicly available data from the United States Census, Philadelphia Department Of Public Health, and the Pennsylvania Department OF Health [45–48].

References

1. American Cancer Society. Key statistics for lung cancer. Atlanta: American Cancer Society; 2022. [updated February 14th, 2022]. https://www.cancer.org/cancer/lung-cancer/about/key-statistics.html#:~:text=The%20American%20Cancer%20Society's%20estimates,men%20and%2061%2C360%20in%20women.
2. Noone AMHN, Krapcho M, Miller D, Brest A, Yu M, Ruhl J, Tatalovich Z, Mariotto A, Lewis DR, Chen HS, Feùer EJ, Cronin KA, (eds). SEER cancer statistics review, 1975–2015. Bethesda, MD: National Cancer Institute; 2017. [updated September 10th, 2018. based on November 2017 SEER data submission, posted to the SEER web site, April 8]. https://seer.cancer.gov/archive/csr/1975_2015/.
3. National Lung Screening Trial Research T, Aberle DR, Adams AM, Berg CD, Black WC, Clapp JD, et al. Reduced lung-cancer mortality with low-dose computed tomographic screening. N Engl J Med. 2011;365(5):395–409.
4. American Lung Association. State of lung cancer. Chicago, IL: American Lung Association; 2022. p. 2022.
5. Giordano R. Where do you live? It may give clues to how old you'll grow, federal data suggests. Philadelphia, PA: The Philadelphia Inquirer; 2018. [updated December 18th, 2018. https://www.inquirer.com/health/life-expectancy-project-philadelphia-new-jersey-census-tract-20181218.html.
6. Fedewa SA, Kazerooni EA, Studts JL, Smith RA, Bandi P, Sauer AG, et al. State variation in low-dose computed tomography scanning for lung cancer screening in the United States. J Natl Cancer Inst. 2020;113(8):1044–52.
7. Odahowski CL, Zahnd WE, Eberth JM. Challenges and opportunities for lung cancer screening in rural America. J Am Coll Radiol. 2019;16(4, Part B):590–5.
8. Liu B, Dharmarajan K, Henschke CI, Taioli E. State-level variations in the utilization of lung cancer screening among Medicare fee-for-service beneficiaries: an analysis of the 2015 to 2017 physician and other supplier data. Chest. 2020;157(4):1012–20.
9. Bryan L, Westmaas L, Alcaraz K, Jemal A. Cigarette smoking and cancer screening underutilization by state: BRFSS 2010. Nicotine Tob Res. 2014;16(9):1183–9.
10. Levy DT, Romano E, Mumford E. The relationship of smoking cessation to sociodemographic characteristics, smoking intensity, and tobacco control policies. Nicotine Tob Res. 2005;7(3):387–96.

11. Ross K, Kramer MR, Jemal A. Geographic inequalities in progress against lung cancer among women in the United States, 1990–2015. Cancer Epidemiol Biomark Prev. 2018;27(11):1261–4.
12. Centers for Disease Control and Prevention. State tobacco activities tracking and evaluation (STATE) system. Atlanta: Centers for Disease Control and Prevention; 2022. https://www.cdc.gov/statesystem.
13. American Lung Association. Smokefree Air Laws [updated November 17th, 2022]. https://www.lung.org/policy-advocacy/tobacco/smokefree-environments/smokefree-air-laws.
14. United States Department of Agriculture: Economic Research Service. Rural poverty & well-being. Washington, DC: United States Department of Agriculture.
15. Centers for Disease Control and Prevention. Geographic Regions and Commercial Tobacco. Health disparities and ways to advance health equity. Atlanta: Centers for Disease Control and Prevention; 2022.
16. Kale MS, Wisnivesky J, Taioli E, Liu B. The landscape of US lung cancer screening services. Chest. 2019;155(5):900–7.
17. Zahnd WE, James AS, Jenkins WD, Izadi SR, Fogleman AJ, Steward DE, et al. Rural–urban differences in cancer incidence and trends in the United States. Cancer Epidemiol Biomark Prev. 2018;27(11):1265–74.
18. Henley SJ, Anderson RN, Thomas CC, Massetti GM, Peaker B, Richardson LC. Invasive cancer incidence, 2004–2013, and deaths, 2006–2015, in nonmetropolitan and metropolitan counties—United States. MMWR Surveill Summ. 2017;66(14):1.
19. Krieger N, Chen JT, Waterman PD, Soobader M-J, Subramanian S, Carson R. Geocoding and monitoring of US socioeconomic inequalities in mortality and cancer incidence: does the choice of area-based measure and geographic level matter? The public health disparities geocoding project. Am J Epidemiol. 2002;156(5):471–82.
20. Beyer KM, Schultz AF, Rushton G. Using ZIP codes as geocodes in cancer research. Geocoding health data: The use of geographic codes in cancer prevention and control, research and practice. Abingdon: Routledge; 2008. p. 37–68.
21. Goodchild MF. Geocoding and geosampling. Spatial statistics and models. Cham: Springer; 1984. p. 33.
22. Rushton G, Armstrong MP, Gittler J, Greene BR, Pavlik CE, West MM, et al. Geocoding in cancer research: a review. Am J Prev Med. 2006;30(2):S16–24.
23. Rushton G, Armstrong MP, Gittler J, Greene BR, Pavlik CE, West MM, et al. Geocoding health data: the use of geographic codes in cancer prevention and control, research and practice. Boca Raton, FL: CRC; 2007.
24. Goldberg DW. A geocoding best practices guide. Springfield, IL: North American Association of Cancer Registries; 2008.
25. Andresen MA, Malleson N, Steenbeek W, Townsley M, Vandeviver C. Minimum geocoding match rates: an international study of the impact of data and areal unit sizes. Int J Geogr Inf Sci. 2020;34(7):1306–22.
26. Zandbergen PA. Ensuring confidentiality of geocoded health data: assessing geographic masking strategies for individual-level data. Adv Med. 2014;2014:1.
27. Richardson DB, Volkow ND, Kwan M-P, Kaplan RM, Goodchild MF, Croyle RT. Spatial turn in health research. Science. 2013;339(6126):1390–2.
28. Brownstein JS, Cassa CA, Mandl KD. No place to hide—reverse identification of patients from published maps. N Engl J Med. 2006;355(16):1741–2.
29. Rey SJ, Arribas-Bel D, Wolf LJ. Geographic data science with python. Boca Raton, FL: CRC; 2020.
30. ArcGIS Pro. Graduated symbols. Redlands, CA: ESRI. https://pro.arcgis.com/en/pro-app/latest/help/mapping/layer-properties/graduated-symbols.htm.
31. ArcGIS. Proportional symbols. Redlands, CA: ESRI. https://pro.arcgis.com/en/pro-app/latest/help/mapping/layer-properties/proportional-symbology.htm.
32. ArcGIS. How kernel density works. Redlands, CA: ESRI. https://desktop.arcgis.com/en/arcmap/10.3/tools/spatial-analyst-toolbox/how-kernel-density-works.htm.
33. ArcGIS. How point density works. Redlands, CA: ESRI. https://desktop.arcgis.com/en/arcmap/10.3/tools/spatial-analyst-toolbox/how-point-density-works.htm.

34. Rosenshein L. Extending your map with spatial analysis. Redlands, CA: ESRI. https://resources.arcgis.com/en/communities/analysis/017z00000015000000.htm.
35. Grubesic T, Murray A. Detecting hot spots using cluster analysis and GIS. 2001.
36. McIntire RK, Lewis E, Zeigler-Johnson C, Shusted C, Barta J, Juon H-S, et al. Estimating eligibility for lung cancer screening by neighborhood in Philadelphia using previous and current USPSTF guidelines. Popul Health Manag. 2022;25(2):254–63.
37. Schootman M, Gomez SL, Henry KA, Paskett ED, Ellison GL, Oh A, et al. Geospatial approaches to cancer control and population sciences. Cancer Epidemiol Biomark Prev. 2017;26(4):472–5.
38. Zeigler-Johnson C, Madsen R, Keith SW, Glanz K, Quinn AM, Giri VN, et al. Testing a prostate cancer educational intervention in high-burden neighborhoods. J Racial Ethn Health Disparities. 2021;9:2477.
39. McIntire RK, Keith SW, Boamah M, Leader AE, Glanz K, Klassen AC, et al. A prostate cancer composite score to identify high burden neighborhoods. Prev Med. 2018;112:47–53.
40. MacQuillan EL, Curtis AB, Baker KM, Paul R, Back YO. Using GIS mapping to target public health interventions: examining birth outcomes across GIS techniques. J Community Health. 2017;42(4):633–8.
41. Ali D, Levin A, Abdulkarim M, Tijjani U, Ahmed B, Namalam F, et al. A cost-effectiveness analysis of traditional and geographic information system-supported microplanning approaches for routine immunization program management in northern Nigeria. Vaccine. 2020;38(6):1408–15.
42. Lofters AK, Gozdyra P, Lobb R. Using geographic methods to inform cancer screening interventions for south Asians in Ontario, Canada. BMC Public Health. 2013;13:395.
43. Sahar L, Douangchai Wills VL, Liu KK, Kazerooni EA, Dyer DS, Smith RA. Using geospatial analysis to evaluate access to lung cancer screening in the United States. Chest. 2021;159(2):833–44.
44. Altaweel M. In: Dempsey C, editor. GIS lounge [Internet]. Santa Clara, CA: Elite CafeMedia; 2018. [cited 2022]. https://www.gislounge.com/gis-cancer-screening/.
45. Environmental Systems Research Institute. ArcGIS Pro (2.9.3). Redlands, CA: ESRI.
46. City Of Philadelphia. Permits, violations & licenses. Tobacco retailers. Philadelphia, PA: City Of Philadelphia.
47. Philadelphia Department of Public Health. 2017 community health assessment (CHA) Philadelphia PA. Philadelphia, PA: Philadelphia Department of Public Health; 2017.
48. Bureau USC. American Community Survey: ACS 5-year estimates. 2020. https://data.census.gov/cedsci/table?t=Income%20and%20Poverty&g=0400000US42%240500000&tid=ACSST5Y2019.S1701.

Chapter 30
The Essential Ingredient of Partnership: The Bristol Myers Squibb Foundation's Collaboration Focused Approach to Health Equity and Lung Cancer Screening

Patricia M. Doykos and Priscilla L. Ko

A Mission Rooted in the Power of Partnerships

The mission of the Bristol Myers Squibb Foundation is to promote health equity and improve the health outcomes of populations disproportionately affected by serious diseases by strengthening healthcare worker capacity, integrating medical care and community-based supportive services, and mobilizing communities in the fight against serious diseases and conditions. The Foundation engages partners to develop, test, and sustain innovative interventions and clinic–community partnerships to help underserved patients access care and support for cancer in the United States, China, Brazil, and nine countries in Africa, and for cardiovascular and immunological diseases in the United States. Funding is provided to create and test health equity innovations that strengthen health systems and community resources for patient engagement and social support. Robust monitoring and evaluation are employed to help grantees demonstrate the effectiveness and value of the programs to stakeholders, such as health system administrators, payers, and policymakers who can enable long-term sustainability and scaling.

The Foundation team identifies areas of high unmet need in populations that are disproportionately affected by the serious diseases of focus and selects partners with expertise and innovative ideas for solutions to improve equitable access to care, quality of care, and health outcomes. In December 2013, the United States Preventive Services Task Force (USPSTF) issued its initial Grade B recommendation of annual screening for lung cancer with low-dose computed tomography (LDCT) for asymptomatic persons aged 55–80 years who have a 30-pack or more per year smoking history and currently smoke or have quit within the past 15 years [1]. This was followed in 2014 by the Center for Medicare and Medicaid Services national coverage

P. M. Doykos (✉) · P. L. Ko
The Bristol Myers Squibb Foundation, New York, NY, USA
e-mail: patricia.doykos@bms.com; Priscilla.ko@utexas.edu

G. C. Kane et al. (eds.), *Lung Cancer Screening*,
https://doi.org/10.1007/978-3-031-33596-9_30

329

determination [2]. In turn, also in 2014, the Foundation launched a lung cancer screening initiative focused on the "tobacco belt" spanning several states in Appalachia and the southeastern United States as well as on other communities with high smoking rates and lung cancer burden including Philadelphia (Fig. 30.1).

The Foundation sought to help ensure that this new standard of care for lung cancer screening and detection was not delayed in reaching high risk communities further widening healthcare and health disparity gaps. Coincident with the issuance of the new screening guidelines, a new and revolutionary era of immuno-oncology treatment was also being ushered in with the potential to improve clinical outcomes and quality of life for cancer patients. This treatment advance further underscored the importance of ensuring equity in annual screening and early detection opportunities for patients at high risk for lung cancer due to their smoking history.

Partnership is the essential ingredient that stands at the center of the Foundation's approach to health equity. The most important partner is the very community that the grantee and implementing partners are looking to positively impact. Consultation

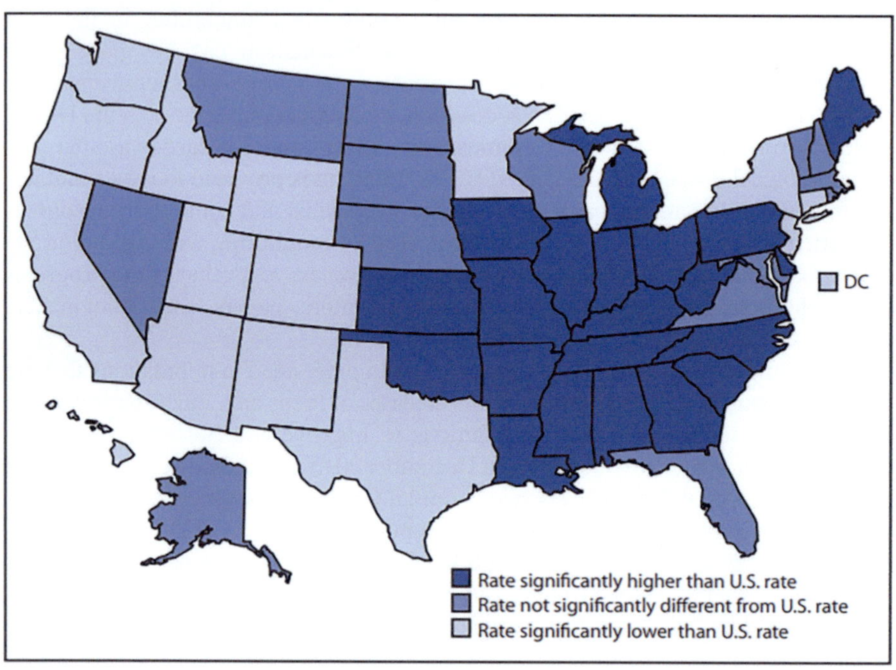

Abbreviation: DC = District of Columbia.

* As underlying cause of death, lung cancer deaths are identified with *International Classification of Diseases, Tenth Revision* codes C33 and C34.

† Deaths per 100,000 population are age-adjusted to the 2000 U.S. standard population, for a U.S. rate of 34.8.

Fig. 30.1 Courtesy of US National Vital Statistics System, 2018

and engagement with the community is critical and seen as part of a broader idea of community mobilization. It is not limited to advising a project prior to implementation, but part of an ongoing process and bidirectional engagement to inform, drive, and ensure aspects of the project including needs assessments, community strength and asset mapping, metrics creation, intervention and service delivery, continuous improvement, communication, and sustainability and scaling strategies. With the heightened and broadened understanding of the social and structural determinants of health driving inequities, there is a demand for meaningful and coordinated action that ties together health and community development actors and non-traditional partners who have strong ties, a long-standing presence, and the trust of communities. The Foundation emphasizes clinic–community partnerships that address barriers that patients face inside and outside the clinic. It supports not only the work of the clinical and community partners to deliver a program or intervention, but also provides for the resources and time needed for new and nontraditional partners to build strong working relationships and co-create operating norms and systems.

Co-Developing Solutions in Lung Health Through Clinic–Community Partnerships

Clinic–community partnerships are interdependent to co-develop solutions and deliver equitable lung cancer treatment, care, and support to underserved populations across the care continuum. Organizations share a common and aligned goal of improving the health of their communities and these linkages help coordinate health care delivery, promote community involvement in health strategies and implementation to reduce and prevent disease [3]. These partnerships allow a shared value and focus on both the medical complexities of lung cancer while also acknowledging the social determinants of health to create a community-centered approach.

Jefferson Health's Lung Cancer Learning Community serves as an exemplary model of clinic–community partnerships in its engagement of diverse stakeholders to increase shared decision making and lung cancer screening in vulnerable populations across Philadelphia. Through partnerships with local community-based organizations and primary care practices, there have been numerous lessons in understanding community needs and how to effectively engage patients from diverse populations including: Blacks/African Americans, Asian immigrants, veterans, and LBGTQ people. It is imperative for clinic–community partnerships to implement lung cancer screening and ensure access for disproportionately affected populations. For instance, some of the local social service providers such as Southeast Asian Mutual Assistance Association Coalition, Cambodian Association of Greater Philadelphia, and African Family Health Organization participated in a community needs assessment and facilitated interviews to describe the knowledge, attitudes, and beliefs of lung cancer and lung cancer screening in diverse communities. These assessments aided the Jefferson Health team to understand the medical and social barriers hindering patients to lung cancer screening and how to design the educational programming to be more culturally humble and linguistically appropriate. The feedback and sharing from the community have allowed a broader conversation of lung health as the model seeks to address the entire continuum of care with lung cancer prevention efforts such as tobacco cessation all the way through to provide treatment, care, and support for patients diagnosed with lung cancer.

Leveraging Best Practices Through a Learning Collaborative Network

Although the project at Jefferson Health focused on an urban initiative for Philadelphia and surrounding counties, its Lung Cancer Learning Community drew in and exchanged lessons with lung cancer screening initiatives delivered in rural settings including two statewide initiatives supported by the Foundation in Kentucky and Maine. With Kentucky ranked first in the country for lung cancer deaths, The Kentucky Lung Cancer Education Awareness Detection and Survivorship (LEADS) Collaborative was the Foundation's first lung cancer grantee. The Kentucky LEADS Collaborative was launched in 2014 as a community-engaged effort forged by the University of Kentucky, the University of Louisville, the Kentucky Cancer Consortium, and the GO2Foundation to educate primary care providers about the new screening guidelines and strengthen tobacco cessation, early detection, and survivorship efforts.

A few years later in 2017, the Maine Lung Cancer Coalition was launched in response to the new annual screening recommendation and Maine's rate of new lung cancer cases being among the highest in the nation. The coalition was a co-funded effort by the Bristol Myers Squibb Foundation, Maine Cancer Foundation, and the Maine Economic Improvement Fund to support the coalition's multi-sector partnership led by the Maine Medical Center Research Institute with two main goals: (1) engaging and educating the public, patients, healthcare providers, payers, and policymakers about evidence-based lung cancer prevention and screening services; and (2) developing and evaluating innovative community-based strategies to increase access to evidence-based lung cancer prevention, screening, and treatment services to the Maine population, focusing on high-risk individuals in rural and underserved communities. Collectively, these programs validate the utility, effectiveness, and replicability of the Learning Community model in both urban and rural settings. Rural populations experience several barriers to healthcare access due to health professional shortages and long distances to receive specialty care. Yet, the need for lung cancer preventative and screening interventions, provider education, and community engagement and mobilization are relevant for all communities. The project partners, geographic area and populations of focus, and intervention descriptions from the three projects are listed in Table 30.1.

Table 30.1 The Bristol Myers Squibb Foundation's partners in lung cancer screening

Grantee/Partners	Geographic area and populations of focus	Description of intervention
Main grantee: Jefferson Health Implementing partners: Philadelphia Chinatown Development Corp, Southeast Asian Mutual Assistance Association Coalition, Cambodian Association of Greater Philadelphia, African Family Health Organization, Veterans Multi-Services Agency, LGBT Elder Initiative, etc.	Philadelphia (citywide/urban) Populations of focus: Blacks/African Americans, Asian immigrants, veterans, and LBGTQ, low SES, elderly	**Aim 1:** Engage a learning community of Jefferson Health patients, providers, community partners, and other stakeholders **Aim 2**: Adapt and implement lung cancer screening program in Jefferson Health primary and specialty care practices **Aim 3**: Evaluate screening program implementation processes, assess program outcomes, and disseminate findings
Main grantee: Maine Lung Cancer Coalition Implementing partners: Maine Medical Center, MaineGeneral Medical Center, MaineHealth, the University of Southern Maine, American Lung Association Funding partners: Maine Cancer Foundation, Maine Economic Improvement Fund	Maine (statewide/rural) Populations of focus: Low SES, uninsured, elderly	**Aim 1:** Engage and educate the public, patients, health care providers, health care payers, and policymakers about evidence-based lung cancer prevention and screening practices **Aim 2:** Develop, implement, and evaluate innovative programs to increase access to evidence-based lung cancer prevention, screening, and treatment services to the entire Maine population, including residents of rural underserved areas
Main grantee: KY LEADS Implementing partners: The University of Kentucky, the University of Louisville, the Kentucky Cancer Consortium, and the GO2Foundation	Kentucky (statewide) Populations of focus: Low SES, Medicaid, uninsured, elderly	**Aim 1**: Educate primary care clinicians to improve their knowledge, generate favorable attitudes, and enhance clinical practice behaviors related to facilitating lung cancer risk reduction, screening, diagnosis, treatment, and survivorship **Aim 2**: Develop a novel precision survivorship care intervention to improve quality of life, facilitate behavior change, and support patient engagement among individuals diagnosed with lung cancer and their caregivers **Aim 3**: Develop, implement, and evaluate the QUILS system, a toolkit incorporating assessment, audit, and feedback, a resource portal designed to enhance quality of lung cancer screening services

More Than Funding to Sustain Partnerships, Services, and Outcomes

In addition to financial resources, the Foundation also supports partners through technical assistance that drive sustainability and advance enabling policies. The Foundation provides grant funding to Harvard Law School's Center for Health Law and Policy Innovation to work one-on-one with grantee partners to sustain their services through policy analysis and research, public payer engagement, and policy-maker education and advocacy efforts. Jefferson Health was a recipient of this technical assistance support leading to a series of interviews with local health systems and health plans on lung cancer screening reimbursement and qualifications. These findings were ultimately published in a 2021 white paper entitled, *Engaging a Learning Community to Achieve the Promise of Lung Cancer Screening* [4].

The Foundation also supports partnership by facilitating a community of practice and actively building community among its grantees, implementing partners and the members of its Expert Advisory Council which is made up of national leaders in health equity, medicine, healthcare delivery, community-based action, patient supportive services, and public policy. Through virtual workshops and an annual grantee summit, the Foundation gathers these partners together to connect, share, learn, and forge independent collaborative efforts. It offers workshops, seminars, and other resources to help partners leverage learnings about what does and does not work and build capacity to better deliver services and care to their community. The annual summit program includes plenary sessions with prominent and inspiring leaders in health equity and social justice, capacity building workshops, grantee presentations on progress and lessons learned, and unstructured social time for grantees to learn more about each other's organizations, goals, and priorities. These convenings also generate camaraderie among partners from hearing one another's challenges, accomplishments, and insights.

Finally, the Foundation seeks to forge and leverage funding and resource partnerships with other foundations and through public–private partnerships. In Philadelphia, the Foundation and Jefferson engaged the Department of Health whose commissioner was prioritizing reduction of smoking related illness and deaths in the city. In Maine, the Foundation served as lead funder and engaged the Maine Cancer Foundation and the Maine Economic Improvement Fund to provide additional funding. In fact, the Maine Cancer Foundation is sustaining the coalition as the "Maine Lung Cancer Coalition – 2nd Generation."

Lessons in Fostering Partnership for Funders

Foundations and other philanthropic funders can enhance the outcomes and impact of their funding through partnership in three important ways:

- Encourage multi-partner proposals for grant funding
- Provide adequate funding and grant terms to allow grant project partners to get to know each other, develop ways of working, and integrate their assets and services to best serve patients and close disparity gaps
- Amplify grant funding and the impact of projects through technical assistance, communities of practice, and grantee convenings
- Reach out to local philanthropic funders and government to draw in additional dollars and leverage resources for grantee projects

In the case of Jefferson Health's Lung Cancer Screening, the grantee took things one step further and itself created a partnership platform for collecting and sharing learnings to further ensure a fair and just opportunity for Philadelphians who are underserved and at risk of lung cancer to access and benefit from annual screening and earlier detection services and achieve their optimal health.

References

1. US Preventive Services Task Force, Krist AH, Davidson KW, Mangione CM, Barry MJ, Cabana M, Caughey AB, Davis EM, Donahue KE, Doubeni CA, Kubik M, Landefeld CS, et al. Screening for lung cancer: US preventative services task force recommendation statement. JAMA. 2021;325(10):962–70.
2. CMS. Medicare Coverage of Screening for Lung Cancer with Low Dose Computer Tomography (LDCT). https://www.cms.gov/medicare-coverage-database/view/ncacal-decision-memo.aspx?proposed=N&NCAId=274. Accessed 5 Feb 2015.
3. Clinical-Community Linkages. Content last reviewed December 2016. Agency for Healthcare Research and Quality, Rockville, MD. https://www.ahrq.gov/ncepcr/tools/community/index.html.
4. Engaging a Learning Community to Achieve the Promise of Lung Cancer Screening. https://www.jefferson.edu/content/dam/tju/jmc/files/medical_oncology/popsci/Jefferson%20LC2%20White%20Paper%2006092021.pdf. Accessed 9 June 2021.

Part VII
On the Horizon: What Lies Ahead in Lung Cancer Screening

Chapter 31
Lung Cancer Screening in Health Systems: Needs, Challenges, and Opportunities

Jennifer Elston Lafata, Christine Neslund-Dudas, and Ronald E. Myers

Background

Health care in the United States (US) is increasingly provided within the context of vertically integrated health systems that include two of more organizations that affiliate to provide health care services, often to defined populations. Health systems play an important role in public health by delivering cancer screening and other care to diverse populations. Schmit et al. (2021) reported that the successful implementation of health system change in cancer-related care is influenced by the alignment of goals among organization leaders, agreement on logistical steps related to implementation, and acceptance of new roles and responsibilities [1]. Health systems have the opportunity to successfully implement lung cancer screening (LCS) programs, a choice that is likely to be accompanied by organizational change. While the alignment of organizational leadership on issues related to LCS is needed to launch different types of LCS programs, factors that facilitate successful implementation of such programs are not well documented. Furthermore, recent studies of organizational change in the context of LCS suggest that health systems that seek to

J. E. Lafata (✉)
Division of Pharmaceutical Outcomes and Policy, Eshelman School of
Pharmacy and UNC Lineberger Comprehensive Cancer Center, University of North Carolina
at Chapel Hill, Chapel Hill, NC, USA
e-mail: JEL@email.unc.edu

C. Neslund-Dudas
Division of Thoracic and Esophageal Surgery, Department of Surgery, Thoms Jefferson
University, Philadelphia, PA, USA
e-mail: Cdudas1@hfhs.org

R. E. Myers
Division of Population Science, Department of Medical Oncology, Thomas Jefferson
University, Philadelphia, PA, USA
e-mail: Ronald.Myers@Jefferson.edu

     339
G. C. Kane et al. (eds.), *Lung Cancer Screening*,
https://doi.org/10.1007/978-3-031-33596-9_31

identify and address a range of factors and also seek to meet community needs [2] are positioned for success.

In this chapter, we review existing health system-based models of LCS and current LCS practices. We also explore the utility of an implementation framework [3] to guide the effective design and implementation of successful LCS programs in health systems. We conclude with a discussion of opportunities to enhance LCS programs and increase LCS equity.

Lung Cancer Screening Process and Existing Care Models

The LCS Process: Lam and Tammemagi [4] describe the "core pathway" to LCS as including patient recruitment, eligibility assessment, discussion of screening risks and benefits, completion of a low dose chest computed tomography (LDCT) scan, and follow-up of screening results. Rendle et al. [5] suggest that implementation of this core pathway requires multiple steps, including patient identification, eligibility assessment, recruitment, education, shared decision making (SDM), provider ordering of and referral for screening, completion of an initial screening test, and follow-up (repeat screening in a year for patients with a normal screening test result or near-term surveillance or diagnostic evaluation for patients with an abnormal screening test result). In the US, health systems and affiliated primary care providers play a central role in making cancer screening, including LCS, available to diverse populations. Wernli et al. [6] have argued that the effective implementation of LCS is more likely in health systems that take steps to identify and engage key stakeholders in the screening process, support the coordination of care across primary care and specialty practices, and use multiple communication channels, including electronic health record (EHR)-based tools and outreach contacts to engage providers and patients in initial screening, repeat screening, and the follow-up of abnormal screening test results.

Decentralized and Centralized LCS Programs. Tabriz et al. [7] described two major types of health system–based LCS programs. In the first type of program, health systems may use a decentralized approach (Fig. 31.1), where "front-end practitioners," often primary care providers, identify patients who are eligible for screening, educate eligible patients about screening, complete SDM, order a screening exam, facilitate follow-up (i.e., annual repeat screening for persons with a normal test result or nearterm surveillance or diagnostic evaluation for those who have an abnormal result), and deliver smoking cessation treatment, as needed.

The second approach (Fig. 31.2) is more centralized. Specifically, health systems encourage front-end practitioners to identify patients eligible for screening, educate eligible patients about screening, determine patient interest in screening, and refer eligible patients to a centralized, health system LCS program. At this point, LCS program personnel reach out to referred patients, complete the shared decision-making process, schedule a screening appointment, arrange for follow-up, and provide referral to or services for tobacco treatment. Some organizations report simultaneously using each type of program independently, or evolving from one type of program to another, or both [7].

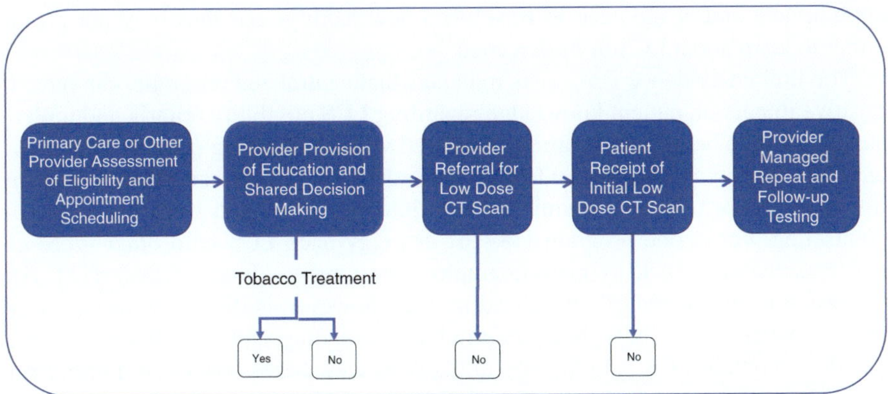

Fig. 31.1 Decentralized lung cancer screening model

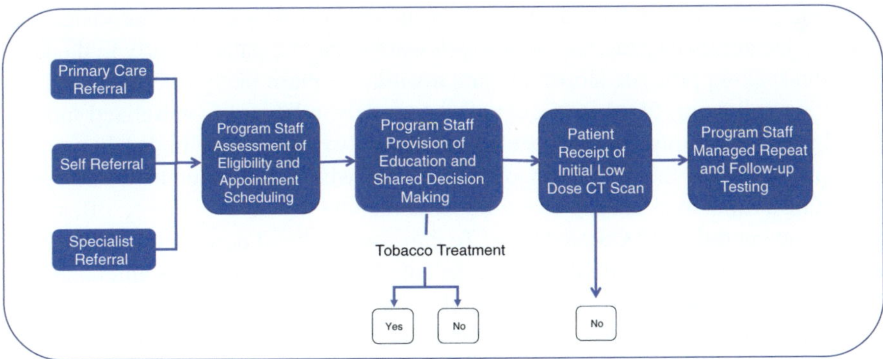

Fig. 31.2 Centralized lung cancer screening model

Currently, there is not consensus among experts regarding which model serves best to promote high quality SDM, increase initial and serial LCS use, and/or advance equity across the LCS continuum [8, 9]. This lack of consensus stems in part from the evidence base surrounding the advantages and disadvantages of these two models which remains in its infancy. When asked, those responsible for overseeing health system–based LCS programs have described a perceived access-quality tradeoff between the two types of programs [7]. Some evidence, albeit limited, now indicates that centralized programs have higher levels of LCS adherence and follow-up [10–12].

Centralized programs are perceived of as offering better SDM quality, relative to decentralized programs (because decision counseling is provided by a relatively small group of highly trained practitioners in centralized programs) [7]. Yet, at the same time, centralized programs are viewed as offering diminished access to LCS relative to decentralized programs [7]. The latter impression is related to the likelihood that only a small number of individuals who are determined to be eligible for LCS are identified and offered screening and because those individuals who are referred for screening face additional access barriers (e.g., an additional appointment and/or the need to travel to a new facility) and thus may not go on either to learn about LCS or be screened.

The limited evidence that exists indicates that centralized programs can have a positive impact on patient knowledge regarding LCS eligibility criteria and understanding of the benefits and harms associated with LCS among patients who present for a screening appointment [13]. Centralized programs can also provide an important opportunity for organizations to integrate SDM and smoking cessation counseling within one program [14–16] or piggy-back LCS onto other types of cancer screening, such as mammography screening for breast cancer [17]. An important disadvantage of centralized models, however, is that SDM occurs only among patients who have been referred for screening and thus likely to have decided to obtain LCS, and thereby unlikely to view SDM when they present for screening as meaningful or beneficial. Ideally, SDM should happen prior to a screening test being ordered, when patients have time to consider the information received, express their preferences, and decide whether or not to undergo screening [8].

Having providers initiate SDM at the time of a primary care office visit, as is done in decentralized programs, is a step toward engaging patients early in the LCS decision-making process. However, patients may be more likely to opt out of LCS screening following SDM in decentralized models, relative to centralized models [13, 18, 19]. Recommended repeat screening is also likely to be higher in centralized programs, as the follow-up of individuals who were adherent to an initial screening is included among the suite of screening services typically offered to patients in centralized LCS programs. To date, only a small number of studies have assessed the impact of centralized and decentralized models on LCS annual adherence and/or follow-up [10–12]. Although adherence was found to be suboptimal across the board, each study found centralized models lead to better adherence. In addition, patients screened by centralized programs were more likely to meet established screening eligibility criteria [12] and centralized screening programs also appeared to ameliorate race disparities in adherence and follow-up relative to that observed in decentralized programs [10].

It is important to note that as currently designed, neither decentralized nor centralized LCS models commonly include any type of routine outreach effort to identify screening-eligible people, educate them about LCS availability, and engage them in SDM. It is, therefore, not surprising that access to LCS is limited in the United States, and the use of LCS is significantly lower than that of other recommended cancer screening tests [20, 21]. Making LCS more accessible, particularly for people who are marginalized because of race, ethnicity, language or otherwise, is vital both to maximizing the benefits from LCS and to minimizing health inequality [22, 23].

Health system support for outreach efforts to identify screening-eligible people, educate them about LCS and its availability, and initiate SDM could have a profound impact on increasing the initial and repeat use of LCS and follow-up. Such methods could also help increase equity in population screening rates, and adherence to recommended follow-up, regardless of the model of LCS program.

LCS Use in Current Practice

Although it has been more than a decade since results of National Lung Screening Trial (NLST) were first reported [24], only a small proportion of the LCS-eligible population has been screened. Studies using data from national surveys, including the 2013 Behavioral Risk Factor Surveillance System [25] and the 2010 and 2015 National Health Interview Survey [26], report rates of self-reported screening with LDCT in the previous 12 months ranging from a low of 3.3% to a high of 14.4%. Kee et al. [27] and Narayan et al. [28], using the 2018 Behavioral Risk Factor Surveillance System survey, found 17.7% and 19.2%, respectively, of eligible smokers reported undergoing LCS. Even studies focusing on health system patient populations report suboptimal screening rates. For example, a study of one large health system in California determined that only 7.8% of eligible patients received at least one order for LCS, between 2014 and 2016 [29]. Collectively, these studies indicate that LCS use is increasing but remains unacceptably low.

Even with low rates of screening uptake, disparities have been observed. Most notably, screening guidelines as issued by the US Preventive Health Services Task Force in 2013 have been shown to be more aligned with the risk profiles of whites and males [30]. Concerns remain, even with the issuance of the Task Force's 2021 guideline [31] although some reports indicate disparities in eligibility for African Americans and women may be reduced [32]. Among screening-eligible adults, studies have found racial/ethnicity, socioeconomic, and/or geographic disparities in the initial uptake of LCS, repeat screening [33, 34], and adherence to follow-up [35, 36], smoking cessation counseling [37], and shift in disease stage as a result of LCS [38].

Clouston et al. [39] have proposed four stages in the social history of disease disparities which are relevant to lung cancer, smoking, and LCS. These stages include: (1) natural mortality, a period in which little to no disparities exist and may even shift; (2) producing inequalities, characterized as unequal diffusion of new tests or treatments; (3) reducing inequalities, a period during which health knowledge is increased; and (4) reduced mortality, when prevention and early detection is widely available. LCS appears to be in stage 2, while it can be argued that smoking cessation straddles stages 2 and 3. How quickly we arrive at stage 4 will, in part, will be dependent on the ways in which integrated health systems implement and integrate LCS and smoking cessation [40].

Enhancing LCS Program Implementation in Health Systems

In a systematic review, Moullin et al. [41] explored the utilization of a four-phase framework known as Exploration, Preparation, Implementation, and Sustainment (EPIS) to change population health. This framework may be useful in specifying a systematic approach health systems can use to develop, operationalize, and evaluate strategies that can be used to change SDM and LCS rates. It also may help to tailor strategies for implementation within local contexts.

According to this framework, the process begins with an *exploration phase* within which an organization identifies evidence-based practices to address needs. Critical to this phase is the identification of an executive sponsor who can facilitate the identification of needed resources and the removal of barriers to change as well as a clinical champion to provide expert knowledge and motivational leadership [2]. Evidence processes for several key steps are needed for a successful LCS program including: (1) identifying, educating, and recruiting people who are eligible for LCS, (2) engaging LCS-eligible people in SDM, and as appropriate smoking cessation counseling, (3) ordering and completing the LDCT scan, (4) communicating and following up with test results (including nodule management/follow-up), and (5) tracking and monitoring LCS performance for continuous improvement. Processes are also needed to support accredited equipment availability and billing.

A recent adaptation of the EPIS framework explicitly acknowledges the need for rapid-cycle testing during implementation [42]. This adaptation considers EPIS, not as a four-step process that progresses in one direction through the four steps, but as a circular wheel in which organizations are continually iterating between steps, and re-cycling through the steps as new information is identified and/or learned. This adaptation is appealing in the context of LCS given the paucity of evidence for many of the core components of the LCS processes, including best practices for identifying those eligible for LCS and implementing SDM.

Once evidence-based procedures have been identified for implementation, the next step in the EPIS framework is the *preparation phase*. This phase includes consideration of the health system's organizational context to identify potential barriers to and facilitators of implementation. Consideration of both the organization's internal characteristics such as available staff and equipment, organizational size and geographical spread, and existing staffing and services as well as the environmental context within which the health system operates is important at this stage. Particularly important in the context of LCS is the identification of existing tobacco counseling services (be those internal or external to the organization) and engagement of clinicians and others who are integral to the core workstreams in the LCS process. These will likely include stakeholders from primary care, radiology, pulmonology, thoracic oncology, and surgery as well as representatives from information technology and/or population health units, and quality or research departments. It is during this stage that organizational-specific internal and external factors might be identified that can support an iterative process of implementation and adaptations to adequately address known implementation barriers as well as to take advantage of likely facilitators.

The EPIS framework next considers the actual *implementation phase* in which different ways to embed core LCS processes within the organization are identified and tested. As highlighted by the adapted EPIS Wheel, this step is likely to be facilitated using rapid-cycle testing [43]. The cycle then continues to a *sustainment phase* in which barriers and facilitators identified during the preparation phase may be reconsidered to enable additional adaptations and ongoing testing. Other frameworks have been proposed for use in the implementation of LCS programs and could be explored for their appropriateness within specific organizational and local contexts [44, 45].

Implementation Challenges and Opportunities

An initial step any health system should take towards implementing an effective LCS program is to constitute an appropriate leadership team with the authority and resources needed to support a comprehensive screening program. LCS leadership teams can engage a range of stakeholders to address the multi-level factors that need to be considered in the process of developing and implementing an effective LCS program [46–49]. Below, we highlight four core work streams this leadership team must address: (1) identifying eligible people for LCS screening, (2) optimizing SDM quality, (3) tracking and monitoring lung nodules, and (4) ensuring equity across the LCS continuum.

Identifying LCS-eligible persons: As Brenner and colleagues have pointed out, one of the key gaps in a health system's capacity to implement LCS is the lack of availability of the smoking history information needed to identify patients who are screening eligible [50]. Studies have repeatedly highlighted shortcomings in smoking-related information within EHRs including implausible changes in smoking status over time (i.e., patients who are documented as "current smokers" who change to "never smokers") [51–53]. LCS eligibility presents additional challenges as screening eligibility is determined not simply based on a person's current tobacco use status, but also by their lifetime cumulative smoking history or "pack years." The calculation of pack years requires knowledge of a person's average cigarette packs smoked per day and the years smoked. This level of detail is rarely documented in the medical record, although EHRs commonly used by health systems have structured tobacco use-related fields, detailed smoking data is often incomplete in these fields. This void in the availability of detailed smoking histories presents a challenge in identifying patients eligible for LCS, but also creates opportunities for innovative approaches to identifying LCS-eligible persons.

Optimizing SDM Quality: LCS decisions are complex. People eligible for LCS must consider the balance of expected benefits (i.e., lung cancer–related mortality reduction) and harms (i.e., risks associated with incidental findings, false-positive results, over-diagnosis, and cumulative radiation exposure) relative to their own personal values and preferences. Because it is well known that people using a decision aid when faced with such complex decision making benefit from improved knowledge, more accurate risk perceptions, more confidence in their decisions, enhanced engagement during the decision-making process, and care receipt that is preference concordant [54–56], CMS and others advocate for the use of SDM and a decision aid when offering LCS. A recent systematic review of tools to promote SDM for LCS supported such recommendations, finding that available LCS tools improved LCS knowledge and reduced decisional conflict [57]. The same review also found that available tools were generally acceptable to patients and providers.

Despite these advantages, physicians often express concerns regarding decision aid practicality [58, 59] and, to date, their use in practice has been limited [48, 59–61]. Findings in the context of LCS are no different. A recent study found that the shared decision-making visit required by CMS was evident in just 10% of Medicare beneficiaries undergoing LDCT [62]. Even when shared decision-making counseling is present prior to screening, concerns regarding the quality of that counseling remain. In the context of LCS, a small qualitative study of office-based patient-physician conversations documented the brevity and universally poor quality of such discussions [63].

When questioned regarding the implementation of SDM for LCS, those overseeing LCS programs have expressed concerns that providers may document SDM as having occurred to meet the criteria for reimbursement, regardless of the quality of counseling provided, even when EHR documentation required the delineation of key SDM steps [7]. Commonly reported barriers to the use of SDM in practice include time constraints and competing demands, a lack of clinician training and clinician belief they are already doing SDM, as well as a lack of organizational support or resources among others [21, 64, 65]. Each of these barriers has been noted in studies specific to LCS [7, 66, 67].

Outside of using a centralized program [13] or telehealth visits [68, 69], there has been little experimentation or innovation yet documented in the published literature regarding the implementation of SDM in the context of LCS. This situation is likely due to CMS requirements that physicians or advanced practice providers deliver SDM, and that SDM occurs in-person. These requirements have recently been changed to include auxiliary providers and telemedicine visits. Such changes should expand options for intervention research and delivery of SDM.

Tracking and Monitoring Lung Nodules: Just as LCS decisions are complex, so are the systems needed to ensure accurate and safe follow-up of screening tests. The type and timing of follow-up needed varies by test result and, depending upon findings, can also involve coordination across several health care providers and facilities. Care received by those with an abnormal finding impacts the ability to diagnose and treat effectively those found to have lung cancer [70, 71], the subsequent use of cancer screening among those found not to have lung cancer [72–78], and the psychological well-being of patients [77, 79, 80].

Organizations implementing LCS programs should establish standardized protocols for follow-up (such as those provided in Lung Imaging Reporting and Data System (Lung-RADS®) assessment categories [81, 82]). Health systems should also adopt tools and systems (e.g., registries and standardized workflows) to support communicating test results to patients, tracking patients across the LCS continuum, and providing the outreach necessary to ensure timely, equitable, and appropriate repeat screening and follow-up. It is important that such systems consider patient barriers to follow-up such as out-of-pocket costs, as once a nodule is detected, follow-up testing is no longer "screening," resulting in patients facing copays and deductibles. Health systems also should go beyond implementing simple automated notifications of abnormal results as, even with alerts, critical imaging results may not receive timely follow-up in the outpatient setting [83].

Ensuring Equity across the LCS Continuum: Another challenge is to ensure equity in who is offered and receives LCS. Programs that rely on in-reach activities only (i.e., programs that target only those people who present to physician office visits) inherently perpetuate existing structural barriers to care access. It is essential that health systems implement proactive outreach contacts to address this problem. Embracing such a population health approach requires shifting the perspective from caring for only people who present for care to having a more complete understanding of the health of the population served.

Systematically identifying and addressing access barriers when designing LCS programs is an important initial step. Such an approach is critical to delivering on the potential of the new LCS guidelines, allowing health systems to address systemic racism and other inequities in care. Horn and Haas [84] have recently advocated for cancer screening dashboards that report data on disparities in screening rates by race and ethnic group, sexual orientation, and gender identity as a first step toward ensuring equity and safety within LCS. The inability to use structured data currently available within most EHRs to identify those eligible for LCS, therefore, constitutes a structural barrier to achieving equity in LCS.

Another barrier is reflected in the health system's capacity to measure the quality of SDM in screening programs. A recent study found that perceived discrimination in medical settings was associated with people reporting not having enough time with their physician and not being as involved in decision-making as they wanted to be [85]. Thus, it is important for health systems to consider not only how to offer persons in marginalized populations the opportunity to learn about LCS, participate in quality SDM, and access to screening and follow-up care, but also to assess the extent to which these goals are achieved.

Conclusions

As suggested by the discussion in the preceding text, implementing a successful LCS program in a health system is a challenge that requires the alignment of leadership along multiple dimensions. Current low screening rates provide evidence that the widespread implementation of effective LCS programs remains a goal not yet achieved. To date, there has been little attention devoted to evaluating the implementation of LCS programs in health systems.

The impact of health system implementation of centralized and decentralized LCS program models, each of which have their strengths and weaknesses, is reflected in low LCS rates observed across the country. This state of affairs presents an important opportunity for health systems to use rapid-cycle testing and other approaches to designing and testing new, more hybrid-type LCS screening models that embrace the advantages found within each of the current LCS models while also addressing their inherent weaknesses. It is important for health system leadership to support concerted efforts to align organizational goals, strategies, and roles related to population engagement in LCS programs.

Health systems should embrace a systematic approach to monitoring the performance of LCS programs and to the identification of effective strategies to expand access to high-quality SDM and LCS across diverse populations. LCS programs are likely to need to consider multiple and varied approaches to outreach, expanded staff roles, explicit linkages with internally and externally operated smoking cessation programs, opportunities to capitalize on emerging telehealth capabilities, and leveraging well-established population health strategies.

Health systems are well positioned to take on leadership roles in developing the EHR infrastructure needed to identify those eligible for LCS (whether via structured fields, artificial intelligence capabilities, or otherwise), designing innovative and effective outreach strategies, and ways for monitoring program quality and equity across the LCS continuum. They also are well positioned to support provider training and add enhanced outreach activities in existing LCS programs. The commitment to reach people who face diverse access barriers is key to maximizing health care quality, equity, and the success of LCS programs. In this effort, it is also important to engage health care payers, community, and advocacy organizations along with other stakeholders from across the LCS care continuum. Health systems that embrace such processes and strive to develop new, innovative LCS models will be positioned to reduce lung cancer morbidity and mortality for all.

References

1. Schmit C, D'Hoore W, Lejeune C, Vas A. Predictors of successful organizational change: the alignment of goals, logics of action, and leaders' roles to initiate clinical pathways. Int J Care Pathw. 2011;15:4–14.
2. Slatore CG, Golden SE, Thomas T, Bumatay S, Shannon J, Davis M. "It's really like any other study": rural radiology facilities performing low-dose computed tomography for lung cancer screening. Ann Am Thorac Soc. 2021;18(12):2058–66.
3. Aarons GA, Hurlburt M, Horwitz SM. Advancing a conceptual model of evidence-based practice implementation in public service sectors. Admin Pol Ment Health. 2011;38(1):4–23.
4. Lam S, Tammemagi M. Contemporary issues in the implementation of lung cancer screening. Eur Respir Rev. 2021;30(161):200288.
5. Rendle KA, Burnett-Hartman AN, Neslund-Dudas C, Greenlee RT, Honda S, Elston Lafata J, et al. Evaluating lung cancer screening across diverse healthcare systems: A process model from the lung PROSPR consortium. Cancer Prev Res (Phila). 2020;13(2):129–36.
6. Wernli KJTL, Brush S, Ehrlich K, Gao H, Anderson ML, Palazzo L. Understanding patient and clinical stakeholder perspectives to improve adherence to lung cancer screening. Perm J. 2021;25(20):1–9.
7. Alishahi Tabriz A, Neslund-Dudas C, Turner K, Rivera MP, Reuland DS, Elston LJ. How health-care organizations implement shared decision-making when it is required for reimbursement: the case of lung cancer screening. Chest. 2021;159(1):413–25.
8. Dobler CC, Midthun DE, Montori VM. Quality of shared decision making in lung cancer screening: the right process, with the right partners, at the right time and place. Mayo Clin Proc. 2017;92(11):1612–6.
9. Goodson JD. POINT: should only primary care physicians provide shared decision-making services to discuss the risks/benefits of a low-dose chest CT scan for lung cancer screening? Yes. Chest. 2017;151(6):1213–5.
10. Kim RY, Rendle KA, Mitra N, Saia CA, Neslund-Dudas C, Greenlee RT, et al. Racial disparities in adherence to annual lung cancer screening and recommended follow-up care: a multicenter cohort study. Ann Am Thorac Soc. 2022;19:1561.
11. Sakoda LC, Rivera MP, Zhang J, Perera P, Laurent CA, Durham D, et al. Patterns and factors associated with adherence to lung cancer screening in diverse practice settings. JAMA Netw Open. 2021;4(4):e218559.
12. Smith HB, Ward R, Frazier C, Angotti J, Tanner NT. Guideline-recommended lung cancer screening adherence is superior with a centralized approach. Chest. 2022;161(3):818–25.

13. Mazzone PJ, Tenenbaum A, Seeley M, Petersen H, Lyon C, Han X, et al. Impact of a lung cancer screening counseling and shared decision-making visit. Chest. 2017;151(3):572–8.
14. Aberle DR. Implementing lung cancer screening: the US experience. Clin Radiol. 2017;72(5):401–6.
15. Mazzone P, Powell CA, Arenberg D, Bach P, Detterbeck F, Gould MK, et al. Components necessary for high-quality lung cancer screening: American College of Chest Physicians and American Thoracic Society Policy Statement. Chest. 2015;147(2):295–303.
16. Iaccarino JM, Duran C, Slatore CG, Wiener RS, Kathuria H. Combining smoking cessation interventions with LDCT lung cancer screening: a systematic review. Prev Med. 2019;121:24–32.
17. Lopez DB, Flores EJ, Miles RC, Wang GX, Mt G, Shepard JO, et al. Assessing eligibility for lung cancer screening among women undergoing screening mammography: cross-sectional survey results from the National Health Interview Survey. J Am Coll Radiol. 2019;16(10):1433–9.
18. Kinsinger LS, Anderson C, Kim J, Larson M, Chan SH, King HA, et al. Implementation of lung cancer screening in the veterans health administration. JAMA Intern Med. 2017;177:399.
19. Reuland DS, Cubillos L, Brenner AT, Harris RP, Minish B, Pignone MP. A pre-post study testing a lung cancer screening decision aid in primary care. BMC Med Inform Decis Mak. 2018;18(1):5.
20. Humphrey LL, Deffebach M, Pappas M, Baumann C, Artis K, Mitchell JP, et al. Screening for lung cancer with low-dose computed tomography: a systematic review to update the US preventive services task force recommendation. Ann Intern Med. 2013;159(6):411–20.
21. Gravel K, Legare F, Graham ID. Barriers and facilitators to implementing shared decision-making in clinical practice: a systematic review of health professionals' perceptions. Implement Sci. 2006;1:16.
22. Huo J, Shen C, Volk RJ, Shih YT. Use of CT and chest radiography for lung cancer screening before and after publication of screening guidelines: intended and unintended uptake. JAMA Intern Med. 2017;177(3):439–41.
23. Legare F, Witteman HO. Shared decision making: examining key elements and barriers to adoption into routine clinical practice. Health Aff (Millwood). 2013;32(2):276–84.
24. National Lung Screening Trial Research T, Aberle DR, Adams AM, Berg CD, Black WC, Clapp JD, et al. Reduced lung-cancer mortality with low-dose computed tomographic screening. N Engl J Med. 2011;365(5):395–409.
25. Zahnd WE, Eberth JM. Lung cancer screening utilization: a behavioral risk factor surveillance system analysis. Am J Prev Med. 2019;57(2):250–5.
26. Jemal A, Fedewa SA. Lung cancer screening with low-dose computed tomography in the United States-2010 to 2015. JAMA Oncol. 2017;3(9):1278–81.
27. Kee D, Wisnivesky J, Kale MS. Lung cancer screening uptake: analysis of BRFSS 2018. J Gen Intern Med. 2021;36(9):2897–9.
28. Narayan AK, Gupta Y, Little BP, Shepard JO, Flores EJ. Lung cancer screening eligibility and use with low-dose computed tomography: results from the 2018 behavioral risk factor surveillance system cross-sectional survey. Cancer. 2021;127(5):748–56.
29. Li J, Chung S, Wei EK, Luft HS. New recommendation and coverage of low-dose computed tomography for lung cancer screening: uptake has increased but is still low. BMC Health Serv Res. 2018;18(1):525.
30. Han SS, Chow E, Ten Haaf K, Toumazis I, Cao P, Bastani M, et al. Disparities of National lung cancer screening guidelines in the US population. J Natl Cancer Inst. 2020;112(11):1136–42.
31. Pinsky PF, Lau YK, Doubeni CA. Potential disparities by sex and race or ethnicity in lung cancer screening eligibility rates. Chest. 2021;160(1):341–50.
32. Ritzwoller DP, Meza R, Carroll NM, Blum-Barnett E, Burnett-Hartman AN, Greenlee RT, et al. Evaluation of population-level changes associated with the 2021 US preventive services task force lung cancer screening recommendations in community-based health care systems. JAMA Netw Open. 2021;4(10):e2128176.

33. Sosa E, D'Souza G, Akhtar A, Sur M, Love K, Duffels J, et al. Racial and socioeconomic disparities in lung cancer screening in the United States: a systematic review. CA Cancer J Clin. 2021;71(4):299–314.

34. Poghosyan H, Fortin D, Moen EL, Quigley KS, Young GJ. Differences in uptake of low-dose CT scan for lung cancer among white and black adult smokers in the United States-2017. J Health Care Poor Underserved. 2021;32(1):165–78.

35. Kunitomo Y, Bade B, Gunderson CG, Akgun KM, Brackett A, Cain H, et al. Racial differences in adherence to lung cancer screening follow-up: a systematic review and meta-analysis. Chest. 2022;161(1):266–75.

36. Nunez ER, Caverly TJ, Zhang S, Glickman ME, Qian SX, Boudreau JH, et al. Adherence to follow-up testing recommendations in US veterans screened for lung cancer, 2015-2019. JAMA Netw Open. 2021;4(7):e2116233.

37. Heffner JL, Coggeshall S, Wheat CL, Krebs P, Feemster LC, Klein DE, et al. Receipt of tobacco treatment and one-year smoking cessation rates following lung cancer screening in the veterans health administration. J Gen Intern Med. 2021;37:1704.

38. Ganesh A, Katipally R, Pasquinelli M, Feldman L, Spiotto M, Koshy M. Increased disparities in patients diagnosed with metastatic lung cancer following lung CT screening in the United States. Clin Lung Cancer. 2021;23:151.

39. Clouston SA, Rubin MS, Phelan JC, Link BG. A social history of disease: contextualizing the rise and fall of social inequalities in cause-specific mortality. Demography. 2016;53(5):1631–56.

40. President's Cancer Panel. Closing gaps in cancer screening: connecting people, communities, and systems to improve equity and access. Bethesda, MD: President's Cancer Panel; 2021.

41. Moullin JC, Dickson KS, Stadnick NA, Rabin B, Aarons GA. Systematic review of the exploration, preparation, implementation, sustainment (EPIS) framework. Implement Sci. 2019;14(1):1.

42. Becan JE, Bartkowski JP, Knight DK, Wiley TRA, DiClemente R, Ducharme L, et al. A model for rigorously applying the exploration, preparation, implementation, sustainment (EPIS) framework in the design and measurement of a large scale collaborative multi-site study. Health Justice. 2018;6(1):9.

43. Edwards Deming W. Out of crisis. Cambridge: MIT Press; 2018.

44. Matlock DD, Fukunaga MI, Tan A, Knoepke C, McNeal DM, Mazor KM, et al. Enhancing success of Medicare's shared decision making mandates using implementation science: examples applying the pragmatic robust implementation and sustainability model (PRISM). MDM Policy Pract. 2020;5(2):2381468320963070.

45. Myers RE, DiCarlo M, Romney M, Fleisher L, Sifri R, Soleiman J, et al. Using a health system learning community strategy to address cancer disparities. Learn Health Syst. 2018;2(4):e10067.

46. Carter-Harris L, Gould MK. Multilevel barriers to the successful implementation of lung cancer screening: why does it have to be so hard? Ann Am Thorac Soc. 2017;14(8):1261–5.

47. Optican RJ, Chiles C. Implementing lung cancer screening in the real world: opportunity, challenges and solutions. Transl Lung Cancer Res. 2015;4(4):353–64.

48. Zeliadt SB, Hoffman RM, Birkby G, Eberth JM, Brenner AT, Reuland DS, et al. Challenges implementing lung cancer screening in federally qualified health centers. Am J Prev Med. 2018;54(4):568–75.

49. Odahowski CL, Zahnd WE, Eberth JM. Challenges and opportunities for lung cancer screening in rural America. J Am Coll Radiol. 2019;16(4 Pt B):590–5.

50. Brenner ACL, Birchard K, Doyle-Burr C, Eick J, Henderson L. Improving the implementation of lung cancer screening guidelines at an academic medical center. J Healthc Qual. 2017;40(1):27–35.

51. Polubriaginof F, Salmasian H, Albert DA, Vawdrey DK. Challenges with collecting smoking status in electronic health records. AMIA Annu Symp Proc. 2017;2017:1392–400.

52. Cole AM, Pflugeisen B, Schwartz MR, Miller SC. Cross sectional study to assess the accuracy of electronic health record data to identify patients in need of lung cancer screening. BMC Res Notes. 2018;11(1):14.

53. Modin HE, Fathi JT, Gilbert CR, Wilshire CL, Wilson AK, Aye RW, et al. Pack-year cigarette smoking history for determination of lung cancer screening eligibility. Comparison of the electronic medical record versus a shared decision-making conversation. Ann Am Thorac Soc. 2017;14(8):1320–5.
54. Stacey D, Bennett CL, Barry MJ, Col NF, Eden KB, Holmes-Rovner M, et al. Decision aids for people facing health treatment or screening decisions. Cochrane Database Syst Rev. 2011;10:CD001431.
55. Stacey D, Legare F, Lewis K, Barry MJ, Bennett CL, Eden KB, et al. Decision aids for people facing health treatment or screening decisions. Cochrane Database Syst Rev. 2017;4:CD001431.
56. Volk RJ, Linder SK, Lopez-Olivo MA, Kamath GR, Reuland DS, Saraykar SS, et al. Patient decision aids for colorectal cancer screening: a systematic review and meta-analysis. Am J Prev Med. 2016;51(5):779–91.
57. Fukunaga MI, Halligan K, Kodela J, Toomey S, Furtado VF, Luckmann R, et al. Tools to promote shared decision-making in lung cancer screening using low-dose CT scanning: a systematic review. Chest. 2020;158(6):2646–57.
58. Graham ID, Logan J, O'Connor A, Weeks KE, Aaron S, Cranney A, et al. A qualitative study of physicians' perceptions of three decision aids. Patient Educ Couns. 2003;50(3):279–83.
59. Brace C, Schmocker S, Huang H, Victor JC, McLeod RS, Kennedy ED. Physicians' awareness and attitudes toward decision aids for patients with cancer. J Clin Oncol. 2010;28(13):2286–92.
60. Jimbo M, Rana GK, Hawley S, Holmes-Rovner M, Kelly-Blake K, Nease DE Jr, et al. What is lacking in current decision aids on cancer screening? CA Cancer J Clin. 2013;63(3):193–214.
61. Elwyn G, Scholl I, Tietbohl C, Mann M, Edwards AG, Clay C, et al. "Many miles to go …": a systematic review of the implementation of patient decision support interventions into routine clinical practice. BMC Med Inform Decis Mak. 2013;13(Suppl 2):S14.
62. Goodwin JS, Nishi S, Zhou J, Kuo YF. Use of the shared decision-making visit for lung cancer screening among medicare enrollees. JAMA Intern Med. 2019;179(5):716–8.
63. Brenner AT, Malo TL, Margolis M, Elston Lafata J, James S, Vu MB, et al. Evaluating shared decision making for lung cancer screening. JAMA Intern Med. 2018;178(10):1311–6.
64. Legare F, Ratte S, Gravel K, Graham ID. Barriers and facilitators to implementing shared decision-making in clinical practice: update of a systematic review of health professionals' perceptions. Patient Educ Couns. 2008;73(3):526–35.
65. Waddell A, Lennox A, Spassova G, Bragge P. Barriers and facilitators to shared decision-making in hospitals from policy to practice: a systematic review. Implement Sci. 2021;16(1):74.
66. Iaccarino JM, Clark J, Bolton R, Kinsinger L, Kelley M, Slatore CG, et al. A National survey of pulmonologists' views on low-dose computed tomography screening for lung cancer. Ann Am Thorac Soc. 2015;12(11):1667–75.
67. Hoffman RM, Sussman AL, Getrich CM, Rhyne RL, Crowell RE, Taylor KL, et al. Attitudes and beliefs of primary care providers in New Mexico about lung cancer screening using low-dose computed tomography. Prev Chronic Dis. 2015;12:E108.
68. Tanner NT, Banas E, Yeager D, Dai L, Hughes Halbert C, Silvestri GA. In-person and telephonic shared decision-making visits for people considering lung cancer screening: an assessment of decision quality. Chest. 2019;155(1):236–8.
69. Fagan HB, Fournakis NA, Jurkovitz C, Petrich AM, Zhang Z, Katurakes N, et al. Telephone-based shared decision-making for lung cancer screening in primary care. J Cancer Educ. 2020;35(4):766–73.
70. Ost DE, Niu J, Elting LS, Buchholz TA, Giordano SH. Determinants of practice patterns and quality gaps in lung cancer staging and diagnosis. Chest. 2014;145(5):1097–113.
71. Ost DE, Niu J, Elting LS, Buchholz TA, Giordano SH. Quality gaps and comparative effectiveness in lung cancer staging and diagnosis. Chest. 2014;145(2):331–45.
72. Dabbous FM, Dolecek TA, Berbaum ML, Friedewald SM, Summerfelt WT, Hoskins K, et al. Impact of a false-positive screening mammogram on subsequent screening behavior and stage at breast cancer diagnosis. Cancer Epidemiol Biomark Prev. 2017;26(3):397–403.

73. Ford ME, Havstad SL, Demers R, Cole JC. Effects of false-positive prostate cancer screening results on subsequent prostate cancer screening behavior. Cancer Epidemiol Biomark Prev. 2005;14(1):190–4.

74. Ford ME, Havstad SL, Flickinger L, Johnson CC. Examining the effects of false positive lung cancer screening results on subsequent lung cancer screening adherence. Cancer Epidemiol Biomark Prev. 2003;12(1):28–33.

75. Defrank JT, Brewer N. A model of the influence of false-positive mammography screening results on subsequent screening. Health Psychol Rev. 2010;4(2):112–27.

76. Salz T, DeFrank JT, Brewer NT. False positive mammograms in Europe: do they affect reattendance? Breast Cancer Res Treat. 2011;127(1):229–31.

77. Taylor KL, Shelby R, Gelmann E, McGuire C. Quality of life and trial adherence among participants in the prostate, lung, colorectal, and ovarian cancer screening trial. J Natl Cancer Inst. 2004;96(14):1083–94.

78. Allen JD, Shelton RC, Harden E, Goldman RE. Follow-up of abnormal screening mammograms among low-income ethnically diverse women: findings from a qualitative study. Patient Educ Couns. 2008;72(2):283–92.

79. Brett J, Austoker J. Women who are recalled for further investigation for breast screening: psychological consequences 3 years after recall and factors affecting re-attendance. J Public Health Med. 2001;23(4):292–300.

80. Wiener RS, Gould MK, Woloshin S, Schwartz LM, Clark JA. What do you mean, a spot?: a qualitative analysis of patients' reactions to discussions with their physicians about pulmonary nodules. Chest. 2013;143(3):672–7.

81. Fleischner Society Recommendations for follow-up of small lung nodules detected incidentally on CT (patients >=35 Years of Age). [cited 2017 March 12]. http://www.snm.org/docs/PET_COE/off_the_wall/Fleis.pdf.

82. Lung-RADS™ Version 1.0 Assessment categories release date: April 28, 2014. https://www.acr.org/~/media/ACR/Documents/PDF/QualitySafety/Resources/LungRADS/AssessmentCategories.pdf.

83. Singh H, Thomas EJ, Mani S, Sittig D, Arora H, Espadas D, et al. Timely follow-up of abnormal diagnostic imaging test results in an outpatient setting: are electronic medical records achieving their potential? Arch Intern Med. 2009;169(17):1578–86.

84. Horn DM, Haas JS. Expanded lung and colorectal cancer screening—ensuring equity and safety under new guidelines. N Engl J Med. 2022;386(2):100–2.

85. Benjamins MR, Middleton M. Perceived discrimination in medical settings and perceived quality of care: a population-based study in Chicago. PLoS One. 2019;14(4):e0215976.

Chapter 32
Across the Landscape: Community-Based Partnerships for Lung Cancer Risk Reduction—From Federal Initiatives to Local Influences

Ana Maria Lopez

Background

Cancer is a global epidemic. Despite progress in cancer detection and treatment, cancer is already exceeding cardiovascular disease mortality in many developed countries [1]. The diagnosis of cancer significantly impacts health and well-being through premature death, cost of illness, lost productivity, and health impact on survivors [2]. With the population aging, further increases in cancer diagnoses are anticipated [3].

In 1981, Doll and Peto published the classic cancer epidemiology paper outlining factors that contribute to cancer risk. In this paper, the role of tobacco use, nutrition, occupational exposure, and infection in cancer development was described. Tobacco was clearly defined as a major cause of cancer-related death [4]. Today, tobacco is linked to nearly 90% of lung cancer deaths in the United States [5]. Globally, the World Health Organization estimates that nearly eight million people meet premature death annually due to tobacco use, with more than a million of these deaths attributed to second-hand exposure [6]. It is estimated that tobacco is the single most avoidable cause of death in the world today [7]. It is not only a carcinogen; tobacco addiction adversely impacts multiple chronic illnesses, increases surgical risk, and complicates cancer survivorship [8, 9]. Tobacco use persists with greater prevalence in many vulnerable populations raising the opportunity for health equity interventions [10].

Cancer is an epidemic, a public health problem. Public health strategies focus on prevention and risk reduction. To be successful, cancer prevention approaches must take place *with* the at-risk well, and *with* the at-risk communities, that is, we need to

A. M. Lopez (✉)
Department of Medical Oncology, Sidney Kimmel Cancer Center, Thomas Jefferson University, Philadelphia, PA, USA
e-mail: AnaMaria.Lopez@jefferson.edu

go where the people are. In this chapter, we will discuss community partnerships as effective lung cancer risk-reduction approaches. Our focus will be on tobacco, including second-hand tobacco smoke exposure. We will focus on risk from the macro, the role of large governmental agencies, to the micro, the individual. For the remainder of this chapter, cancer risk-reduction will be used instead of cancer prevention due to the awareness that although we may have some control regarding risks and risk reduction, fully preventing cancer is not likely in the individual's control.

Community Partnerships as a Cancer Risk-Reduction Strategy: Rationale

Although tobacco exposure may be viewed as an individual act, that is, an individual chooses to smoke, tobacco exposure has a high risk of addiction, obviating choice, and is often socially mediated. Individuals live within an ecology of social structures that support or discourage specific behaviors and norms. Socially acceptable behavior is a product of these social norms. There has been a shift in the acceptability of tobacco use in the United States since its post-War peak acceptability in the 1950s. An accompanying shift in cultural norms has generally supported major significant policy changes supporting smoke-free environments. For example, simply lighting a cigarette would not be acceptable in many group settings without first asking permission from others present [11].

Given the role of our social structures in supporting tobacco use, communities, broadly speaking, emerge as potential partners in cancer risk-reduction. Community voices may be amplified in collective advocacy. These partnerships raise opportunities to go beyond the "usual suspects" and think more expansively. This work engages the needs of non-smokers to prevent the onset of smoking and of smokers to support smoking cessation and early detection of disease.

Community Partnerships for Lung Cancer Risk-Reduction

National Cancer Institute

The National Cancer Institute (NCI) established the Cancer Information Service Partnership Program, which included more than 900 community organizations and focused on the needs of medically underserved populations. Partnerships supported networking, education, and program development. An evaluation in 2007 demonstrated collaboration and benefits to the partnerships [12].

Current NCI community efforts include the National Outreach Network (NON), a network of health educators across the country focused on program development, education, and research embedded in cancer centers. Additional NCI-focused community engagement partnerships are part of the Center to Reduce Cancer Health Disparities—the Community Networks Program Centers, the Minority Institution Cancer Center Partnership, and the Patient Navigation Research Program. Additional partnership efforts are housed in the Minority Based Community Clinical Oncology Program, the Community Cancer Centers Program, and the NCI Cancer Centers. These community network partnerships can bring clinical trials to communities.

Legislative Partnerships: Advocacy and Policy

The epidemiology of lung cancer reveals that it was once considered rare. Tobacco use, prevalence, and acceptability increased as costs decreased. Free or subsidized cigarettes were distributed in the military during World War I, normalizing tobacco use [13]. Physician and celebrity "recommendations" for tobacco use were common in the mid-twentieth century [14]. This was concurrent with the confluence of studies that demonstrated the connection between cigarette use and the increasing rates of lung cancer. Advocacy resulted in legislation that impacted public health.

The Federal Cigarette Labeling and Act of 1965 required a package warning label and banned smoking on domestic airline flights of 2 h or less. The Public Health Cigarette Smoking Act of 1969 modified the package warning label: "Warning: The Surgeon General Has Determined that Cigarette Smoking Is Dangerous to Your Health," prohibited cigarette advertising on television and radio, and prevented states or local governments from regulating cigarette advertising for health reasons. The Little Cigar Act of 1973 banned little cigar advertising on television and radio. The Comprehensive Smoking Education Act of 1984 requires four rotating health warning labels on packages and ads. The Comprehensive Smokeless Tobacco Education Act of 1986 established three rotating health warning labels. Public Law 100-202 (1987) banned smoking on domestic airline flights with a flight time of 2 h or less. Public Law 101-164 (1989) banned smoking on domestic airline flights with a flight time of 6 h or less. The Synar Amendment to the Alcohol, Drug Abuse, and Mental Health Administration (ADAMHA) Reorganization Act of 1992 required states to adopt and enforce restrictions on tobacco sales to minors to be eligible for block grant funding to address substance abuse. The Pro-Children Act of 1994 required all federally funded children's services to be smoke-free. The Family Smoking Prevention and Tobacco Control Act of 2009 gave the Food and Drug Administration (FDA) the authority to regulate tobacco products. The Consolidated Appropriations Act of 2020, Amending the Federal Food, Drug, and Cosmetic Act, and the Public Health Service Act prohibited tobacco product sales to all persons under the age of 21, and required states to assess these sales to be eligible for substance abuse block grant funds [15].

Advocacy efforts at the state and local levels have resulted in additional restrictions on who can smoke and where smoking can take place. Regional differences in tobacco use in public spaces, schools, colleges, universities, workplaces, restaurants, and bars exist within the United States and globally. Advocacy strategies center on decreasing access to tobacco products. This is especially effective in reducing exposure in young people for addiction prevention [16]. Costs are an effective deterrent in limiting access. Increased taxation has been an effective means to discourage tobacco use [17]. Costs, however, remain a concern on military bases [18] and on American Indian reservations, where costs tend to be lower [19, 20].

Messaging and Marketing Partnerships

The tobacco industry has multiple commercial products in its portfolio, for which profit maximization is the goal, as demonstrated by pro-tobacco product messaging and marketing campaigns. Targeting non-smokers who may be most susceptible to these messages and thus most likely to initiate tobacco use may be a successful marketing strategy [11]. Multiple studies have documented increased pro-tobacco marketing in communities where persons historically intentionally excluded from educational and employment opportunity reside [21–26]. Marketing strategies serve to normalize tobacco use, mark tobacco initiation as a natural transition to adulthood, associate tobacco use with glamor, enhanced social status, and as an effective tool for relaxation [11]. Digital communication efforts can counter messaging with "counter-marketing" and serve as opportunities for tobacco education and risk-reduction programming [27]. As outlined earlier, advocacy strategies and community partnerships have successfully limited marketing to children and historically excluded communities.

School-Based Partnerships

High school dropout rates in the United States have been stable at less than 10% over the last decade [28]; Since young persons under the age of 18 can be found in schools [28], schools are opportune tobacco education risk-reduction partners. School-based tobacco interventions are intended to reduce intent to initiate, initiation itself, and prevalence. A systematic review of school-based partnership programs demonstrates success in these three areas in the short term (less than 12 months). Some of the efforts reviewed had long-term impact up to 15 years and others had an even more enduring impact up to 18 years. Success was related to attaining refusal skills in a social influence model and peer support, in addition to age-appropriate learnings about the risks of tobacco use. Additional efforts include tobacco-free school policies, education and training for educators, parental engagement, and smoking cessation care for students, school staff, and parents [29, 30]. Improved efficacy may be associated with behavioral reinforcement via a community program [31]. These studies point to the importance of going beyond information sharing related to risk. Partnerships whose interventions include practicing behaviors that support smoking cessation and diminish initiation risk and that are accompanied by peer support, tobacco-free school policies, parental engagement, and smoking cessation for the adults proximal to the student have a greater chance for success.

Workplace Partnerships

Partnerships with employers have generally resulted in effective policy interventions [32]. The impact of smoke-free worksite policies has been demonstrated to be favorable to smoking cessation and to preventing smoking initiation. Analyses regarding economic impact reveal savings to the employer, decreased absenteeism, improved productivity, and health benefits for the employee who stops smoking and for those at risk for second-hand exposure due to averted healthcare costs. The estimated net benefit of smoke-free workplace policies was noted to be $48 billion to $89 billion annually [33]. Many workplaces offer health insurance discounts to non-smokers and smoking cessation programs for smokers. A Cochrane review examined workplace-based practices to support modifiable risk factors for chronic disease that included tobacco use and identified few studies suggesting the need for implementation science research in this area [34].

Home-Based Partnerships

People often spend large amounts of time at their residence. Community-based partnerships focused on the individual's home have generally targeted environmental exposure control. Tobacco exposure is often one of many exposures being addressed, and the health target is often an acute respiratory exacerbation of asthma. Morgan et al. demonstrated the benefit of such an intervention that successfully achieved behavior change in the home. This successful approach included modeling the behavior, rehearsing the behavior, and verifying and reinforcing the person's ability to achieve the desired behavior to decrease environmental tobacco smoke and exposure to indoor allergens. The authors demonstrated that behavioral change requires support [35]. Focusing exclusively on tobacco smoke exposure, a recent meta-analysis identified success in decreasing tobacco smoke pollution in the home through individual action; however, persistence of the pollutant was noted. These findings suggest a possible benefit to regulatory approaches and expansion of smoke-free areas in closer living conditions [36]. Immediate minute-by-minute feedback on levels of particulate matter in the environment was especially effective in behavior change support [37].

Peer-Led Partnerships

Peers are a major behavioral influence as the peer-group often models what is normal or to be expected. For tobacco smoking initiation prevention and cessation, peer-led interventions may be particularly effective. Most studies are small and include other addictive substances making long-term impact evaluation for the partnership on tobacco difficult [38]. When tailored interventions are used, benefit emerges. Most studies randomize the participants to a peer-led group where the group leader has received specific training. In a tailored approach, the participant is asked which group leader is preferred. Group assignments are based on the participant's preference [39]. Additional peer-based efforts may focus on social media interactions. Social media reaches people where they are with tailored interventions based on age and gender [40].

Community Partnerships for Lung Cancer Early Detection

Lung Cancer Screening

A lung cancer screening recommendation is dependent on smoking history. Although guidelines have been published, implementation is lagging even as we enter the second decade after publication of the National Lung Screening Trial (NLST). Clinician-based factors resulting in lagging implementation may include lack of awareness of the guideline or the misconception that only visits slated for lung cancer screening should address lung cancer screening. Patient-based factors may include shame regarding ongoing tobacco use or history of use and fear and guilt of what the screening may reveal. Community-based efforts to overcome these efforts may include education, facilitating access to screening and treatment, and tobacco cessation support. One effort being studied engages community health workers (CHWs), trusted community members to educate and facilitate lung cancer screening [41]. Bringing education and screening services to the at-risk well at shopping centers that people frequent has demonstrated efficacy [42].

Community Partnerships: Principles

Community-based participatory research takes time and requires coalition-building and investment for success [43]. Clinicians, health systems, and academic systems must demonstrate staying power and trustworthiness for community partnerships to be successful. Usual assessments of community programs may demonstrate quasi success because our usual model for implementation is autocratic and unidimensional instead of democratic, meeting people where they are with respect, and multidimensional, acknowledging that people's lives are complex and guided by multiple priorities. Persons live in communities and experience multiple experiences that may influence the person toward tobacco use or against. Lung cancer risk reduction strategies must similarly target these multiple influences. We have outlined several opportunities for intervention—in the home, with the peer-group, in the schools, in the workplace, with media and marketing, and at the legislative level. Strategies cannot be effective as singular one-time events that seek to immunize the at-risk individual from tobacco risk, but as a series of ecological influences that also target ambient messages.

Factors essential for community partnership success include respect, an open heart to learn, humility to acknowledge what we do not know, and cultural humility to be guided by the community's priorities, needs, and experiences. The opportunity for community partnership may be guided by the following processes [44]:

- Seek partners with similar values.
- Include respected community leaders.
- Establish, practice, and commit to equity (contributions may vary; all contributions are valued).
- Model commitment.
- Understand that trust takes time.
- Work with a trusted community liaison who can facilitate communication, collaboration, and conflict.

Conclusion

Addressing tobacco use is a critical factor in lung cancer risk reduction that can impact numerous chronic and acute illnesses. Supporting tobacco cessation and preventing smoking initiation are opportunities ripe for community partnership from the individual level to legislative policy. How we engage with communities over time and collaborate across different efforts will be the most significant factors in supporting success equitably.

References

1. Dagenais GR, Leong DP, Rangarajan S, Lanas F, Lopez-Jaramillo P, Gupta R, et al. Variations in common diseases, hospital admissions, and deaths in middle-aged adults in 21 countries from five continents (PURE): a prospective cohort study. Lancet. 2020;395(10226):785–94.
2. NCI. The importance of cancer Public health research. Public health research and cancer. Frederick, MD: NCI; 2022. https://www.cancer.gov/research/areas/public-health
3. NCI. Age and cancer risk. Cancer causes and prevention. Frederick, MD: NCI; 2021. https://www.cancer.gov/about-cancer/causes-prevention/risk/age.
4. Doll R, Peto R. The causes of cancer: quantitative estimates of avoidable risks of cancer in the United States today. J Natl Cancer Inst. 1981;66(6):1192–308.

5. CDC. What are the risk factors for lung cancer? In: Lung cancer. Atlanta: CDC; 2022. https://www.cdc.gov/cancer/lung/basic_info/risk_factors.htm.
6. WHO. Tobacco. Geneva: WHO; 2022. https://www.who.int/news-room/fact-sheets/detail/tobacco.
7. Proctor RN. Tobacco and the global lung cancer epidemic. Nat Rev Cancer. 2001;1(1):82–6.
8. Yoshikawa R, Katada J. Effects of active smoking on postoperative outcomes in hospitalised patients undergoing elective surgery: a retrospective analysis of an administrative claims database in Japan. BMJ Open. 2019;9(10):e029913.
9. US Department of Health and Human Services. The health consequences of smoking—50 years of progress: a report of the surgeon general. Washington DC: US Department of Health and Human Services; 2014.
10. Sakuma KLK, Pierce JP, Fagan P, Nguyen-Grozavu FT, Leas EC, Messer K, et al. Racial/ethnic disparities across indicators of cigarette smoking in the era of increased tobacco control, 1992–2019. Nicotine Tob Res. 2021;23(6):909–19.
11. Bonnie RJ, Lynch BS. Growing up tobacco free: preventing nicotine addiction in children and youths. Washington DC: National Academies Press; 1994.
12. La Porta M, Hagood H, Kornfeld J, Treiman K. Partnership as a means for reaching special populations: evaluating the NCI's CIS Partnership program. J Cancer Educ. 2007;22(2):S35–40.
13. Proctor RN. The history of the discovery of the cigarette–lung cancer link: evidentiary traditions, corporate denial, global toll. Tob Control. 2012;21(2):87–91.
14. Tobacco stops with me. https://stopswithme.com/history-tobacco-marketing-scary-story/.
15. CDC. Selected laws enacted by the U.S. government regarding the regulation of tobacco sales, marketing, and use (excluding laws pertaining to agriculture or excise tax). Smoking and tobacco use. Atlanta: CDC; 2022. https://www.cdc.gov/tobacco/basic_information/policy/legislation/index.htm.
16. Elders MJ, Perry CL, Eriksen MP, Giovino GA. The report of the surgeon general: preventing tobacco use among young people. Am J Public Health. 1994;84(4):543–7.
17. Ellis Lisa. Evidence-based strategies to reduce global tobacco use. 2021. https://www.hsph.harvard.edu/ecpe/evidence-based-strategies-to-reduce-global-tobacco-use/.
18. Kong AY, Golden SD, Ribisl KM, Krukowski RA, Vandegrift SM, Little MA. Cheaper tobacco product prices at US air force bases compared with surrounding community areas, 2019. Tob Control. 2021;31(e2):e169–74.
19. DeCicca P, Kenkel D, Liu F. Reservation prices: an economic analysis of cigarette purchases on Indian reservations. Natl Tax J. 2015;68(1):93–118.
20. Soulakova JN, Pack R, Ha T. Patterns and correlates of purchasing cigarettes on Indian reservations among daily smokers in the United States. Drug Alcohol Depend. 2018;192:88–93.
21. Wilkinson AV, Vandewater EA, Carey FR, Spitz MR. Exposure to pro-tobacco messages and smoking status among Mexican origin youth. J Immigr Minor Health. 2014;16(3):385–93.
22. Stevens EM, Vázquez-Otero C, Li X, Arya M, Vallone D, Minsky S, et al. Tobacco messages encountered in real-time among low socio-economic position groups: a descriptive study. BMC Public Health. 2021;21(1):1–6.
23. Cruz TB, Rose SW, Lienemann BA, Byron MJ, Meissner HI, Baezconde-Garbanati L, et al. Pro-tobacco marketing and anti-tobacco campaigns aimed at vulnerable populations: a review of the literature. Tob Induc Dis. 2019;17:17.
24. Zhu J, Li J, He Y, Li N, Xu G, Yu J. The influence and interaction of exposure to pro-smoking and anti-smoking messaging on youth smoking behaviour and susceptibility. Tob Induc Dis. 2019;17:86.
25. Public Health Law Center. The Tobacco Industry and the Black Community. 2021. https://www.publichealthlawcenter.org/sites/default/files/resources/Tobacco-Industry-Targeting.pdf.
26. Keller-Hamilton B, Stevens EM, Wedel AV, LaPolt DT, Miranda A, Wagener TL, Patterson JG. Associations of race and ethnicity with tobacco messaging exposures and tobacco use among bisexual and pansexual women. Prev Med Rep. 2022;25:101657.

27. Elser H, Hartman-Filson M, Alizaga NM, Vijayaraghavan M. Exposure to pro-and anti-tobacco messages online and off-line among people experiencing homelessness. Prev Med Rep. 2019;15:100944.
28. National Center for Education Statistics. Status dropout rates. Annual reports. Washington, DC: National Center for Education Statistics; 2022. https://nces.ed.gov/programs/coe/indicator/coj/status-dropout-rates.
29. Dobbins M, DeCorby K, Manske S, Goldblatt E. Effective practices for school-based tobacco use prevention. Prev Med. 2008;46(4):289–97.
30. Thomas RE, McLellan J, Perera R. Effectiveness of school-based smoking prevention curricula: systematic review and meta-analysis. BMJ Open. 2015;5(3):e006976.
31. Koplan J, Kolbe L, Eriksen M. Guidelines for school health programs to prevent tobacco use and addiction. Morb Mortal Wkly Rep. 1994;43(2):1–18.
32. Hopkins DP, Razi S, Leeks KD, Kalra GP, Chattopadhyay SK, Soler RE, Task Force on Community Preventive Services. Smokefree policies to reduce tobacco use: a systematic review. Am J Prev Med. 2010;38(2):S275–89.
33. Mudarri DH. In: The costs and benefits of smoking restrictions: an assessment of the smoke-free environment act of 1993 (HR 3434). Indoor air division 6607J, Office of Radiation and Indoor Air, US Environmental Protection Agency; 1994.
34. Wolfenden L, Goldman S, Stacey FG, Grady A, Kingsland M, Williams CM, et al. Strategies to improve the implementation of workplace-based policies or practices targeting tobacco, alcohol, diet, physical activity and obesity. Cochrane Database Syst Rev. 2018;11:CD012439.
35. Morgan WJ, Crain EF, Gruchalla RS, O'Connor GT, Kattan M, Evans R III, et al. Results of a home-based environmental intervention among urban children with asthma. N Engl J Med. 2004;351(11):1068–80.
36. Rosen LJ, Myers V, Winickoff JP, Kott J. Effectiveness of interventions to reduce tobacco smoke pollution in homes: a systematic review and meta-analysis. Int J Environ Res Public Health. 2015;12(12):16043–59.
37. Wilson I, Semple S, Mills LM, Ritchie D, Shaw A, O'Donnell R, et al. REFRESH—reducing families' exposure to secondhand smoke in the home: a feasibility study. Tob Control. 2013;22(5):e8.
38. Mac Arthur GJ, Harrison S, Caldwell DM, Hickman M, Campbell R. Peer-led interventions to prevent tobacco, alcohol and/or drug use among young people aged 11–21 years: a systematic review and meta-analysis. Addiction. 2016;111(3):391–407.
39. Valente TW, Hoffman BR, Ritt-Olson A, Lichtman K, Johnson CA. Effects of a social-network method for group assignment strategies on peer-led tobacco prevention programs in schools. Am J Public Health. 2003;93(11):1837–43.
40. Haines-Saah RJ, Kelly MT, Oliffe JL, Bottorff JL. Picture me Smokefree: a qualitative study using social media and digital photography to engage young adults in tobacco reduction and cessation. J Med Internet Res. 2015;17(1):e4061.
41. Williams LB, McCall A, Joshua TV, Looney SW, Tingen MS. Design of a community-based lung cancer education, prevention, and screening program. West J Nurs Res. 2019;41(8):1152–69.
42. Crosbie PA, Balata H, Evison M, Atack M, Bayliss-Brideaux V, Colligan D, et al. Implementing lung cancer screening: baseline results from a community-based 'lung health check' pilot in deprived areas of Manchester. Thorax. 2019;74(4):405–9.
43. Butterfoss FD, Lachance LL, Orians CE. Building allies coalitions: why formation matters. Health Promot Pract. 2006;7(2_suppl):23S–33S.
44. Drits-Esser D, Coulter H, Mannello MC, Sunada G, Alder SC, Davis PFA, et al. The community faces model: community, university and health department partners thriving together for effective health education. Collaborations (Coral Gables). 2019;2(1):10.

Chapter 33
Where Do We Go from Here?

Julie A. Barta and Karen E. Knudsen

Background

The field of lung cancer screening (LCS) and early detection has undergone tremendous growth over the past decade, generating a multitude of additional unanswered questions [1]. Current gaps in knowledge exist in optimizing selection criteria for lung cancer screening, leveraging technology including the electronic health record (EHR) for LCS, and expanding implementation strategies for high-quality LCS. It is known that the balance of harms and benefits lies in favor of screening among high-risk individuals with few life-limiting comorbidities. However, the optimal strategy for defining lung cancer risk remains unknown, and efforts to refine existing risk models and eligibility criteria will need to take into account diverse populations so that LCS can be offered using an equitable approach. Second, although leveraging the EHR and other technology-based approaches may provide greater access to eligible patient and more efficient processes for carrying out LCS, optimal platforms and workflows are not yet known. Finally, ongoing focus on improving LCS uptake and implementing pathways for high-quality screening are also critical to realizing the promise of LCS.

Though lung cancer incidence has been declining for both men (since the mid-1980s) and women (since the mid-2000s), lung cancer is still quite prevalent. There will be an estimated 236,740 new cases of lung cancer in 2022 in the United

J. A. Barta (✉)
Department of Medicine, Thomas Jefferson University, Philadelphia, PA, USA
e-mail: Julie.barta@jefferson.edu

K. E. Knudsen
Sidney Kimmel Cancer Center, Thomas Jefferson University, Philadelphia, PA, USA

American Cancer Society, Atlanta, GA, USA
e-mail: Karen.knudsen@cancer.org

States, and 130,180 estimated deaths. From 2014–2018, the incidence rate was 57.3 per 100 K, and from 2015–2019, the death rate was 36.7 for 100 K [2]. According to the American College of Radiology Lung Cancer Screening public reports, the lung cancer screening rate was 6.6% in 2019 in the United States, and 6.5% in 2020 [3].

Optimizing Selection Criteria for Lung Cancer Screening

Multiple studies have demonstrated clearly that low-dose CT (LDCT) for LCS prevents the greatest number of deaths among participants at greatest risk for 5-year lung cancer death [4]. Subsequent studies have shown that using an individual risk-based model for selection for LCS may prevent more lung cancer deaths than categorical age and smoking-based eligibility criteria [5]. Specifically, the Prostate, Lung, Colorectal, and Ovarian Cancer Screening Trial ($PLCO_{m2012}$) model, Lung Cancer Risk Assessment (LCRAT) and Lung Cancer Death Risk Assessment (LCDRAT), and the Bach models have been noted to most accurately predict lung cancer risk and demonstrate superior performance in selecting individuals for LCS [5–8]. Moreover, risk prediction models can identify individuals who develop lung cancer with higher sensitivity, as well as greater cost effectiveness compared with United States Preventive Services Task Force criteria [6, 9, 10]. However, these risk models often select for individuals with the heaviest cigarette smoking histories, who may have competing causes of death including comorbid pulmonary or cardiovascular disease or other cancers. In this population, the balance of harms and benefits related to LCS may differ from that among individuals without comorbid conditions [11]. Currently, it is not known how best to integrate lung cancer risk and potential screening harms into defining eligibility for LCS. One approach to identifying an optimal threshold for LCS benefit is to measure life-years gained or quality-adjusted life-years gained. For example, using a risk-based prediction model to select individuals for LCS may lead to increased screening efficiency [12, 13]. However, these methods have not yet been tested prospectively or rigorously compared to current strategies.

Although individual risk-based prediction to identify eligible patients for LCS may improve reductions in lung cancer mortality, this hypothesis has not been tested in real-world cohorts with diverse racial, cultural, and geographic backgrounds. Current risk models have been derived from LCS trials including 5% or fewer Black/African-American individuals, potentially limiting their accuracy in vulnerable populations [14, 15]. For example, one centralized LCS program reported that 6-year lung cancer risk calculated using the $PLCO_{m2012}$ model was not aligned with lung cancer diagnoses among Black/African-American participants in LCS [16]. Moreover, subgroup analyses of the National Lung Screening Trial and NELSON suggest that Black/African-Americans and women may receive greater lung cancer mortality reduction from LCS compared with men [17, 18]. This and other similar studies suggest that our current understanding of lung cancer risk is incomplete [19].

In addition to improving the accuracy of existing clinical models, future research should test integrated clinical, radiologic, and molecular biomarkers for lung cancer risk stratification. Risk models can be combined with LDCT results to predict future lung cancer risk, which in turn could potentially inform screening intervals [20, 21]. Alternatively, clinical risk factors can be combined with blood-based biomarkers for personalized lung cancer risk assessment. For example, Fahrmann and colleagues reported statistically significant improvements in sensitivity and specificity for lung cancer prediction when combining the $PLCO_{m2012}$ model with a four-protein serum panel [22]. In the future, advances in incidental lung nodule management may be extended to screen-detected nodules as well; combined clinical variables, radiomic signatures, and blood biomarkers have been demonstrated to improve non-invasive diagnosis of indeterminate lung nodules [23].

Future research should also be directed toward populations with lung cancer risk factors that have not been well defined. For example, lung cancer incidence rate ratios have increased among young women born since 1965 compared to men, and this pattern is not fully explained by sex differences in smoking behavior [24]. Similarly, while individuals with low-intensity and nondaily smoking have increased risk for mortality and lung cancer diagnosis, the quantitative impact is not fully understood [25–27]. Finally, never-smokers may have other known or suspected risk factors that can eventually be quantified for lung cancer risk prediction [28].

Leveraging Technology for High-Quality Lung Cancer Screening

Technologic advancements in the healthcare arena have allowed for greater connectivity among providers, patients, and health systems. These connections can be leveraged to implement high-quality LCS. The electronic health record (EHR) has the capacity to improve identification and tracking of screen-eligible individuals, while telemedicine and social media strategies can increase knowledge and access to LCS.

The EHR offers strategies for addressing structural barriers, for example, by offering systematic reminders for providers to offer screening to eligible individuals for whom LDCT remains underutilized [1, 29]. Presently, many health systems have been unable to optimize the strengths of the EHR, and in some cases the EHR can even hinder LCS. For instance, electronic data are frequently inaccurate and/or inadequate to determine eligibility for screening, which diminishes referrals for LDCT [30–33]. These eligibility assessments must remain accurate even as eligibility guidelines undergo revision [34, 35]. There is also inconsistent use of the EHR for screening referrals and standardized templates or procedure codes, even among institutions within a single health system [36]. Finally, measurement of screening outcomes is complicated by unstructured and incomplete information stored in the EHR [37]. These data demonstrate that there are major knowledge gaps about the methods to harness the EHR for improving screening effectiveness.

Although multiple studies have demonstrated variability in identifying, reporting, tracking, and managing lung nodules across providers, institutions, and health systems, several strategies for leveraging the EHR have shown promise in mitigating variability in managing lung nodules [38–41]. For instance, the EHR can be utilized to promote screening through clinical decision support and electronic prompts [42]. In addition, novel approaches for patient communication using the EHR or other technological tools can improve cancer screening rates and patient decision support [43, 44]. Lung CT Screening Reporting and Data System (Lung-RADS) categories can be entered as discrete data, allowing for systematic alerts for nodules that require surveillance. Many centers have implemented multidisciplinary lung nodule clinics to develop approaches for expediting evaluation of suspicious nodules while limiting unnecessary procedures [45–47]. Other novel strategies – for example, integrating quantitative imaging features, clinical parameters, and genomic analyses through convolutional neural networks and other machine learning methods – may allow for discrimination of benign versus neoplastic nodules [48–50]. Therefore, identification of strategies to leverage the EHR's strengths has significant potential to reduce barriers and improve LCS, as well as other population-based health interventions.

Patient-facing communication strategies are also critical to increasing LCS uptake and adherence. We and others have shown that cost and convenience barriers are important factors for LCS program participants, and reasons for non-participation in screening can include distance of travel, lack of available public transportation, and cost of transportation or parking [51–53]. Telemedicine has the potential to mitigate these barriers, but few studies have examined the impact of telemedicine as a routine part of LCS implementation [54]. Other strategies for harnessing technology for direct communication with patients can include use of EHR messaging, text messaging, and social media. For example, smoking cessation programs delivered via mobile phone text messaging may improve not only short term self-reported quit rates, but also smoking cessation rates at 6 months [55]. Text messaging can also be utilized to increase screening uptake, as demonstrated in studies focused on breast, cervical, and colorectal cancer screening [43, 56]. Social media can also be leveraged to improve knowledge about lung cancer screening, and educational posts or advertisements can be targeted to eligible individuals [57]. Future research will need to define implementation strategies – including testing messaging among diverse, non-English-speaking populations – so that patient communication can be delivered equitably and effectively to all groups.

Expanding Implementation Strategies for Lung Cancer Screening

LCS is a complex process that involves a series of highly coordinated steps, from performing shared decision-making and standardized LDCT reporting, evaluating suspicious nodules, and managing incidental findings, to maximizing screening adherence [1]. Each of these steps may be implemented differently among centralized or decentralized LCS programs, and health systems or hospitals with varying resource availability and patient needs may carry out these steps using a variety of methods. Research is needed in multiple areas including defining strategies for increasing LCS uptake, integrating tobacco treatment counseling into LCS, and maximizing adherence with annual scans and short-interval follow-up [1]. Once feasible and effective strategies are developed, standardized approaches can be adopted by programs seeking to offer high-quality LCS. The inclusion of LCS-focused quality metrics in platforms such as the Health Effectiveness and Data Information Set, developed and reported by the National Committee for Quality Assurance, can further promote transparency and create accountability.

Prior to the expanded United States Preventive Services Task Force (USPSTF) eligibility criteria in 2021, studies reported a wide range of LCS rates up to 15%, with significant discordance between lung cancer mortality and state-level screening as well as large variability in geographic accessibility to LCS [58, 59]. With a larger denominator of individuals now eligible for LCS, estimated uptake is far lower [60]. Processes for improving LCS uptake are complex and require multilevel interventions to address patient-, provider-, and systems-related barriers [61]. Effective community engagement requires the development of culturally and linguistically appropriate educational materials, leveraging relationships with community stakeholders, and facilitating convenient access for shared decision-making and LDCT scans. Furthermore, community health workers can be effective in increasing LCS awareness and knowledge among underserved populations [62]. Outreach approaches will need to be tailored to local needs, with geographic information systems mapping providing one potential way of identifying areas of vulnerability [59, 63].

Future research should also identify implementation strategies for LCS programs to strengthen critical components of the screening pathway [64]. For example, the optimal approaches to integrating tobacco treatment counseling into LCS are not currently known. Although LCS is a teachable moment for smoking cessation and positive LDCT results have been associated with increased quit rates in retrospective analyses, some randomized clinical trials have not demonstrated statistically significant differences in short- or long-term abstinence rates [65, 66]. An additional area of needed investigation is in defining methods for increasing adherence with annual LCS and short-interval follow-up scans. Multiple studies have demonstrated that increased LCS adherence may be associated with individual-level factors such as age, smoking status, and education level, as well as LDCT results and LCS program structure [52, 67, 68]. What remains unknown is how barriers to participation can be addressed to improve LCS adherence. Ongoing work in the field includes development of adherence toolkits, as well as studies of telemedicine utilization to improve convenience in LCS [69, 70]. Other critical steps in the screening pathway where research gaps remain include implementation of shared decision-making, characterizing harms of LCS, and defining strategies for patient coordination, navigation, and tracking to ultimately improve patient-centered screening outcomes. Development of standardized definitions and quality metrics in the field will be crucial to moving forward in these areas.

Conclusion

The landscape of lung cancer screening is growing exponentially, with near-constant advances in epidemiology and population health, implementation science, and biomarker research. Increased recognition of lung cancer screening investigation as a funding priority is critical for continuing these rapid advances in the field. Additionally, ongoing support from research consortia, professional societies, advocacy organizations, and cross-cutting multidisciplinary groups is crucial. These organizations should focus on bringing high-quality lung cancer screening to all individuals at risk for lung cancer, with particular attention to providing equitable screening for under-represented groups. Vulnerable populations can include those experiencing disparities related to race, sexual orientation, geography, socioeconomic status, and psychiatric and/or substance use disorders. Future gains in lung cancer survival depend on a comprehensive and inclusive approach to research in early detection.

References

1. Mazzone PJ, Silvestri GA, Souter LH, Caverly TJ, Kanne JP, Katki HA, et al. Screening for lung cancer: CHEST guideline and expert panel report. Chest. 2021;160(5):e427–94.
2. Siegel RL, Miller KD, Fuchs HE, Jemal A, et al. Cancer statistics 2022. CA Cancer J Clin. 2022;72:7–33.
3. Fedewa SA, Bandi P, Smith RA, Silvestri GA, Jemal A, et al. Lung cancer screening rates during the COVID-19 pandemic. Chest. 2021;161:587–8.
4. Kovalchik SA, Tammemagi M, Berg CD, Caporaso NE, Riley TL, Korch M, et al. Targeting of low-dose CT screening according to the risk of lung-cancer death. N Engl J Med. 2013;369(3):245–54.
5. Katki HA, Kovalchik SA, Berg CD, Cheung LC, Chaturvedi AK. Development and validation of risk models to select ever-smokers for CT lung cancer screening. JAMA. 2016;315(21):2300–11.
6. Katki HA, Kovalchik SA, Petito LC, Cheung LC, Jacobs E, Jemal A, et al. Implications of nine risk prediction models for selecting ever-smokers for computed tomography lung cancer screening. Ann Intern Med. 2018;169(1):10–9.
7. Oken MM, Hocking WG, Kvale PA, Andriole GL, Buys SS, Church TR, et al. Screening by chest radiograph and lung cancer mortality: the prostate, lung, colorectal, and ovarian (PLCO) randomized trial. JAMA. 2011;306(17):1865–73.
8. Bach PB, Kattan MW, Thornquist MD, Kris MG, Tate RC, Barnett MJ, et al. Variations in lung cancer risk among smokers. J Natl Cancer Inst. 2003;95(6):470–8.
9. Tammemägi MC, Ruparel M, Tremblay A, Myers R, Mayo J, Yee J, et al. USPSTF2013 versus PLCOm2012 lung cancer screening eligibility criteria (international lung screening trial): interim analysis of a prospective cohort study. Lancet Oncol. 2022;23(1):138–48.
10. Cressman S, Peacock SJ, Tammemägi MC, Evans WK, Leighl NB, Goffin JR, et al. The cost-effectiveness of high-risk lung cancer screening and drivers of program efficiency. J Thorac Oncol. 2017;12(8):1210–22.
11. Rivera MP, Tanner NT, Silvestri GA, Detterbeck FC, Tammemägi MC, Young RP, et al. Incorporating coexisting chronic illness into decisions about patient selection for lung cancer screening. An official American Thoracic Society Research Statement. Am J Respir Crit Care Med. 2018;198(2):e3–e13.

12. Kumar V, Cohen JT, van Klaveren D, Soeteman DI, Wong JB, Neumann PJ, et al. Risk-targeted lung cancer screening. Ann Intern Med. 2018;168(3):161–9.
13. Meza R, Jeon J, Toumazis I, ten Haaf K, Cao P, Bastani M, et al. Evaluation of the benefits and harms of lung cancer screening with low-dose computed tomography: modeling study for the US preventive services task force. JAMA. 2021;325(10):988–97.
14. Aberle DR, Adams AM, Berg CD, Black WC, Clapp JD, Fagerstrom RM, et al. Reduced lung-cancer mortality with low-dose computed tomographic screening. N Engl J Med. 2011;365(5):395–409.
15. Tammemagi MC, Katki HA, Hocking WG, Church TR, Caporaso N, Kvale PA, et al. Selection criteria for lung-cancer screening. N Engl J Med. 2013;368(8):728–36.
16. Shusted CS, Evans NR, Juon H-S, Kane GC, Barta JA. Association of race with lung cancer risk among adults undergoing lung cancer screening. JAMA Netw Open. 2021;4(4):e214509.
17. Tanner NT, Gebregziabher M, Hughes Halbert C, Payne E, Egede LE, Silvestri GA. Racial differences in outcomes within the National lung screening trial. Implications for widespread implementation. Am J Respir Crit Care Med. 2015;192(2):200–8.
18. de Koning HJ, van der Aalst CM, de Jong PA, Scholten ET, Nackaerts K, Heuvelmans MA, et al. Reduced lung-cancer mortality with volume CT screening in a randomized trial. N Engl J Med. 2020;382:503–13.
19. Pasquinelli MM, Tammemägi MC, Kovitz KL, Durham ML, Deliu Z, Rygalski K, et al. Risk prediction model versus United States preventive services task Force lung cancer screening eligibility criteria: reducing race disparities. J Thorac Oncol. 2020;15:1738–47.
20. Tammemägi MC, ten Haaf K, Toumazis I, Kong CY, Han SS, Jeon J, et al. Development and validation of a multivariable lung cancer risk prediction model that includes low-dose computed tomography screening results: a secondary analysis of data from the National lung screening trial. JAMA Netw Open. 2019;2(3):e190204.
21. Robbins HA, Cheung LC, Chaturvedi AK, Baldwin DR, Berg CD, Katki HA. Management of lung cancer screening results based on individual prediction of current and future lung cancer risks. J Thorac Oncol. 2022;17(2):252–63.
22. Fahrmann JF, Marsh T, Irajizad E, Patel N, Murage E, Vykoukal J, et al. Blood-based biomarker panel for personalized lung cancer risk assessment. J Clin Oncol. 2022;40(8):876–83.
23. Kammer MN, Lakhani DA, Balar AB, Antic SL, Kussrow AK, Webster RL, et al. Integrated biomarkers for the management of indeterminate pulmonary nodules. Am J Respir Crit Care Med. 2021;204(11):1306–16.
24. Jemal A, Miller KD, Ma J, Siegel RL, Fedewa SA, Islami F, et al. Higher lung cancer incidence in young women than young men in the United States. N Engl J Med. 2018;378(21):1999–2009.
25. Inoue-Choi M, Christensen CH, Rostron BL, Cosgrove CM, Reyes-Guzman C, Apelberg B, et al. Dose-response Association of low-intensity and nondaily smoking with mortality in the United States. JAMA Netw Open. 2020;3(6):e206436.
26. Thomson B, Tapia-Conyer R, Lacey B, Lewington S, Ramirez-Reyes R, Aguilar-Ramirez D, et al. Low-intensity daily smoking and cause-specific mortality in Mexico: prospective study of 150 000 adults. Int J Epidemiol. 2021;50(3):955–64.
27. Balte P, Bhatt S, Chaves P, Couper D, Freedman N, Jacobs D Jr, et al. Association of low-intensity smoking with respiratory and lung cancer mortality. Eur Respir J. 2020;56(suppl 64):4389.
28. Kerpel-Fronius A, Tammemägi M, Cavic M, Henschke C, Jiang L, Kazerooni E, et al. Screening for lung cancer in individuals who never smoked: an International Association for the Study of Lung Cancer early detection and screening committee report. J Thorac Oncol. 2022;17(1):56–66.
29. Fathi JT, White CS, Greenberg GM, Mazzone PJ, Smith RA, Thomson CC. The integral role of the electronic health record and tracking software in the implementation of lung cancer screening; a call to action to developers: a white paper from the National lung cancer roundtable. Chest. 2020;157(6):1674–9.

30. Cole AM, Pflugeisen B, Schwartz MR, Miller SC. Cross sectional study to assess the accuracy of electronic health record data to identify patients in need of lung cancer screening. BMC Res Notes. 2018;11(1):14.
31. Tarabichi Y, Kats DJ, Kaelber DC, Thornton JD. The impact of fluctuations in pack-year smoking history in the electronic health record on lung cancer screening practices. Chest. 2018;153(2):575–8.
32. Wilshire CL, Fuller CC, Gilbert CR, Handy JR, Costas KE, Louie BE, et al. Electronic medical record inaccuracies: multicenter analysis of challenges with modified lung cancer screening criteria. Can Respir J. 2020;2020:7142568.
33. Modin HE, Fathi JT, Gilbert CR, Wilshire CL, Wilson AK, Aye RW, et al. Pack-year cigarette smoking history for determination of lung cancer screening eligibility. Comparison of the electronic medical record versus a shared decision-making conversation. Ann Am Thorac Soc. 2017;14(8):1320–5.
34. Force USPST. Draft recommendation statement: lung cancer, screening. 2020. https://www.uspreventiveservicestaskforce.org/uspstf/draft-recommendation/lung-cancer-screening-2020#fullrecommendationstart;2020July.
35. Force USPST. Screening for lung cancer: US preventive services task force recommendation statement. JAMA. 2021;325(10):962–70.
36. Gould MK, Sakoda LC, Ritzwoller DP, Simoff MJ, Neslund-Dudas CM, Kushi LH, et al. Monitoring lung cancer screening use and outcomes at four cancer research network sites. Ann Am Thorac Soc. 2017;14(12):1827–35.
37. Rai A, Doria-Rose VP, Silvestri GA, Yabroff KR. Evaluating lung cancer screening uptake, outcomes, and costs in the United States: challenges with existing data and recommendations for improvement. J Natl Cancer Inst. 2019;111(4):342–9.
38. Tanner NT, Porter A, Gould MK, Li XJ, Vachani A, Silvestri GA. Physician assessment of pretest probability of malignancy and adherence with guidelines for pulmonary nodule evaluation. Chest. 2017;152(2):263–70.
39. Tanner NT, Aggarwal J, Gould MK, Kearney P, Diette G, Vachani A, et al. Management of pulmonary nodules by community pulmonologists: a multicenter observational study. Chest. 2015;148(6):1405–14.
40. Gould MK, Donington J, Lynch WR, Mazzone PJ, Midthun DE, Naidich DP, et al. Evaluation of individuals with pulmonary nodules: when is it lung cancer? Diagnosis and management of lung cancer, 3rd ed: American College of Chest Physicians evidence-based clinical practice guidelines. Chest. 2013;143(5 Suppl):e93S–120S.
41. MacMahon H, Naidich DP, Goo JM, Lee KS, Leung ANC, Mayo JR, et al. Guidelines for management of incidental pulmonary nodules detected on CT images: from the Fleischner society 2017. Radiology. 2017;284(1):228–43.
42. Patel MS, Navathe AS, Liao JM. Using nudges to improve value by increasing imaging-based cancer screening. J Am Coll Radiol. 2020;17(1):38–41.
43. Mougalian SS, Gross CP, Hall EK. Text messaging in oncology: a review of the landscape. JCO Clin Cancer Inform. 2018;2:1–9.
44. Fukunaga MI, Halligan K, Kodela J, Toomey S, Furtado VF, Luckmann R, et al. Tools to promote shared decision making in lung cancer screening using low-dose computerized tomography: a systematic review. Chest. 2020;156:A1732.
45. Roberts TJ, Lennes IT, Hawari S, Sequist LV, Park ER, Willers H, et al. Integrated, multidisciplinary management of pulmonary nodules can streamline care and improve adherence to recommendations. Oncologist. 2020;25(5):431–7.
46. Verdial FC, Madtes DK, Cheng G-S, Pipavath S, Kim R, Hubbard JJ, et al. Multidisciplinary team-based management of incidentally detected lung nodules. Chest. 2020;157(4):985–93.
47. Madariaga ML, Lennes IT, Best T, Shepard J-AO, Fintelmann FJ, Mathisen DJ, et al. Multidisciplinary selection of pulmonary nodules for surgical resection: diagnostic results and long-term outcomes. J Thorac Cardiovasc Surg. 2020;159(4):1558–66.e3.

48. Baldwin DR, Gustafson J, Pickup L, Arteta C, Novotny P, Declerck J, et al. External validation of a convolutional neural network artificial intelligence tool to predict malignancy in pulmonary nodules. Thorax. 2020;75(4):306.
49. Massion PP, Antic S, Ather S, Arteta C, Brabec J, Chen H, et al. Assessing the accuracy of a deep learning method to risk stratify indeterminate pulmonary nodules. Am J Respir Crit Care Med. 2020;202(2):241–9.
50. Wang J, Gao R, Huo Y, Bao S, Xiong Y, Antic SL, et al. Lung cancer detection using co-learning from chest CT images and clinical demographics. Proc SPIE Int Soc Opt Eng. 2019;10949:109491G.
51. Raju S, Khawaja A, Han X, Wang X, Mazzone PJ. Lung cancer screening: characteristics of nonparticipants and potential screening barriers. Clin Lung Cancer. 2020;21(5):e329–36.
52. Barta JA, Shusted CS, Ruane B, Pimpinelli M, McIntire RK, Zeigler-Johnson C, et al. Racial differences in lung cancer screening beliefs and screening adherence. Clin Lung Cancer. 2021;22(6):570–8.
53. Ali N, Lifford KJ, Carter B, McRonald F, Yadegarfar G, Baldwin DR, et al. Barriers to uptake among high-risk individuals declining participation in lung cancer screening: a mixed methods analysis of the UK lung cancer screening (UKLS) trial. BMJ Open. 2015;5(7):e008254.
54. Henderson LM, Benefield T, Bosemani T, Long JM, Rivera MP. Impact of the COVID-19 pandemic on volumes and disparities in lung cancer screening. Chest. 2021;160(1):379–82.
55. Free C, Knight R, Robertson S, Whittaker R, Edwards P, Zhou W, et al. Smoking cessation support delivered via mobile phone text messaging (txt2stop): a single-blind, randomised trial. Lancet. 2011;378(9785):49–55.
56. Kerrison RS, Shukla H, Cunningham D, Oyebode O, Friedman E. Text-message reminders increase uptake of routine breast screening appointments: a randomised controlled trial in a hard-to-reach population. Br J Cancer. 2015;112(6):1005–10.
57. Strong A, Renaud M. Using social media as a platform for increasing knowledge of lung cancer screening in high-risk patients. J Adv Pract Oncol. 2020;11(5):453–9.
58. Fedewa SA, Kazerooni EA, Studts JL, Smith RA, Bandi P, Sauer AG, et al. State variation in low-dose computed tomography scanning for lung cancer screening in the United States. J Natl Cancer Inst. 2020;113:1044–52.
59. Sahar L, Douangchai Wills VL, Liu KK, Kazerooni EA, Dyer DS, Smith RA. Using geo-spatial analysis to evaluate access to lung cancer screening in the United States. Chest. 2020;159:833–44. https://doi.org/10.1016/j.chest.2020.08.2081.
60. Rivera MP, Katki HA, Tanner NT, Triplette M, Sakoda LC, Wiener RS, et al. Addressing disparities in lung cancer screening eligibility and healthcare access. An official American Thoracic Society Statement. Am J Respir Crit Care Med. 2020;202(7):e95–e112.
61. Wang GX, Baggett TP, Pandharipande PV, Park ER, Percac-Lima S, Shepard J-AO, et al. Barriers to lung cancer screening engagement from the patient and provider perspective. Radiology. 2019;290(2):278–87.
62. Williams LB, Shelton BJ, Gomez ML, Al-Mrayat YD, Studts JL. Using implementation science to disseminate a lung cancer screening education intervention through community health workers. J Community Health. 2021;46(1):165–73.
63. Le T, Miller S, Berry E, Zamarripa S, Rodriguez A, Barkley B, et al. Implementation and uptake of rural lung cancer screening. J Am Coll Radiol. 2022;19(3):480–7.
64. Lam S, Tammemagi M. Contemporary issues in the implementation of lung cancer screening. Eur Respir Rev. 2021;30(161):200288.
65. Brain K, Carter B, Lifford KJ, Burke O, Devaraj A, Baldwin DR, et al. Impact of low-dose CT screening on smoking cessation among high-risk participants in the UK lung cancer screening trial. Thorax. 2017;72(10):912.
66. Tremblay A, Taghizadeh N, Huang J, Kasowski D, MacEachern P, Burrowes P, et al. A randomized controlled study of integrated smoking cessation in a lung cancer screening program. J Thorac Oncol. 2019;14(9):1528–37.

67. Lopez-Olivo MA, Maki KG, Choi NJ, Hoffman RM, Shih Y-CT, Lowenstein LM, et al. Patient adherence to screening for lung cancer in the US: a systematic review and meta-analysis. JAMA Netw Open. 2020;3(11):e2025102.
68. Sakoda LC, Rivera MP, Zhang J, Perera P, Laurent CA, Durham D, et al. Patterns and factors associated with adherence to lung cancer screening in diverse practice settings. JAMA Netw Open. 2021;4(4):e218559.
69. Roy UB, Byrne M, McCoy J, Blair C, Studts J. P2.11-32 project ACTS (adherence to CT screening): developing patient engagement tools to support lung cancer screening adherence. J Thorac Oncol. 2019;14(10):S805–S6.
70. Shusted CS, Juon HS, Ruane BM, Jackson B, Zeigler-Johnson C, McIntire R, et al. A comparison of sociodemographic characteristics of patients undergoing lung cancer screening during the COVID-19 pandemic with pre-COVID patients. B8 B008 LUNG CANCER 2021: ADVANCES IN TARGETS, SCREENING, AND DIAGNOSIS. American Thoracic Society international conference abstracts: American Thoracic Society; 2021. p. A1080-A.

Chapter 34
Imagining an Equitable Lung Cancer Screening Landscape

Gregory C. Kane, Julie A. Barta, Nathaniel R. Evans III, and Ronald E. Myers

Imagining the Following

Current lung cancer screening (LCS) guidelines from the United States Preventive Services Task Force (USPSTF) and the Centers for Medicare and Medicaid Services (CMS) make screening available, beginning at age 50 for persons who have a smoking history of 20 or more pack-years and have not quit in the previous 15 years [1]. When compared to earlier USPSTF and CMS screening guidelines, these changes will have the effect of substantially increasing the number of women and persons in minority populations who are eligible for LCS [2–5]. While increasing the number of persons in vulnerable populations who are eligible for screening is a positive step, this change alone may not have a beneficial effect on achieving greater equity in LCS and related outcomes [5, 6]. Health systems must take steps to help ensure more significant equity in initial and repeat screening uptake as well as in the follow-up of abnormal screening results.

As documented throughout the book, a critical step in ensuring equity across the care continuum is guaranteeing the patient fully understands the impact of undergoing screening and the potential downstream tests and procedures that may accompany an abnormal scan. To assist patients, who often may not have a high degree of health literacy, high quality shared decision making (SDM) about LCS

G. C. Kane (✉) · J. A. Barta
Department of Medicine, Thomas Jefferson University, Philadelphia, PA, USA
e-mail: Gregory.Kane@Jefferson.edu; Julie.barta@jefferson.edu

N. R. Evans III
Department of Surgery, Thomas Jefferson University, Philadelphia, PA, USA
e-mail: Nathaniel.Evans@Jefferson.edu

R. E. Myers
Medical Oncology, Thomas Jefferson University, Philadelphia, PA, USA
e-mail: Ronald.Myers@Jefferson.edu

© The Author(s), under exclusive license to Springer Nature Switzerland AG 2023
G. C. Kane et al. (eds.), *Lung Cancer Screening*,
https://doi.org/10.1007/978-3-031-33596-9_34

is imperative. SDM must include patient education about screening as well as clarification of patient values and preferences related to screening. Unfortunately, this does not routinely occur in clinical practice. Several tools exist to assist primary care providers and other clinicians to work through SDM about lung cancer, one option discussed in earlier chapters is a free, online, self-directed LCS SDM program developed by leading experts from the National Lung Cancer Roundtable, Thomas Jefferson University, the American College of Chest Physicians, and the Go2 Foundation. Health systems that wish to increase the likelihood that patient–provider conversations about LCS occur in a structured manner that minimizes bias should encourage providers to consider completing an SDM training program.

Health systems are indeed prepared to enter an "Era of Health Equity" in Medicine after prior eras of "Expansion," "Cost Containment," and "Assessment and Accountability" [7]. It is also clear that the new generation of healthcare leaders are prepared to lead this charge. In imagining the future landscape of LCS, we do indeed see the prospect of expanding this screening service in scope to match mammography and colonoscopy, as well as to address health equity, not as an afterthought but as the primary goal of this effort. Moreover, the uptake of LCS has been sporadic across states and regions of the United States and has not been aligned with lung cancer mortality [8]. By comparison, breast and colon cancer, which have lower overall mortality in the United States, have screening rates of approximately 70% [9]. We must and will meet this level of uptake by the end of the 2020s.

A crucial step toward expanding LCS to the likes of mammography and colonoscopy: engaging organizational leaders, health plan representatives, primary care providers, patients from vulnerable populations, community organization advocates, and other stakeholders in a learning community dedicated to increasing LCS and equity is a must. In our experience, this health system–based learning community at Jefferson Health not only developed an effective LCS population outreach and SDM strategy, but also put in motion a "call to action" aimed at engaging vulnerable populations, healthcare systems, and health plans alike through a white paper. Specifically, health systems are encouraged to organize lung cancer learning communities, adopt a systematic approach to identifying and engaging patients in SDM and LCS at multiple touchpoints, conduct cost analyses related to the screening effort, and advocate for increased public and private investment in strategies that can increase screening and equity. While this may require an up-front investment, the potential for downstream revenue from additional diagnostic testing, biopsies, surgeries, and treatment for tumors identified at earlier stages should provide substantial revenue for hospitals and health systems and most importantly should provide an opportunity for cure from early detection and reduction in smoking rates.

Perhaps the greatest potential of utilizing a health system-wide learning community is to present a framework for provider support and patient outreach for all individuals touched by the healthcare system, with a particular focus on underserved and often overlooked peoples. As members of such a community, the editors of this book can attest to the power of the learning community model: continuous adaption to the changing landscape of screening, testing new initiatives, as well as learning and publishing as we move forward toward building a more equitable LCS process within our own system and sharing our insights along the way. This possibility has been enhanced by new partnerships with philanthropic organizations, which have catalyzed further research and new funding. In a remarkable essay in the New Yorker [10], Atul Gawande presents a philosophical argument that incrementalism in modern medicine is the pathway to gradual and iterative advances in outcomes for patients. We agree. The iterative process in this new field of endeavor (LCS) is being catalyzed by the learning community model and the willingness of thought leaders to imagine a more just future. However, there is a need for urgency if we are to realize the goal of increased and more equitable rollout of LCS to match the screening uptake of mammography and colonoscopy by the end of this decade.

One modern tool that was not historically available in generations past to address health equity is the electronic health record (EHR). While ridiculed as a "billing machine" with a patient note feature attached [11], the more recent versions of EHRs have provided public health tools that may help us transform patient outreach and management [12–15]. The growing use of the EHR for public health applications may be its most important and, not quite yet fulfilled, application.

This process may be further accelerated by the use of geographic information systems and geographic analyses, which can add a new dimension to outreach and be enhanced by overlaying patient-level data with geographic data. These analyses allow for the identification and characterization of areas with a high burden of lung cancer risk factors while determining where patients impacted by the program reside. Investigation utilizing geographic analyses allows for data visualization in a way never before possible. Such data visualization at the community and health district level could allow for focusing on areas of greatest need: namely, areas of high smoking-associated mortality.

Health systems should embrace the opportunity to raise screening rates and increase equity by developing, implementing, evaluating, and sustaining strategies intended to support primary care providers and provide patient outreach contact interventions. Specifically, health systems are encouraged to support provider efforts to identify patients eligible for LCS, train providers in high-quality SDM, and facilitate patient referral and appointment scheduling. Regarding patient outreach, health systems are encouraged to prepare direct care coordinators to contact eligible patients and engage them in SDM about LCS.

Recent studies on organizational change suggest that health systems motivated to address community needs and that choose to develop and implement innovative strategies to engage relevant stakeholders in efforts to increase LCS can position themselves for success. Throughout the book, we highlighted decentralized and centralized models of health system-based LCS programs, as well as current program LCS practices, and explored the utility of an implementation framework that can guide the development of programs within health systems that can increase screening and equity. Health systems are encouraged to use rapid cycle testing and other approaches to designing and testing new LCS screening models that take advantage of the strengths of current LCS models and address the inherent weaknesses of the models in their capacity to increase equity.

Equity in the Conduct of Screening and Follow-Up

Amidst these large-scale efforts to improve rates of LCS, optimizing the balance of harms and benefits must remain a priority. Simply increasing the number of eligible individuals who undergo LCS will undermine the larger goal of reducing lung cancer mortality if we fail to define the population for whom early detection of lung cancer provides the greatest benefits [3]. Ongoing research in this area includes risk model-based selection of individuals for LCS, as well as refining methods for measuring quality-adjusted life-years gained through screening. As the field moves forward, it is critical to remember that lung cancer risk factors may carry different levels of significance for different groups, and that unique moderators and mediators may impact various vulnerable or underserved populations to a different extent. For a more comprehensive understanding of lung cancer risk, we need to include more racial, geographic, socioeconomic, and other diverse subgroups of individuals in clinical trials and research studies.

Once patients enter the door for LCS, a myriad of additional barriers may stand in the way of successful screening completion. It is imperative that we provide education, navigation, and other resources to facilitate the complex process of LCS. Multidisciplinary, centralized programs, for example, can provide comprehensive guidance for patients from shared decision-making through low-dose Computed Tomography screening (LDCT) scheduling, results review, and evaluation of positive screening findings. Prior work from our group and others has demonstrated that vulnerable populations have lower rates of LCS completion and longer time to follow-up [15, 16]. Providing navigation support to underserved individuals may be one method of facilitating LCS, although this has not been demonstrated in a prospective clinical trial as yet [17]. Annual adherence with subsequent LDCT screening and management of incidental findings are additional outcomes where centralized LCS programs may provide benefits to individuals undergoing screening [18]. To ensure equity in the conduct of screening, it is critical for programs to demonstrate a racially and culturally sensitive, non-stigmatized approach to welcoming individuals at high risk for lung cancer. In all of this, the organizational structure of the LCS program may prove pivotal, in part because the process of LCS is so different from other cancer screening services. While centralized programs are more resource-intensive, such resources can free primary care physicians to focus on managing chronic health conditions and responding to acute patient complaints.

This author team, in many ways, is characteristic of the effectiveness of a diverse healthcare team in addressing healthcare disparities. Coming from different racial, ethnic, and professional backgrounds, and importantly representing different disciplines of Medicine, Surgery, and Public Health, we can each bring a perspective to solving this problem that is unique and greater than any of us alone could contribute. This perspective needs to be developed more prominently in our US healthcare systems, but especially in academic medical centers where we train the next generation of learners and disseminate ideas through our scholarship of discovery. Jordan Cohen, MD, an Internist and former President of the Association of American

Medical Colleges (AAMC), made a strong case for a diverse healthcare workforce two decades ago, emphasizing the need to reform the pre-college educational system [19]. Unfortunately, recent data, while showing a positive trend toward increased numbers of underrepresented minorities in medicine, still has not shown a substantial change in the numbers of underrepresented trainees in Internal Medicine [20].

Approaching LCS with awareness of the social determinants of health will empower healthcare organizations to consider multifaceted determinants of health as they relate to housing (and its influence on lung cancer risks such as radon or asbestos exposure), transportation (and its effect on high-risk individuals to present for lung cancer screening, as well as how health systems choose to locate their facilities including CT scans and physicians' offices), the digital divide (including access to electronic health records), and of course racial and ethnic disparity – with special attention to culturally and health literacy appropriate communication tools (such specific outreach can help us target populations that have the highest mortality) [21]. Daniel and others have highlighted the complexities of the social determinants of health [21]. Now, it will be the chance for healthcare entities, including Federally Qualified Healthcare Centers (FQHC), Community Health Organizations, private as well as not-for-profit healthcare entities, health systems, and academic health centers to be proactive with regard to these issues. A number of authors who penned this book have been focal in addressing systemic racism as it relates to LCS, so that we can move "beyond equal guidelines" to capture true disparities, without leaving anybody behind [2]. Implicit in the social determinants of health is access to health insurance and health coverage. Fortunately, since the Affordable Care Act, gaps in coverage have been narrowing in the United States. Coverage is an essential element; based upon confidence from the gains of the Affordable Care Act, these authors look forward to a future of healthcare insurance coverage in the United States that leaves fewer Americans behind – including those from zip codes with high smoking-related mortality [22].

One area emphasized in this treatise is the need for ongoing clinical trials to focus more intently on disparities in our clinical research. Acknowledging the limited enrollment of diverse persons in the National Lung Screening Trial (NLST) was lacking, and we must commit to a more equitable analysis of attitudes and perceptions of LCS acceptance among various communities and vulnerable populations if we expect to address the disparities in our midst [23].

A final barrier to an equitable and substantial increase in LCS is addressing stigma and fatalism. We placed an important chapter in an early section of this book because of the role that stigma and fatalism play in affecting not just smokers but all lung cancer patients [24]. In Chap. 3, the authors describe the fundamental stigma of smoking as a behavior and modifiable risk factor [25, 26]. It is clear that to encourage eligible Americans to join in LCS, we must mitigate this stigma and allow eligible individuals to seek care without blame or stress. Unfortunately, there has been little research on this topic, but recent investigations are beginning to chip away at this obstacle [27, 28]. Not to be underemphasized is the need for lung cancer clinicians – internists, pulmonologists, surgeons, oncologists, radiation therapists, and advanced practice providers (APPs), to take ownership of the history of stigmatism and do everything in their power to overcome this unfortunate perception among patients. A recent communication module has shown an important impact, specifically in addressing this issue in lung cancer [29]. While stigma may interfere with presenting for screening or initial symptoms evaluation, fatalism can impact therapy selections of patients already diagnosed with lung cancer [30]. Certainly, our hope is that through a shared decision making approach every patient will freely choose the best type of therapy for them as individuals. Our hope is also, however, that fatalism will not prevent them from making certain decisions that could prove helpful or even curative, because of a premature sense that they are going to die regardless of the plan of care. The simple truth is that current advances in lung cancer therapeutics can offer hope, even for patients with advanced-stage disease. From the perspective of equity, it is important to underscore that black and Hispanic persons were more likely than whites to exhibit fatalistic beliefs [31]. Again, it is incumbent of physicians caring for lung cancer patients to remain current with the clinic science of lung cancer treatment and to be sure that all patient recommendations are based on objective facts and not influenced by fatalism or pessimism [32].

We can envision a more equitable implementation of LCS if we have the commitment and partnerships to succeed. Using, again, the convention outlined by Richard Rothstein in his landmark book entitled *The Color of Law*, the term "we" will refer to the collective of the members of the health care system, including administrative and clinical leaders, physicians, nurses, respiratory therapists, medical assistants, navigators, and public health professionals [33]. *We* have the responsibility to expand LCS informed by public health science and with a commitment to ensuring the expanded implementation is equitable across zip codes, communities, and US regions. The public health approach outlined in this treatise can serve as a roadmap to guide health systems and communities toward a future of a more equitable lung screening reality that can address the mortality across all populations with no racial, ethnic, or demographic groups left behind. All that this will take is the application of our energy and imaginations!

References

1. Moyer VA. Screening for lung cancer: US preventive services task force recommendation statement. Ann Intern Med. 2014;160(5):330–8.
2. Robbins HA, Landy R, Ahluwalia JS. Achieving equity in lung cancer screening for black individuals requires innovation to move beyond "equal" guidelines. JAMA Oncol. 2022;8:514.
3. Tanner NT, Gebregziabher M, Hughes Halbert C, Payne E, Egede LE, Silvestri GA. Racial differences in outcomes within the National Lung Screening Trial. Implications for widespread implementation. Am J Respir Crit Care Med. 2015;192(2):200–8.
4. Rivera MP, Katki HA, Tanner NT, Triplette M, Sakoda LC, Wiener RS, et al. Addressing disparities in Lung cancer Screening eligibility and healthcare access. An official American Thoracic Society statement. Am J Respir Crit Care Med. 2020;202(7):e95–e112.
5. Horn DM, Haas JS. Expanded lung and colorectal cancer screening—ensuring equity and safety under new guidelines. N Engl J Med. 2022;386(2):100–2.

6. Pu CY, Lusk CM, Neslund-Dudas C, Gadgeel S, Soubani AO, Schwartz AG. Comparison between the 2021 USPSTF lung cancer screening criteria and other lung cancer screening criteria for racial disparity in eligibility. JAMA Oncol. 2022;8(3):374–82.

7. Relman AS. Assessment and accountability: the third revolution in medical care. N Engl J Med. 1988;319(18):1220–2.

8. Fedewa SA, Kazerooni EA, Studts JL, Smith RA, Bandi P, Sauer AG, et al. State variation in low-dose computed tomography scanning for Lung cancer Screening in the United States. J Natl Cancer Inst. 2021;113(8):1044–52.

9. Anon. QuickStats: death rates* from colorectal cancer,(†) by age group—United States, 1999–2019. MMWR Morb Mortal Wkly Rep. 2021;70(35):1233.

10. Gawande A. The heroism of incremental care, vol. 23. New York: The New Yorker; 2017.

11. Mearian L. Poorly designed systems make doctors 'a slave to their EHR' 2019 [updated May 22nd, 2019, March 27th, 2021]. https://www.computerworld.com/article/3397039/poorly-designed-systems-make-doctors-a-slave-to-their-ehr.html.

12. Fathi JT, White CS, Greenberg GM, Mazzone PJ, Smith RA, Thomson CC. The integral role of the electronic health record and tracking software in the implementation of Lung cancer Screening-a call to action to developers: a white paper from the National Lung Cancer Roundtable. Chest. 2020;157(6):1674–9.

13. Shekelle PG, Pane JD, Agniel D, Shi Y, Rumball-Smith J, Haas A, et al. Assessment of variation in electronic health record capabilities and reported clinical quality performance in ambulatory care clinics, 2014-2017. JAMA Netw Open. 2021;4(4):e217476.

14. Kern LM, Barrón Y, Dhopeshwarkar RV, Edwards A, Kaushal R. Electronic health records and ambulatory quality of care. J Gen Intern Med. 2013;28(4):496–503.

15. Lake M, Shusted CS, Juon HS, et al. Black patients referred to a lung cancer screening program experience lower rates of screening and longer time to follow-up. BMC Cancer. 2020;20:561.

16. Sakoda LC, Rivera MP, Zhang J, Perera P, Laurent CA, Durham D, et al. Patterns and factors associated with adherence to lung cancer screening in diverse practice settings. JAMA Netw Open. 2021;4(4):e218559.

17. Smith HB, Ward R, Frazier C, Angotti J, Tanner NT. Guideline-recommended lung cancer screening adherence is superior with a centralized approach. Chest. 2022;161(3):818–25. https://doi.org/10.1016/j.chest.2021.09.002. Epub 2021 Sep 15.

18. Mazzone PJ, Silvestri GA, Patel S, Kanne JP, Kinsinger LS, Wiener RS, Soo Hoo G, Detterbeck FC. Screening for Lung cancer: CHEST guideline and expert panel report. Chest. 2018;153(4):954–85. https://doi.org/10.1016/j.chest.2018.01.016. Epub 2018 Feb 17.

19. Cohen JJ, Gabriel BA, Terrell C. The case for diversity in the health care workforce. Health Aff (Millwood). 2002;21(5):90–102.

20. Liao J, Nishath T, Thevuthasan S, Nieblas-Bedolla E, Christophers B, Starks H, et al. Race/ethnicity trends among US internal medicine residency applicants and Matriculants: a cross-sectional study. Ann Intern Med. 2022;175:611.

21. Daniel H, Bornstein SS, Kane GC, Carney JK, Gantzer HE, Henry TL, et al. Addressing social determinants to improve patient care and promote health equity: an American College of Physicians Position Paper. Ann Intern Med. 2018;168(8):577–8.

22. Artiga S, Orgera K, Damico A. Changes in health coverage by race and ethnicity since the ACA, 2010–2018. San Francisco, CA: Kaiser Family Foundation; 2020.

23. National Lung Screening Trial Research Team, Aberle DR, Adams AM, Berg CD, Black WC, Clapp JD, et al. Reduced lung-cancer mortality with low-dose computed tomographic screening. N Engl J Med. 2011;365(5):395–409.

24. Hamann HA, Ostroff JS, Marks EG, Gerber DE, Schiller JH, Craddock Lee SJ. Stigma among patients with lung cancer: a patient-reported measurement model. Psychooncology. 2014;23(1):81–92.

25. Evans-Polce RJ, Castaldelli-Maia JM, Schomerus G, Evans-Lacko SE. The downside of tobacco control? Smoking and self-stigma: a systematic review. Soc Sci Med. 2015;145:26–34.

26. Stuber J, Galea S, Link BG. Smoking and the emergence of a stigmatized social status. Soc Sci Med. 2008;67(3):420–30.
27. Hamann HA, Williamson TJ, Studts JL, Ostroff JS. Lung cancer stigma then and now: continued challenges amid a landscape of progress. J Thorac Oncol. 2021;16(1):17–20.
28. Chambers SK, Morris BA, Clutton S, Foley E, Giles L, Schofield P, et al. Psychological wellness and health-related stigma: a pilot study of an acceptance-focused cognitive behavioural intervention for people with lung cancer. Eur J Cancer Care (Engl). 2015;24(1):60–70.
29. Banerjee SC, Haque N, Bylund CL, Shen MJ, Rigney M, Hamann HA, et al. Responding empathically to patients: a communication skills training module to reduce lung cancer stigma. Transl Behav Med. 2021;11(2):613–8.
30. Sharf BF, Stelljes LA, Gordon HS. 'A little bitty spot and I'm a big man': patients' perspectives on refusing diagnosis or treatment for lung cancer. Psychooncology. 2005;14(8):636–46.
31. Bergamo C, Lin JJ, Smith C, Lurslurchachai L, Halm EA, Powell CA, et al. Evaluating beliefs associated with late-stage lung cancer presentation in minorities. J Thorac Oncol. 2013;8(1):12–8.
32. Schroen AT, Detterbeck FC, Crawford R, Rivera MP, Socinski MA. Beliefs among pulmonologists and thoracic surgeons in the therapeutic approach to non-small cell lung cancer. Chest. 2000;118(1):129–37.
33. Rothstein R. The color of law: a forgotten history of how our government segregated America. New York, NY: Liveright Publishing Corporation; 2020.

Index